DEVELOPING POWER

SECOND EDITION

T0285582

National Strength and Conditioning Association

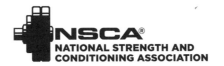

NSCA®
NATIONAL STRENGTH AND
CONDITIONING ASSOCIATION

Paul Comfort

EDITOR

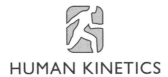

HUMAN KINETICS

Library of Congress Cataloging-in-Publication Data

Names: Comfort, Paul, editor. | National Strength & Conditioning
   Association (U.S.), sponsoring body.
Title: Developing power / Paul Comfort, editor.
Description: Second edition. | Champaign, IL : Human Kinetics, [2025] |
   Series: NSCA's Sport Performance Series | Includes bibliographical
   references and index.
Identifiers: LCCN 2024011591 (print) | LCCN 2024011592 (ebook) | ISBN
   9781718220461 (paperback) | ISBN 9781718220478 (epub) | ISBN
   9781718220485 (pdf)
Subjects: LCSH: Physical education and training. | Muscle strength. |
   Weight training. | Bodybuilding. | Physical fitness--Physiological
   aspects. | BISAC: SPORTS & RECREATION / Bodybuilding & Weightlifting |
   HEALTH & FITNESS / Exercise / General
Classification: LCC GV711.5 .D474 2025 (print) | LCC GV711.5 (ebook) |
   DDC 613.7/11--dc23/eng/20240606
LC record available at https://lccn.loc.gov/2024011591
LC ebook record available at https://lccn.loc.gov/2024011592

ISBN: 978-1-7182-2046-1 (print)

The web addresses cited in this text were current as of February 2024, unless otherwise noted.

Senior Acquisitions Editor: Roger W. Earle; **Managing Editor:** Kevin Matz; **Copyeditor:** Jennifer MacKay; **Proofreader:** Mary Elisabeth Frediani; **Indexer:** Michael Ferreira/Ferreira Indexing, Inc.; **Permissions Manager:** Laurel Mitchell; **Graphic Designer:** Denise Lowry; **Cover Designer:** Keri Evans; **Cover Design Specialist:** Susan Rothermel Allen; **Photograph (cover):** © Human Kinetics; **Photographs (interior):** © Human Kinetics, unless otherwise noted; **Photo Asset Manager:** Laura Fitch; **Photo Production Specialist:** Amy M. Rose; **Photo Production Manager:** Jason Allen; **Senior Art Manager:** Kelly Hendren; **Illustrations:** © Human Kinetics, unless otherwise noted; **Printer:** Versa Press

We thank Matthew Sandstead, NSCA-CPT,*D, Scott Caulfield, MA, CSCS,*D, TSAC-F,*D, RSCC*E, and the National Strength and Conditioning Association (NSCA) in Colorado Springs, Colorado, for overseeing (Matthew and Scott) and hosting (NSCA) the photo shoot for this book.

Human Kinetics books are available at special discounts for bulk purchase. Special editions or book excerpts can also be created to specification. For details, contact the Special Sales Manager at Human Kinetics.

Printed in the United States of America   10 9 8 7 6 5 4 3 2 1

The paper in this book is certified under a sustainable forestry program.

Human Kinetics
1607 N. Market Street
Champaign, IL 61820
USA

United States and International
Website: **US.HumanKinetics.com**
Email: info@hkusa.com
Phone: 1-800-747-4457

Canada
Website: **Canada.HumanKinetics.com**
Email: info@hkcanada.com

E9041

DEVELOPING POWER

SECOND EDITION

Contents

Introduction

The ability to produce maximal muscular power is important in sport performance. One only needs to look at a basketball player performing a slam dunk or a rugby player changing direction in a game to realize the importance of power for optimal athletic performance. Maximal muscular power refers to the highest level of power (work divided by time) that can be achieved during concentric muscle actions. In the applied setting of sport performance, maximal power can be thought of as representing the greatest instantaneous power during a single movement performed, although it is necessary to understand how the power output has been generated, because relative force production (i.e., relative to the mass being accelerated) determines acceleration, and the duration over which this force is applied (i.e., relative mean force × time = relative impulse) determines the resulting velocity (see chapters 1 and 2). It is this relative impulse that determines the takeoff velocity during a jump or the release of an object being thrown. This is of utmost importance when considering movements such as sprinting, jumping, throwing, changing direction, and striking; therefore, power can be considered a critical aspect of many sports.

This book discusses the latest evidence-based guidelines for the assessment and training of muscular power, using case studies from a range of areas along with relevant research regarding the assessment and development of power. It provides strength and conditioning professionals with the latest information on how to assess power, but more importantly, it provides examples for using this information to design programming. The first chapter sets the scene by introducing the key concepts and underlying science of muscular power. The correct terminology for describing the components of power are outlined. The chapter also explores the biological and mechanical basis of power, including morphological factors, neural factors, and muscle mechanics. The strong relationship between maximal strength, rapid force production, and power is another critical theme in the first chapter and throughout the book.

A variety of testing methods are available to practitioners to assess power; however, it is important to consider the validity, reliability, and measurement error associated with these tests and to understand the differences between testing methodologies. Therefore, practitioners should not implement strength and power tests simply for the sake of testing. It is also important to examine the tests used and to avoid choosing them solely because they have been used previously or because the equipment and the expertise are available. These concepts form the basis of chapter 2, which provides the reader with an advanced explanation of the assessment of power.

The connection between assessment and programming is critical when designing training programs to develop power. In other words, how are testing results used to determine programming? A key purpose of athlete assessment is to obtain insight into the athlete's training needs. This is an important theme in the book and requires an in-depth understanding of program design. Chapter 3 explains training principles in relation to power development, but more importantly, it explores how these should be implemented in a sequential approach via periodization.

It is not just in sports that power is important. Increasing evidence shows that other populations, such as older adults, also experience meaningful benefits from increasing strength and power. In addition, as resistance training becomes a more integral part of training programs for youth athletes, strength and conditioning professionals increasingly need to be aware of the role of power training. Practitioners working with different client populations need to know how to assess and develop muscular power in their clients effectively. Chapter 4 explains the application of power testing and training for two populations with whom strength and conditioning coaches and exercise scientists are increasingly working: youth athletes and older adults. The benefits of power development are now well recognized for these groups, and practitioners can apply the principles discussed in this chapter across a wide range of populations.

For practitioners to be able to train power well, it is critical that they have a range of effective exercises to use with their athletes. A series of chapters provides a technical breakdown of exercises and teaching progressions that develop power. Chapter 5 discusses upper body exercises; chapter 6, lower body exercises; chapter 7 (which is a new chapter), core power development; and chapter 8, power exercises for the whole body, including weightlifting exercises and their derivatives. Being able to coach and also to perform exercises effectively and safely is an important part of the exercise prescription process. Using a range of methods to develop power and choosing appropriate exercises are critical for strength and conditioning professionals, and some methods for doing so are introduced in chapters 3 and 4. Chapter 9 extends these discussions by examining more advanced methods of developing power, such as complex training and the use of variable resistance, in more detail.

An often overlooked aspect of improving muscular power is where it fits into the design of a training program. It is important for practitioners to realize that power is not developed in isolation; it also needs to be considered as part of the overall training program, especially considering that acceleration is underpinned by relative force. As such, power is discussed throughout the book in the context of complete program preparation rather than as an isolated component. For example, it is well known that developing maximal strength and rapid force production forms the basis of optimal power development, and this is an important theme of the book. The final two chapters provide sample training programs that develop power, both for team sports, such as rugby union, basketball, volleyball, soccer, American football, baseball, softball, field hockey, and lacrosse (chapter 10), and individual sports, such as swimming, rowing, track and field, golf, tennis, surfing, skateboarding, combat sports, and winter sports (chapter 11). A key feature of these two final chapters is that they highlight the link between the assessment of power and how assessment can be used to develop training programs.

The contributors to this book consist of some of the best practitioners and researchers in the field of strength and conditioning and sport science. They have been invited to contribute because of their research expertise and their extensive practical experience working with high-level athletes. They also have the ability to communicate evidence-based information effectively and to apply the latest research in a practical manner. The overall goal of this book is to provide strength and conditioning professionals with the most cutting-edge and accurate information on power development for improved sport performance. This book will be a valuable addition to the libraries of strength and conditioning professionals, sport scientists, coaches, and athletes who are interested in evidence-based power training.

The second edition of this book has been substantially updated throughout, based on the most up-to-date research findings, with the application of such findings presented by some of the world's leading strength and conditioning professionals. The underpinning physiology and biomechanics of power development are explored in detail. In addition, extensive revisions and critiques of testing methods used to assess power have been included to ensure practitioners are able to make evidence-informed decisions regarding the needs of their athletes and the methods best suited to enhance physical development. A new chapter on the development of core power (chapter 7) has been introduced, along with additional sports used as examples within the later chapters (e.g., field hockey, lacrosse, surfing, and skateboarding).

CHAPTER 1

The Nature of Producing Power

Paul Comfort
Paul A. Jones
John J. McMahon
Jeffrey McBride*

Examining power from its inception at the molecular level provides valuable information when designing an optimal training program. From a mechanical context, *power* is the amount of work performed (i.e., net force × displacement) divided by the time in which it was performed (power = net force × displacement ÷ time). Given that velocity = Δ displacement ÷ Δ time, power can also be represented as force multiplied by velocity. Power is therefore influenced by both force and time (i.e., impulse = force × time). The impulse generated determines the velocity of movement (impulse–momentum theorem). For example, during a countermovement jump, if an athlete applies a greater propulsive force over a given propulsive phase duration, the resulting impulse will increase, producing greater acceleration (change in velocity) and therefore a higher velocity at takeoff, leading to an increased jump height. These variables should also be put in the context of the constantly changing system in which this phenomenon is examined in terms of muscle lengths (i.e., force–length relationship), joint angles, and concentric, eccentric, and stretch-shortening cycle patterns of muscle function. Examining power provides a valuable context in which to develop effective ways to maximize athletic performance.

ENERGY

Availability of adenosine triphosphate (ATP) has been considered the primary constituent of the ability to generate power (20, 127) (figure 1.1a). Research-

*Paul Comfort, Paul A. Jones, and John J. McMahon were contracted to author this chapter; Jeffrey McBride's name was added to acknowledge his significant contribution partially retained from the previous edition.

ers have shown that energy within the body is derived from the hydrolysis (unbinding) of ATP, which uses the bond energy between the third phosphate group (γ) and the adjacent phosphates (129). The energy within these bonds is obtained through the metabolism of energy substrates—primarily carbohydrates and lipids, for prolonged activities—which are ingested through natural food sources (25, 72). Because power is work per unit of time, motions or activities that consist of maximal power appear to involve relatively short time frames (12), and as such, the primary energy sources are those that tend to be the most rapidly available. These sources consist of stored ATP within muscle tissue and the short-term rapid formation of ATP through the donation of phosphate groups from phosphocreatine, which is stored in muscle tissue (61). The additional sources of energy to rephosphorylate adenosine diphosphate (ADP) to reform ATP may be derived from the anaerobic processing of glucose (carbohydrate) stored within muscle tissue and the liver. Energy for sustained levels of small to moderate power output for long-term endurance activities could be derived from either the subsequent processing of the end products of anaerobic glycolysis (pyruvate) or beta oxidation of fatty acids (lipids, stored within the body in adipocytes) and anaerobic respiration (the Krebs cycle and the electron transport chain) (63, 152).

The process of generating external power appears to begin with a muscle action (usually concentric) to produce force (124) (figure 1.1*b* and *c*). This muscle shortening could result in limb motion, which is referred to as *internal work*; this internal work relative to time is, then, internal power (figure 1.1*d*) (114). The motion of the limbs can allow for the generation of external forces (forces applied to the ground or external objects through the arms and legs), which often results in the subsequent movement of the whole body's center of mass (COM). *External work* is the external force generated times the displacement of the COM (work = force × displacement), and relative to time (power = work ÷ time), it is external power (figure 1.1*e*) (84). This external power is a possible indicator of performance in activities (e.g., how fast athletes can run or how high they can jump) (117); however, while power is associated with jump height, it is relative net propulsive impulse (i.e., the net propulsive impulse relative to body mass) that determines jump height (85, 106), based on the impulse–momentum relationship. In the case of endurance or activities performed repeatedly, *mechanical efficiency* (the ratio of energy created per unit of time relative to external power) may be the primary variable of concern (73, 104). The main component of the process of generating power is the ability to generate force, and more importantly, to generate force rapidly, because velocity is determined by relative impulse. It is also important to note that the duration for force production in many sporting tasks is limited (commonly <250 milliseconds), further highlighting the importance of rapid force production.

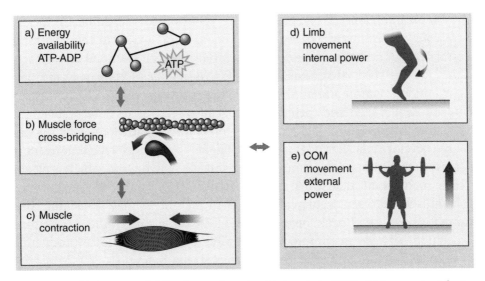

Figure 1.1 *(a)* Energy availability from adenosine triphosphate (ATP), *(b)* force output from actin–myosin crossbridging, *(c)* muscle contraction, *(d)* limb movement and internal power, and *(e)* whole-body center of mass (COM) movement and external power.

FORCE

The ability to generate force within the body's skeletal muscle tissue is quite a miraculous process. In some respects, skeletal muscle could be considered similar to an electric motor but in a molecular form (102). This skeletal muscle "molecular motor" takes chemical energy (ATP) and uses it to perform mechanical work, just as an electric motor uses electricity to perform mechanical work. More specifically, in skeletal muscle, the hydrolysis of ATP, or the removal of the γ-phosphate group, and the subsequent conformational change of myosin (swivel) creates mechanical work (15). Within the context of a single crossbridge, or myosin–actin interaction, the amount of force developed has been reported as approximately 4 piconewtons (10). Thus, in the context of squatting a 220 pound (100 kg) mass, about 981 trillion piconewtons, or 245 trillion crossbridges, may be required. There appear to be approximately 300 molecules of myosin in each thick myosin filament protein, with each molecule consisting of two heads that attach to, swivel, and detach from actin filaments to produce force (139). It has been reported that these thick filaments are arranged in a pattern to form a *sarcomere*, the smallest repeating functional unit in a muscle. Some data indicate there are 2,000 to 2,500 sarcomeres per 0.4 inches (1 cm) of muscle fiber length. While muscles have quite a variation in length, this provides a general construct of the massive number of crossbridges per fiber, per motor unit, and ultimately, per muscle (13, 24, 151).

The regulatory mechanisms for force output may be vital in determining the amount of work performed per crossbridge and in what time frame this occurs.

Various combinations of mechanisms are reported to determine the power output of a whole muscle. The regulatory mechanisms appear to begin with the central nervous system and the action potentials (i.e., the electrical signals) sent to the muscles (100, 113). Skeletal muscles are regulated via *motor units* (i.e., a single motor neuron and all the muscle fibers it innervates). The number of motor units recruited and their firing rates (also referred to as *rate coding*) are key factors that determine peak force and, more importantly for power, the rate of force development (RFD) (45, 57, 130). Higher firing rates appear to result in increased RFD through the summation of muscle twitch force, which typically occurs as the result of a single action potential (45). Thus, the rate at which these muscle twitches occur with respect to each other may determine their summative pattern of peak force and RFD (39). Interestingly, there is a strong association between maximum force production and rapid force production (3, 4, 26, 57), highlighting the importance of strength development to increase rapid force production and power development (32, 34, 35, 37).

The results of numerous studies indicate that inherent capabilities within humans generate action potentials in control of force production, which can be modified by training (41-43, 148). However, beyond the scope of rate coding, several possible subsequent processes also determine what the peak force and RFD for a muscle may be. The other areas of regulation may include the neuromuscular junction or gap, which consists of neurotransmitter (acetylcholine) release and the generation of action potentials along the membrane of the muscle fibers themselves (44) (figure 1.2). Researchers have shown that within a muscle fiber, the release and sequestering of calcium from the sarcoplasmic reticulum, which is both rate-controlled and a trainable phenomenon, may be rate-limiting (78). In addition, there may still be a limiting factor in terms of crossbridge kinetics (111). This may be prescribed by the rate-limiting steps of ATP hydrolysis, the myosin conformational changes, and the detachment–reattachment rates of the myosin head to actin. Thus, a multitude of considerations exists for how force is created within the neuromuscular system, and subsequently, how work is performed. This force should be put in the context of the actual displacement that occurs within the sarcomere, the muscle fiber, and the whole muscle when considering the expression of mechanical work.

DISPLACEMENT AND VELOCITY

Understanding the various aspects of displacement of the internal system (crossbridges, sarcomeres, muscle fibers, and whole muscle) and their translation into the more external aspects of displacement and the velocity of the body's limbs, and then of external objects or the whole body (figure 1.1c through e), is important to understanding power. Beginning from an internal perspective, the conformational change in myosin may result in a lever-type system of rotation around

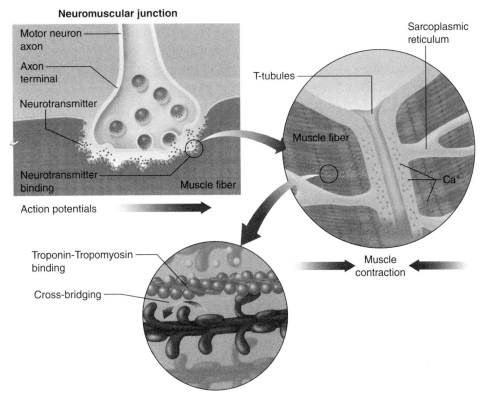

Figure 1.2 Process of muscle contraction, from the axon terminal to the neurotransmitter release at the neuromuscular junction to the sarcoplasmic reticulum release of calcium, actin–myosin crossbridging, and muscle contraction.

a fixed point through an angle of approximately 70 degrees (19); this has been referred to as the *working stroke* (129). The amount of actual displacement for a single crossbridge interaction has been reported as approximately 5.3 nanometers (86). Within the context of a single muscle contraction, millions of crossbridge interactions translate into length changes within sarcomeres, and subsequently, the whole muscle. A sarcomere has been reported as the smallest functional unit within skeletal muscle and often the starting point for the examination of the force–length change relationship that exists in muscle (122). The resting length of a sarcomere has been reported to be 2 to 3 μm, shortening to 1 to 1.5 μm and lengthening to 3.5 to 4 μm. Sarcomeres are arranged in series, and thus, the shortening of the whole muscle represents the collective shortening of multiple sarcomeres. Two possibilities of sarcomere shortening have been reported: One could assume that all sarcomeres shorten the same amount within the context of a single concentric muscle action (segment-controlled model), or it is possible that various sarcomeres shorten different amounts (fixed-end model), resulting in different possible force–length relationships (122). Variation in the number of sarcomeres in a series might also affect the shape and scope of the force–length relationship and is possibly influenced by the type of training in which an athlete engages (122). Changes in whole-muscle length during contraction occur within a range of 0.4 to 0.8 inches (10.2 to 20.3 mm) (74).

FACTORS THAT AFFECT FORCE PRODUCTION

A variety of elements influence the amount of force that an individual can produce. Muscle length affects force output in a hyperbolic pattern, with maximal force at optimal length due to myosin-actin overlap. Velocity influences force production, decreasing with concentric actions but potentially exceeding norms during stretch-shortening cycles. Eccentric actions show a unique force-velocity relationship, with force increasing initially but plateauing at high velocities, potentially leading to muscle damage. Muscle fiber arrangement, particularly pennation, affects force production by increasing cross-sectional area and allowing for variable anatomical gear ratios influenced by training. Tendon insertion points determine joint movement and torque production, with pros and cons regarding proximal versus distal locations.

Muscle Length

Force output across the range of muscle-length change does not appear to be a constant (figure 1.3a). The length changes may result in various states of myosin–actin overlap, and thus, different numbers of actual crossbridges. Force output appears to occur in a hyperbolic pattern of decreased force output either at very short (ascending limb) or long (descending limb) lengths, with maximal force production occurring at some optimal length between these two points (plateau region) (122). There may be an active force production component of a muscle caused by crossbridge interactions but also passive force production, particularly during lengthening, that could be the result of stretching large structural proteins, such as titin, which appear to connect myosin to the Z-line of the sarcomere (149). This passive force production (or tension) should be a consideration, especially during stretch-shortening cycles within a muscle that commonly occur during athletic movement patterns such as running or jumping (38).

Velocity

To add to the complexity of this process, a velocity-dependent component may result in force production within a muscle (figure 1.3b). Force output decreases with concentric muscle actions as the velocity of shortening increases inversely (6). Thus, a muscle may not be able to produce the same force during an isometric muscle action as it can during a high-velocity muscle action. However, levels of force production during the concentric phase may exceed this standard pattern during stretch-shortening cycles because of various possible mechanisms initiated during the eccentric (i.e., loading) phase due to the stretch reflex, stored elastic energy (i.e., titin), and crossbridge potentiation (51).

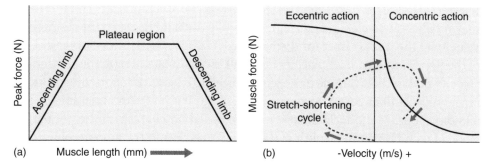

Figure 1.3 *(a)* Muscle force varies as a function of length, increasing (ascending limb), reaching a plateau, and then subsequently decreasing (descending limb) in a lengthened position. *(b)* Muscle force during a concentric, an eccentric, and a stretch-shortening cycle muscle action.

The eccentric phase of the force–velocity relationship appears to be the opposite in that with increasing velocity, force output increases to a certain level and then plateaus or decreases during extremely high eccentric velocities (active muscle lengthening) (88). This is because the force might be generated in two distinct ways during concentric versus eccentric muscle actions. Concentric force production may be caused by crossbridge swiveling and the attachment–detachment pattern as a result of ATP hydrolysis, as previously discussed. Conversely, force production during eccentric muscle actions may occur from forced detachment of the myosin head from actin because of tension-induced lengthening of the muscle. This may be why eccentric muscle actions have been reported to be associated with muscle damage resulting from forced detachment of myosin heads and the forced lengthening of structural proteins (i.e., actin, myosin, tropomyosin, and troponin) as well (120, 121). During multijoint exercises, higher velocity during the lowering phase does not result in higher force production until deceleration or braking occurs. For example, during a squat, a higher eccentric velocity requires a reduction in agonist muscular force production so that gravity accelerates the athlete during the descent; however, for deceleration to commence, the force must exceed the mass of the system, and a resulting braking impulse equal to the athlete's momentum is required to stop motion.

Muscle Fiber Arrangement

One other factor that may determine the relationship between the sarcomere, or muscle fiber, and force output relative to velocity of the contraction is the pattern of muscle fiber arrangement relative to the whole muscle–tendon unit (50). Most muscles have a pennate design, in which the muscle fibers are at an angle to the tendon line of the origin and insertion points of the whole muscle (*pennation angle*). This phenomenon may serve two purposes. First, it may allow for an increased cross-sectional area of muscle fibers within a given volume, referred to as the *physiological cross-sectional area*. Second, muscle pennation also may result in an *anatomical gear ratio*, which is the ratio between the shortening velocity of the muscle fiber (or displacement) relative to the shortening velocity of the whole muscle (or displacement) (8, 9). In a pennate design, the shortening velocity of the whole muscle has been reported to exceed the shortening velocity of the muscle fiber based on the amount of pennation (pennation angle). The anatomical gear ratio for a muscle may be based on changes in the pennation angle, depending on the length of the whole muscle and the amount of tension within the muscle. The primary benefit of this variable anatomical gear ratio might be that it extends the range of shortening velocity (at higher velocities) at which the muscle can produce substantial levels of force (18). Both the physiological cross-sectional area and the anatomical gear ratio might be independently influenced by the type of training that an athlete performs (1, 8, 47).

Variations in Tendon Insertion

Ultimately, the process of whole-muscle shortening appears to result in joint movement based on the orientation of the origin and the insertion point of the tendons of the muscle (71). The origin and insertion points may also play a role in the amount of angular displacement and the velocity of the corresponding limb (11). Joint *torque* (the angular effect of force) is a product of the whole-muscle level of force and its corresponding moment arm. A *moment arm* is defined by the length of a straight line identified from the joint axis of rotation to a point perpendicular to the line of muscle action (an artificial extension of the force vector from the respective whole-muscle contraction). Moment arm lengths are influenced both by the origin and insertion points of a particular muscle and by the joint angle at which a specific activity takes place (2). Different muscles within the body have various origin and insertion points, most likely based on their required function within the context of a specific joint. Pros and cons are associated with more distal or more proximal origin and insertion locations (122). For example, a more distal origin or insertion might result in greater torque production (due to a greater moment arm) but through a more limited range of joint motion. More proximal locations may result in less torque (due to a smaller moment arm) but a broader spectrum of torque production across larger joint angles. The other aspect of a distal location is that the velocity of the whole-muscle contraction might need to be higher to result in a higher movement velocity of the most distal portion of the limb, such as the hand or foot (122). A more proximal location might result in the opposite condition.

This could influence the velocity of the limb in terms of its interaction with external objects such as a ball or the ground itself and also the amount of force applied to these objects (5, 128). This might be the most important aspect of the concepts of displacement and velocity as they apply to the COM displacement and velocity of the whole body (i.e., jumping or running).

The vertical displacement of the COM of the whole body, for example, represents an athlete's jump height, and the horizontal velocity of the COM of the whole body represents running velocity (49, 67). Athletic performances might be derived from the internal displacement and velocity capabilities of crossbridges, sarcomeres, muscle fibers, whole muscles, joint movements, and the external values of concern relating to displacement and velocity of the COM of the whole body (67). The external magnitude of force production, most often referred to as *ground reaction forces* (GRFs), and the duration over which force is applied (i.e., impulse [net force × time]) determine the characteristics of the displacement and velocity of the COM of the whole body. Thus, force, displacement, and time can be measured and used to determine power output. However, before referring directly to power, force and displacement must be put in the context of work (force × displacement).

WORK AND TIME

As mentioned previously, the goal of a molecular motor is to convert chemical energy (i.e., ATP) to perform mechanical work (force production and displacement) (48). This is the working stroke. Force production is a product of crossbridge interaction and the subsequent sliding (or displacement) of actin, resulting in sarcomere shortening followed by muscle fiber shortening and, finally, whole-muscle shortening—thus, mechanical work (14). The myosin–actin interaction has been reported to result in approximately 20 to 50 kJ/mol of free energy, which is assumed to be translated into usable work (working stroke) (81). An important aspect of using free energy derived from crossbridge interactions may be the ratio between this free energy and the subsequent amount of mechanical work that is actually performed (48, 81). This has been described as the *mechanical efficiency* of the system. We also may derive free energy from a crossbridge interaction as a result of the hydrolysis of ATP, which, as mentioned previously, is formed within the body through mechanisms of processing primarily carbohydrate and lipids. Energy production might be, to a certain extent, determined by changes in lactate concentration (from pyruvate generated in anaerobic glycolysis) and the amount of oxygen transported into the body (aerobic respiration: the Krebs cycle and electron transport chain) (46, 89). Lactate can be measured from the blood, and oxygen consumption can be measured by monitoring the amount that enters the body ($\dot{V}O_2$) (107). A method for estimating energy expenditure is to measure inspired oxygen amounts and express this certain level of energy expenditure as 20,202 J/L of oxygen (46).

Blood lactate levels used as an estimate of energy expenditure are 60 J × body mass × Δblood lactate (126).

The other aspect of calculating mechanical efficiency is the mechanical work performed. Calculating work at the muscle level for an athlete may not be possible with current technology. In vitro models of preparations of a single muscle fiber or whole muscle have been used to calculate work (145). However, at a higher level of function, some investigations have labeled internal work—the summation of individual body segment movements—as a reflection of the process of whole-muscle contractions around their respective joints (123) (figure 1.4). This process involves assumptions, and the processing occurs through a series of analyses that track body-segment movements through videography and GRF measurements. Energy changes (and thus, internal work) are a measure of the collective changes in potential and kinetic energies of the components of the system (body segments) (150). Another form of assessment is external work (7, 21, 22, 140). This is the summation of the changes in potential and kinetic energies of the COM of the whole body. For the purposes of assessing mechanical efficiency in terms of athletic performance, the measure of external work might be the most practical and the most relevant to athletic performance.

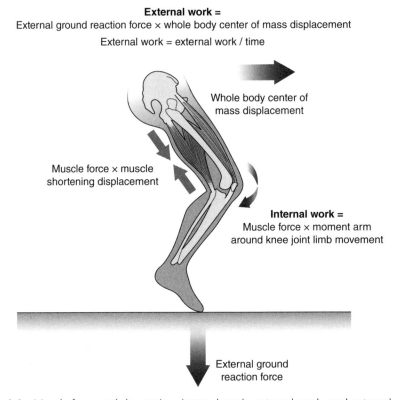

External work =
External ground reaction force × whole body center of mass displacement
External work = external work / time

Whole body center of mass displacement

Muscle force × muscle shortening displacement

Internal work =
Muscle force × moment arm around knee joint limb movement

External ground reaction force

Figure 1.4 Muscle force and shortening, internal work, external work, and external power.

Thus, the most meaningful aspect of athletic performance may be the ratio between energy expenditure (lactate and $\dot{V}O_2$) and external work. This ratio has been reported in the literature and may be a trainable phenomenon that has an impact on athletic performance (89, 90, 107), especially as it relates to the capability to produce greater work in a given time period (i.e., greater power) for endurance-related activities (75). Calculation of external work may also have the most significance for athletic performance in terms of understanding the importance of power (84). Many researchers have examined the relationship between power and performance (see chapter 2). What these researchers refer to is work performed by the COM of the whole body relative to time. These measures have been calculated from GRFs (force plate measurements) during jumping and running (52, 79). Thus, an athlete's ability to alter kinetic and potential energies (work) could be important in understanding how to improve these variables with respect to time, resulting in increased power (98).

POWER

Power is defined as the rate of performing work, and work is the product of force and displacement. Another way to think about power is as the amount of force produced during an activity at a given velocity. However, some biomechanists have questioned the use of this simplification of power (87, 153), even though the equation power = work ÷ time can easily be rearranged to power = force × velocity. It was previously mentioned that a myosin–actin interaction (crossbridge) has been referred to as the *working stroke*. Another common, and maybe more relevant, term is the *power stroke* (53). Power is the culmination of the variables previously discussed: force, displacement, and time. These three variables may be the essence of athletic performance and thus why power has been extensively researched and discussed by both scientists and practitioners (62, 92, 93, 95). Ballistic or semiballistic movement patterns, such as the jump squat and the power clean, have been reported to result in higher power outputs in comparison to a heavy-weight squat (performed at a higher percentage of the 1-repetition maximum [1RM]) (33, 59, 60, 105). Although a heavy squat requires relatively high force production, the velocity of the movement is lower than during a jump squat or a power clean. This lower velocity (and, therefore, an increase in movement duration) results in lower values of power (33, 105). This can also be viewed in the context of power being work divided by time; because the duration of a squat compared to a jump squat or power clean is noticeably longer, this also partly explains the lower power level, even when the work performed is higher than that of the jump squat or power clean.

Activities performed at a very high velocity also appear to result in lower power levels because force is low, according to the previous discussion of the force–velocity relationship in the muscle. However, a condition of very high velocity (enough to severely limit power) is not a naturally occurring condition in human movements unless they are performed in a zero-gravity or microgravity environment (23). It has been reported that running and jumping within the earth's environment results in relatively high-power outputs because athletes must move their whole body to run or jump against the gravitational force of the planet (their body weight) (23, 110, 125). This means that moderate levels of velocity and force may occur simultaneously, as reflected in data from the jump squat using body mass, for example (33, 76, 105). This interesting concept was initially presented by a study involving jumping in simulated zero-gravity or microgravity environments (23). If an athlete performs a maximal squat, power output appears to be low (high force, low velocity). If athletes jump or run on the earth, their power appears to be high (moderate force, moderate velocity), but if they were to jump on the moon, their power would appear to be low (low force, high velocity). This hyperbolic relationship may assist in establishing concepts of where and why power occurs in human movement and how to train to maximize athletic performance.

Similarly, practitioners and researchers have explored the use of assisted (e.g., using elastic resistance to aid in acceleration and deceleration) and resisted (e.g., using additional load) jumping to enhance jump performance and power development. While these methods appear to be beneficial by increasing power and jump performance, they do not appear to result in any greater improvements in performance compared to traditional ballistic and plyometric training (101).

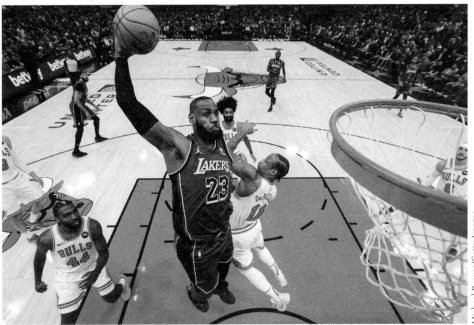

Michael Reaves/Getty Images

Power is essential for athletes like Lebron James.

Importance of Power

Power is an essential quality for running fast and jumping high (77, 94, 96, 97). An organism's ability to generate power might be a product of its evolution in the context of the environment in which it evolves (gravity, atmospheric pressure, and so on) (23, 110, 125). For the purposes of humans, this might be the evolution of the body in the context of the earth's gravitational field. It appears that if athletes want to jump high or run fast, they must generate maximal force through a maximal displacement in a short period of time (59, 60, 125). In addition, they must do this by moving their own body mass against gravity (mass × g) to generate power. Thus, a crossbridge, a muscle fiber, a whole muscle, a joint movement, and a GRF may be optimized in the context of this environmental arrangement (16, 17, 67, 69, 111).

The concepts of maximal force, velocity, and power production might be observed from the level of an individual muscle fiber, of a whole muscle, of a joint, and finally, of the whole body itself (111, 119). Due to the strong associations between strength and power (32, 35, 37) and between maximal and rapid force production (3, 4, 26, 58), power output capability might be a product of the maximal force a system can produce, highlighting the importance of strength development (136, 137). As mentioned previously, this could even be brought back to the molecular motor itself. Hydrolysis of ATP has been reported to result in free energy, and thus, mechanical work, all in the context of a certain period of time. However, the production of force, whether it be in a single crossbridge or a whole muscle, must be placed in the context of what the maximal force production capability of the system is, especially regarding velocity. This is because power is a product of force and velocity; thus, the optimal intersection between these two variables might provide an understanding of both where power occurs and how it can be optimized (99, 119).

Maximal Power

An examination of a single muscle fiber indicates that the maximal power exhibited may occur at 15% to 30% of its maximal force capabilities (53). This also might translate to the whole muscle (68, 69, 111, 112), and even more amazingly, to the force output of the whole body (68, 69, 111, 112). If an athlete weighs 841 Newtons (N) (189 pounds [85.7 kg]) and can generate 1,647 N (370 pounds [167.8 kg]) of maximal force with the legs in a vertical direction, then the external load at which the athlete can create the most power vertically (jump squat) appears to be 33.8% of this total value ([841 N + 1,647 N] × 33.8% = 840.9 N). The solution to this equation, 840.9 N, is approximately the weight of the athlete and 33.8% of the total value (2,488 N), which is similar to the values of 15% to 30% of maximal force production reported in studies of single muscle fibers (53, 54, 69, 145). This means that apparently athletes can generate the most power when they are moving a load approximately equal to their own body weight (31, 33, 40, 103, 105) (figure 1.5).

It appears that when the load the athlete trains with increases (1.0-1.5 × body weight [BW]), peak force increases, with coincidental decreases in peak velocity and, therefore, peak power (105), based on the load–velocity relationship. This is why ballistic power training (e.g., jump squats) might be characterized by training with lower resistance (high peak power, usually ≤40% of the 1RM) and heavy resistance training might be characterized by training with higher resistance (high peak force, usually ≥80% of the 1RM) (131). This relationship appears to be slightly altered when using the squat (nonballistic) or power clean (semiballistic) as a modality for power training (28, 33, 131), in that the loading is heavier and expressed as a percentage of how much weight the athlete lifts (bar weight or 1RM). In the case of the squat, it might be approximately 56% of the 1RM, and in the power clean, it might be 80% ± 10% of the 1RM (33, 105, 131).

Sometimes, the expressions of load are different between the jump squat and the squat or the power clean. The loading for the jump squat, as discussed earlier, is in the context of using the athlete's body weight as the load (1.0 × BW) or the athlete's body weight plus some level of additional external loading (1.5 × BW). The loading for the squat or the power clean typically has been placed in the context of how much load is on the bar that the athlete lifts (1RM). In figure 1.5, a load of 1.0 × BW would be equal to 0% of the 1RM, or no external load. If an athlete's mass is 180 pounds (81.8 kg) and he or she has a squat 1RM of 300 pounds (136.4 kg), for example, a load of 1.5 × BW would be equal to 90% of the 1RM (1.5 × 180 pounds [81.8 kg] = 270 pounds [122.7 kg]; 270 pounds [122.7 kg] ÷ 300 pounds [136.4 kg] = 0.90). One can see that in the jump squat, a much lower intensity (load) might be used (0% of the 1RM), and in the squat (56% of the 1RM) and the power clean (80% of the 1RM), a much higher intensity (load) might be used to attain peak power output (33, 105, 131), although this load varies across weightlifting exercises and their derivatives (28, 135) (table 1.1).

During a squat, a large portion of the concentric phase results in deceleration to ensure that the athlete does not leave the ground and perform a jump. As such, when performing the squat to enhance power production, it may be more suitable to emphasize strength development rather than using a load that acutely elicits the greatest power (34-36). In addition, training at the load that elicits peak power during an exercise may not result in the greatest improvement in performance in sporting tasks, with no changes in sprint and jump performance when training involves jumping with either the individual's maximal power load (20%-43.5% of the 1RM) or high loads (80% of the 1RM) (70). Moreover, numerous experts have suggested that a mixed-methods approach to power development is most appropriate, ensuring that training loads cover a spectrum of loads but emphasize either the force or velocity end of the force–velocity continuum (65, 115, 116, 146, 147).

Table 1.1 Example Load Ranges to Maximize Power Output During Weightlifting Exercises and Their Derivatives

Exercise	Load range	References
Clean	70%-90% 1RM clean	(55, 56)
Snatch	60%-80% 1RM snatch*	(56, 64)
Power clean	60%-80% 1RM power clean	(27, 29, 33)
Power snatch	≥80% 1RM power snatch*	(56, 118)
Hang power clean	60%-80% 1RM power clean	(82, 83, 133, 138, 141, 142)
Mid-thigh power clean	60%-80% 1RM power clean	(20)
Clean pull from the floor	~120% 1RM power clean	(66)
Clean pull (from the knees)	100%-140% 1RM power clean	(108)
Hang clean pull	100%-140% 1RM power clean	(108)
Mid-thigh pull	60%-100% 1RM power clean	(109)
Countermovement shrug	80%-140% 1RM power clean	(109)
Hang high pull	30%-65% 1RM hang power clean	(134, 138, 142)
Jump shrug	30%-45% 1RM hang power clean	(132, 138)

1RM = 1-repetition maximum.

*There may be some differences in the load that elicits peak power when calculated based on barbell velocity, as performed by Pennington et al. (118), Hadi et al. (64), and Flores et al. (55, 56), compared to when calculated based on system velocity (30, 91, 105).

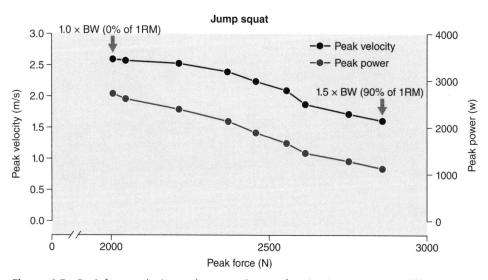

Figure 1.5 Peak force, velocity, and power when performing jump squats at different loads, from 1.0 × body weight (BW) (0% of the 1-repetition maximum [1RM]) to 1.5 × BW (90% of the 1RM).

CONCLUSION

When jumping and running, athletes must move their own body weight. Because jumping, running, and most other field-based activities seem to be ballistic in nature, the concepts identified by research using a jump squat model, in terms of force, velocity, and power, seem plausible. Therefore, when athletes jump or run with their own body weight, it could possibly be considered power training (i.e., $1.0 \times$ BW or 0% of the 1RM). Performing power cleans or their derivatives could supplement jumping and running to develop power, possibly using higher loads, depending on the power clean variation used (see table 1.1).

Researchers have indicated that training with a load that maximizes power may result in the greatest improvements in power during that exercise (80, 143, 144); thus, using appropriate loading for each exercise might be an important consideration for programming. Furthermore, it appears that in general, training with multiple loads may be ideal for improving muscle power and velocity across the whole force–velocity spectrum (65, 115, 116, 146, 147) using appropriate combinations of exercises and loads. Power may be the essence of maximizing athletic performance. The information covered in this chapter, from a molecular level to the context of jumping and running, provides some evidence to support such claims. Athletes use their bodies to run, jump, swim, ride, and climb. This is the nature of power.

CHAPTER 2

Assessing Power and Individual Training Needs

John J. McMahon
Paul A. Jones
Paul Comfort
Sophia Nimphius*

Power has become one of the most discussed aspects of human performance within the strength and conditioning literature. However, measuring power, as well as the colloquialized term *power*, have been criticized for being misused or wrongly interpreted (36, 85). The true definition and appropriate context for using the term *power* should be understood before assessing power (see chapter 1). In the strength and conditioning literature, power has been measured through a variety of modes (e.g., isokinetic, isoinertial, and ballistic), using various loads, and during a variety of exercises (16, 54). These tests and measurements were typically performed to describe human muscular performance. However, the traditional methods of measuring power output have often occurred during repeated maximal efforts over a distance or for a certain amount of time, as with a stair-climbing test or Wingate power test (71).

Nowadays, the strength and conditioning community often measures power output during ballistic exercises, commonly defined as throwing, jumping, and weightlifting activities that allow the athlete to accelerate either the bar (or other external implement) or the body through the entire range of motion (2, 54). Ballistic exercises themselves are not power activities exclusively but instead tend to be activities in which external mechanical power or system power (i.e., the power applied to the body's center of mass [COM] or the body

*John J. McMahon, Paul A. Jones, and Paul Comfort were contracted to author this chapter; Sophia Nimphius' name was added to acknowledge her significant contribution partially retained from the previous edition.

plus any external implement's COM) is expected to be of a higher value than in other activities that occur at lower velocities (40). The most common variable measured during ballistic exercises is the net power of the system, which is the summed coordinated effort of the power of the individual joints (55, 75). Such a measurement has practical advantages (e.g., time, equipment, and cost) over direct assessment of individual joint powers.

It is important to understand that power is a measurement and correlates well with typical measures of athletic performance (e.g., sprint time or vertical jump height). For example, the use of power as a measure of performance in jumping is ill advised (36, 40, 77), because the explained variance between system power and performance (in this case, jump height) is not large in either male or female athletes (40, 60, 62). Two individuals who attained the same jump height (performance) but with different magnitudes of power may benefit from different exercise programs (see case study examples later). This chapter outlines factors that are critical to understand when measuring system power within the context of strength and conditioning, including the definition of power, calculation of power, validity and reliability, common direct (laboratory-based) and indirect (field-based) assessments of power, and examples of data interpretation from data collected during common ballistic assessments.

DEFINING THE TERM *POWER* IN STRENGTH AND CONDITIONING

The colloquial use of the term *power* as a generic trait is commonly misunderstood and misinterpreted (36, 85). Power is, by definition, the rate of doing work. The unit of measure for work is the joule and the unit of measure for power is the watt (W), defined as 1 joule per second. Coaches often indicate that athletes are powerful by describing their movements as occurring at a high velocity relative to the force they must produce or the load they must overcome during the movement. Therefore, movements that occur at lower velocities because of external loads that must be moved (e.g., another person during a tackle or a weighted jump squat) may still be described as powerful because the velocity is high relative to the force required or the mass being accelerated. The colloquial use of the term *powerful* is likely a loose interpretation of the mathematical definitions of power. The following mathematical equations associated with power and work can be arranged several ways to derive the various equations for power.

$$\text{Power (W)} = \frac{\text{work (J)}}{\text{time (s)}}$$

Because work is a product of force and displacement, substitution leads to the following equation:

$$\text{Power (W)} = \frac{\text{force (N)} \times \text{displacement (m)}}{\text{time (s)}}$$

Simplified further (because velocity = displacement ÷ time), the equation can once again be rearranged to what is commonly used or expressed by strength and conditioning practitioners as the equation for power:

$$\text{Power (W)} = \text{force (N)} \times \text{velocity (m/s)}$$

Power can be expressed as the mean, termed *mean power* (P_{mean}), or as the highest peak of instantaneous power, termed *peak power* (P_{peak}), over an entire movement or within a specific phase of a movement. As such, the P_{mean} will always be a lower value and represents the power across the entire movement or phase, whereas the P_{peak} is the highest power produced during a discrete time point. For example, the P_{mean} during a countermovement jump was reported as 765 W, while the P_{peak} was reported as 5,014 W (9). The discrete time point within which the P_{peak} occurs depends on the sample frequency of the device being used to assess power. Thus, if using a force plate sampling at 1,000 Hz (i.e., 1 sample recorded every 0.001 s), which is suggested to be the criterion approach (63), the P_{peak} reported simply represents the highest power value recorded within a 1-millisecond time frame of the movement being assessed. The P_{mean} and P_{peak} can also be reported at the level of the body (if performing a task involving body mass alone), an external implement (such as a barbell), or the entire system (if quantifying power applied to a combination of both the body and the external implement). Thus, the term *system power* is often used to describe power produced by athletes during loaded ballistic jumps and weightlifting variations. A representative force–time curve produced during the countermovement jump and its associated phases is shown in figure 2.1. In figure 2.2, the corresponding force–, velocity–, power–, and displacement–time curves between the commencement of unweighting (i.e., the

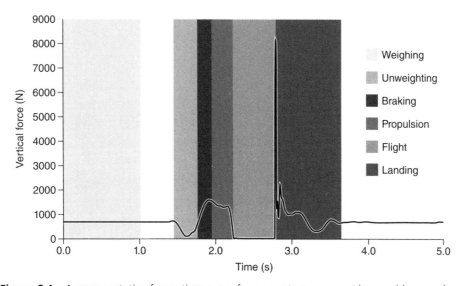

Figure 2.1 A representative force–time curve for a countermovement jump with a graphical representation that shows the weighing, unweighting, braking, propulsion, flight, and landing phases of the jump.

start of the countermovement jump) and takeoff that were obtained from the representative force–time curve shown in figure 2.1 are displayed, along with the individual occurrences of the peak value for each variable.

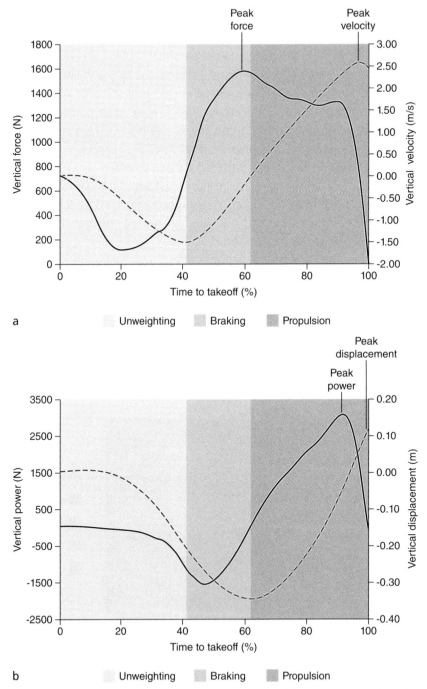

Figure 2.2 Representative force– and velocity–time curves (*a*) and power– and displacement–time curves (*b*) during the unweighting, braking, and propulsion phases of the countermovement jump, with corresponding peak values for each variable labeled.

The current trend among strength and conditioning professionals to measure and report P_{mean} or P_{peak} has led to the development of ballistic assessments (e.g., bench press throw and vertical jumps) (54). During ballistic assessments, power is often calculated to understand the force–velocity profile of an athlete. However, ballistic assessments should not be considered the measurement of power. For example, jump height is often incorrectly assumed to be an indirect measure of leg power, but it is the net impulse (if deconstructing the jump using the impulse–momentum theorem) and the mechanical work (if deconstructing the jump using the work–energy theorem—see chapter 1) produced during the propulsive phase of the jump that dictates jump height (40). Previously reported moderate to large correlations between propulsion power and jump height are artificially inflated due to the almost perfect association ($r = 0.83$-0.94) between the propulsion velocity that coincides with the instant of the P_{peak} and the subsequent jump height (40). Accordingly, a higher propulsion velocity at the instant of the P_{peak} will lead to a greater velocity at takeoff, which in turn directly dictates vertical jump height (35, 45). Thus, instead, the P_{mean} or P_{peak} may be measured during ballistic activities. In fact, system power could technically be measured during any activity except for those that are isometric, where velocity is zero and power is therefore zero. Furthermore, when measuring power, it is critical to fully describe the methods of measurement (discussed in the next section) so that the results can be interpreted within the correct context. Other variables, such as force and velocity, should also be presented, because power is the mechanical construct of force and velocity (49). Therefore, to correctly interpret power as a measured variable, it is necessary to understand the combination of force and velocity changes that elicit the measured power output.

MEASUREMENT OF POWER

Much of the strength and conditioning research involving the measurement of system power has focused on the P_{peak} and P_{mean} produced during a variety of single, maximal-effort movements (e.g., squat, jump squat, bench press throw, or weightlifting) (36) instead of continuous movements such as cycling or rowing, where power output is measured over repeated efforts. A criticism of using and calculating power only during these discrete movements is that the value does not explain or predict actual performance (36). However, what may be of interest to many practitioners is the change in the P_{peak} or P_{mean} during single, maximal-effort movements, which can reflect adaptations to training when interpreted in conjunction with other variables, such as force or velocity and performance measures such as jump height.

Figure 2.2 provides the information needed to understand the interactions between force, velocity, displacement, and power. To understand how the figure relates to aspects of the jump, consider the phases shown in figures 2.1 and 2.2. The weighing phase occurs when the athlete is standing still and upright and immediately before he or she performs the fast countermovement portion of the jump, which comprises the unweighting and braking phases as the athlete flexes the ankles, knees, and hips to lower himself or herself (see that the end of the braking phase coincides with the peak negative vertical displacement in figure 2.2). The athlete then aims to jump to maximum height by extending the hips, knees, and ankles as forcefully as possible during the propulsion phase of the jump. Specifically, the takeoff velocity (which is slightly lower than the peak velocity, as shown in figure 2.2) determines the maximal jump height attained during the flight phase, which is followed by landing (re-flexing the ankles, knees, and hips to decelerate) and then returning to standing height. With this understanding of the phases of the jump, it will be easier to consider phase-specific power or any other variable presented in figures 2.1 and 2.2. For example, this athlete attains peak force prior to takeoff during the braking phase (i.e., while still lowering the COM), but peak power and velocity occur during the propulsion phase (i.e., while raising the COM). An applied review article by McMahon and colleagues provides further information on the phases of the countermovement jump (53).

Jump Phases

The phases of the jump are often described as the portions of the jump with negative change of displacement (i.e., downward movement) or positive change of displacement (i.e., upward movement) (11). The unweighting and braking phases of the jump (i.e., the countermovement portion) have a negative P_{peak} and P_{mean} and commence when the force begins to decrease below a predetermined threshold (figure 2.1). The countermovement ends when velocity goes from negative to positive (crosses zero), as shown in figure 2.2. Simultaneously, this indicates the start of the propulsion phase that subsequently ends at takeoff or when force is at zero or falls below a predetermined threshold just above zero (depending on signal noise) (31).

To derive the power curve shown in figure 2.2, the force and velocity data for each sample (i.e., each 0.001 second when sampling at 1,000 Hz) are multiplied. The power curve is shown in figure 2.2 (right panel), where the occurrence of the P_{peak} is labeled. It is easy to identify the P_{peak} during the braking phase (it is the lowest power value prior to takeoff) and to calculate the P_{mean} during any phase by using the average value of power produced within it (figure 2.2). The actual calculation of power is relatively simple when force is directly measured during the task and the net force (force less the body or system weight) is then divided by body mass (or system mass, if performing a loaded jump) across the entire sample and subsequently numerically integrated to yield velocity; however, as will be discussed, many methods of measurement can be used to derive or estimate the power curve, each with its own advantages and disadvantages.

Validity and Reliability

Validity and reliability are concepts not only critical to testing in general but also important in understanding the measurement of system power. Power produced during a variety of physical performance tests has been reviewed extensively in the literature from a validity and reliability perspective (10, 22, 29, 77). Validity can be described as how well a test measures the criterion of performance it is intended to measure, while reliability can be described as the ability to reproduce results repeatedly, or the consistency of the measure (29). Before the assessment of validity, a measure must be reliable to be worth confirming the validity. All measures of power presented in this chapter are considered to have acceptable reliability; however, with respect to validity, the power measures are split into direct (more valid) and indirect (less valid) measures of system power. When attempting to obtain a valid and reliable measurement of power, even when using direct measures of power, all methodologies are not equal, and the chosen method can still affect the validity and reliability of the measure.

Variables that should be controlled, or held constant, to increase the reliability of testing include the testing equipment and the method of calculation, the instructions to the athlete, the time of day, the athlete's fatigue status and familiarity with the testing protocol, the athlete's experience or training status, the temperature of the testing environment, the warm-up protocol before testing, and the order of testing (if other tests are also being performed).

The more controlled the testing environment, the higher the reliability of the testing, which influences the magnitude of change required to be considered a meaningful change (i.e., beyond measurement error) in performance. In other words, increasing the reliability of the measure improves the precision, allowing a practitioner to identify smaller changes in athlete performance. Statistically, the smallest worthwhile change can be calculated by multiplying the between-athlete standard deviation by 0.2 for any performance variable (28). In practical terms, this represents the smallest magnitude of change that would have to occur before the change could be considered meaningful (28).

Direct and Indirect Power Measurement

Increasing emphasis has been placed on the assessment of power during ballistic activities in strength and conditioning research and practice; therefore, the following description will focus on power assessment during ballistic activities. However, mechanical power output is often measured using a variety of other tests, such as those performed on a cycle ergometer (e.g., the Wingate test). Additionally, power has been measured during weightlifting exercises and their derivatives, but because of the unique nature of these exercises and the separate interaction of the bar with the COM of the athlete, special considerations are required when measuring or calculating power during these exercises (30, 32, 44) and even during a back squat (39). System power output during ballistic activities is often measured using two broad types of assessment: direct and indirect. From a practical perspective, the decreased cost and increased availability of force plates and linear position transducers (LPTs) has led to an increase in the number of practitioners measuring and reporting system power output across a wide variety of tasks using direct measurement. Of note, assessing velocity using a single LPT can lead to inflated estimations of power, because the velocity of the barbell is greater than that of the body or system (30, 32, 39, 44). Figure 2.3 outlines considerations for developing a sport-based assessment battery that includes methodological factors.

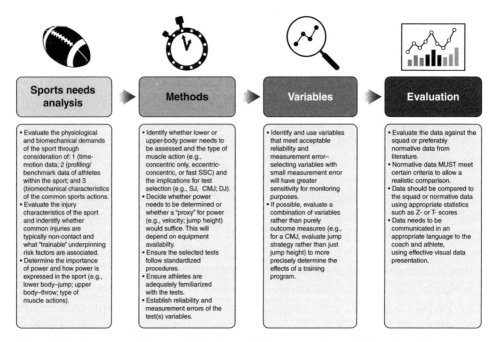

Sports needs analysis	Methods	Variables	Evaluation
• Evaluate the physiological and biomechanical demands of the sport through consideration of: 1 (time-motion data; 2 (profiling/benchmark data of athletes within the sport; and 3 (biomechanical characteristics of the common sports actions. • Evaluate the injury characteristics of the sport and indentify whether common injuries are typically non-contact and what "trainable" underpinning risk factors are associated. • Determine the importance of power and how power is expressed in the sport (e.g., lower body–jump; upper body–throw; type of muscle actions).	• Identify whether lower or upper-body power needs to be assessed and the type of muscle action (e.g., concentric only, eccentric-concentric, or fast SSC) and the implications for test selection (e.g., SJ, CMJ; DJ). • Decide whether power needs to be determined or whether a "proxy" for power (e.g., velocity; jump height) would suffice. This will depend on equipment availabilty. • Ensure the selected tests follow standardized procedures. • Ensure athletes are adequately familiarized with the tests. • Establish reliability and measurement errors of the test(s) variables.	• Identify and use variables that meet acceptable reliability and measurement error–selecting variables with small measurement error will have greater sensitivity for monitoring purposes. • If possible, evaluate a combination of variables rather than purely outcome measures (e.g., for a CMJ, evaluate jump strategy rather than just jump height) to more precisely determine the effects of a training program.	• Evaluate the data against the squad or preferably normative data from literature. • Normative data MUST meet certain criteria to allow a realistic comparison. • Data should be compared to the squad or normative data using appropriate statistics such as Z- or T- scores • Data needs to be communicated in an appropriate language to the coach and athlete, using effective visual data presentation.

Figure 2.3 A proposed framework for determining tests or "power" based on the sport, individual, context, and equipment availability. CMJ = countermovement jump; DJ = drop jump; SJ = squat jump; SSC = stretch-shortening cycle.

For an indirect assessment of power, several equations have been derived to predict power output during jumping (table 2.1). However, it is recommended to use jump height as the performance variable rather than reporting power output by using predictive equations. This is because predicted power has greater error, and therefore, the smallest worthwhile change must be larger to state with certainty that two athletes produced different magnitudes of power (77). For reference, some of the commonly used equations for the prediction of power from a single jump (24, 68) or multiple jumps (4) are listed in table 2.1.

Table 2.1 Common Equations and Methodologies Used for Predicting System Power Output During Jumping

Name (reference)	Methodology considerations	Formula
Bosco formula (4)	• Repeated jumps during a given time (15-60 s). • Test is performed on a contact mat, and countermovement depth should be controlled (~90 degrees of flexion), which can be difficult. • Hands should be kept on hips.	Mean power (W) = $$\frac{\text{flight time} \times \text{test duration} \times g^2}{4 \times \text{number of jumps} \times (\text{test duration} - \text{total flight time})}$$ where flight time = summation of flight time of all jumps.
Harman formula (24)	• Single jump for maximal height. • Originally developed for squat jump; can use countermovement jump, but this may increase inaccuracy.	Peak power (W) = $(61.9 \times \text{jump height [cm]})$ + $(36.0 \times \text{body mass [kg]}) + 1822$ Mean power (W) = $21.2 \times \text{jump height [cm]}$ + $23.0 \times \text{body mass [kg]} + 1393$
Sayers formula (68)	• Single jump for maximal height. • May use squat jump or countermovement jump.	Peak power (W) = $(60.7 \times \text{jump height [cm]})$ + $(45.3 \times \text{body mass [kg]}) - 2055$
Lewis formula (22)	• Single jump for maximal height. • Considered least accurate, but widely used.	Power (W) = $\sqrt{(4.9 \times \text{body mass [kg]})}$ $\times \sqrt{(\text{jump height [m]})} \times 9.81$

Practitioners should avoid using different activities (modes of movement) or comparison of indirect (e.g., Bosco jump test) and direct (e.g., Wingate cycle ergometer test) measures of power. For example, the multiple-jump Bosco test results in a power output different from that measured during a Wingate cycle ergometer test of the same duration on the same group of tested individuals (24). Recommended best practice is to compare power only within the same type of activity and with the same method of power calculation to ensure valid conclusions. Although a difference in results between the Bosco jump test and Wingate cycle ergometer test for the P_{mean} could be explained by differences in stored elastic energy during jumping, one cannot conclude how much of this difference is also a function of comparing direct and indirect measures of power, and doing so is therefore ill advised. Because some practitioners will not have access to the equipment required for direct assessments, a comprehensive list of upper body, lower body, total body, and rotational direct and indirect assessments of power is presented in table 2.2. A similar recommendation against equating displacement to power should be followed for the listed indirect tests of power. Instead, the performance measure reported and used for comparison for an athlete or between athletes should be the jump distance (e.g., broad jump or long jump) or toss and throw distances.

Table 2.2 Common Methods for Direct and Indirect Assessment of Power

Exercise or test	Purpose	Brief methodology	Variations
UPPER BODY			
Medicine ball chest pass	Upper body explosiveness with indirect (distance) measure of power	The individual either sits upright, with the back supported and legs directly in front, or on a weight bench with the feet on the floor and the bench inclined to 45 degrees. The mass of the medicine ball should be relevant to individual's age or sex (body mass). The individual holds a medicine ball in both hands at the chest, and without additional movement, tosses the ball for maximal distance (instruct and familiarize the individual as to angle of toss).	• Mass of medicine ball • Angle of trunk position
Bench press throw	Upper body assessment with direct measure of power*	The individual assumes the same positioning as in a bench press while in a Smith machine.* If available, use a magnetic brake to stop the weight after the throw; otherwise, the individual should be familiar with both the throw and catch before maximal attempts. Choose between performing a concentric-only throw or allowing a countermovement (similar to that of a static or countermovement jump).	• Static • Countermovement • Absolute loading profile • Relative loading profile
Upper body Wingate test	Anaerobic capacity with direct measure of power*	The individual sits in a chair facing a cycle ergometer modified for the upper body.* Feet are flat on the floor. Following a warm-up, the individual pedals the arm crank to maximal cadence; then 0.05 kg of load per kg body mass is added as resistance. Maximal effort will then commence for the required amount of time (typically 30 s).	• Length of test
LOWER BODY			
Countermovement jump (CMJ)	Lower body assessment with stretch-shortening cycle with indirect (height) measure of power	The individual performs a maximal jump using an arm swing. Measure the maximal reach of a single arm overhead, then have the individual jump as high as possible. The individual performs the jump with a self-selected countermovement depth. Subtract distance between total jump height and reach height to determine jump height.	• Single-leg variation

Exercise or test	Purpose	Brief methodology	Variations
LOWER BODY			
Squat (static) jump (SJ)	Lower body assessment without stretch-shortening cycle with indirect (height) measure of power	The individual performs this test the same as the CMJ, except that he or she lowers to the self-selected depth and holds that position. Upon jumping, the individual should only move up. If a countermovement is made, negate the trial.	• Single-leg variation
Broad jump (horizontal jump)	Lower body assessment with stretch-shortening cycle with indirect (distance) measure of power	The individual stands with his or her toes behind a line and then jumps forward as far as possible. The individual should use the arms and land under control on both feet. Measure distance from takeoff line to heel of closest foot.	• Repeated jumps or hops • Single-leg variations
Countermovement jump (CMJ)	Lower body assessment with stretch-shortening cycle with direct measure of power	Instructions are the same as for the indirect CMJ; however, the individual can place his or her hands either on the hips or on a wooden dowel (or bar, where appropriate) so that the power measured is indicative of the lower body. This placement also minimizes variation of results caused by changes in arm swing.	• Body weight • Single-leg variation • Absolute loading profile • Relative loading profile
Squat (static) jump (SJ)	Lower body assessment without stretch-shortening cycle with direct measure of power*	Instructions are the same as for the indirect SJ; however, the individual can place his or her hands either on the hips or on a wooden dowel (or bar, where appropriate) so that the power measured is indicative of the lower body and minimizes variation of results caused by changes in arm swing.	• Body weight • Single-leg variation • Absolute loading profile • Relative loading profile
Lower body Wingate test	Anaerobic capacity with direct measure of power	The individual performs this on a Monark cycle ergometer.* The bike is adjusted so the knee is just short of full extension at the bottom of the pedal stroke. Following a warm-up, the individual pedals to maximal cadence; then 0.075 kg of load per kg body mass is added as resistance. Maximal effort then commences for the required amount of time (typically 30 s).	• Length of test

(continued)

Table 2.2 Common Methods for Direct and Indirect Assessment of Power *(continued)*

Exercise or test	Purpose	Brief methodology	Variations
TOTAL BODY			
Medicine ball toss (overhead or underhand)	Total-body assessment with indirect (distance) measure of power	Numerous methodologies are available that require use of the total body or coordinated movement of the total body to toss or throw a medicine ball for maximal distance. Variations include the standing overhead toss, similar to a soccer throw-in or rugby lineout toss, or an underhand toss, performed either toward the direction of the toss or backward and overhead behind the individual. All variations should be performed with maximal total-body effort.	• Various release positions • Mass of medicine ball
Olympic lifts (snatch, clean, and jerk) and derivatives	Total body assessment (primarily lower body) with direct measure of power*	Measure hang variations directly, as described in table 2.3 and chapter 7. The individual should be proficient in the techniques before performing these exercises.	• Exercise variations (e.g., hang clean) • Absolute loading profile • Relative loading profile
ROTATIONAL			
Rotational medicine ball toss	Rotational assessment with indirect measure of power	This is commonly performed by athletes in sports with a high rotational component, such as baseball and softball. From a side-on stance, The athlete tosses the ball for maximal distance. The ball should be in both hands and start behind the athlete at a height between the waist and shoulders, similar to a batting stance.	• Mass of medicine ball

Note: Individuals should perform these tests only after appropriate familiarization and warm-up, in line with suggestions for improving reliability of testing.

*Direct measures of power use one of the methodologies that directly assess variables to calculate system power, as described in table 2.3.

Consistent with the information provided thus far on power measurement, if possible, practitioners should not exclusively use the equations in table 2.1 or any indirect (predictive) measure of power. The direct measurement of system power is considered the most valid measure capable of effectively detecting minimal differences or smallest worthwhile changes in system power following a training block or for comparison between athletes. Considering the types of direct measures used to report power output (10, 14, 54), the reliability and validity of these methodologies should also be considered. An understanding of the advantages and disadvantages of various methodologies for the direct assessment of power is described in table 2.3.

Table 2.3 Advantages and Disadvantages of Various Direct Measures of System or Mechanical Power

Equipment	Advantages	Disadvantages
2 (or 4) LPTs and FP	Direct measure of force and displacement (to calculate velocity). Includes measurement of horizontal displacement (or velocity) during movements that are not fully linear (vertical or horizontal only).	Most expensive setup and requires designated space because of equipment requirements.[a]
1 LPT and FP	Direct measure of both force and displacement (to calculate velocity). Combination is a valid assessment of power based on the bar velocity during ballistic movements.	Assumption that movements are fully linear (e.g., not ideal for Olympic variations) and bar velocity is representative of center-of-mass velocity.[a]
FP only	Highly reliable and valid for both weightlifting (from hang positions) and ballistic movements. Valid assessment of power based on the center-of-mass velocity.	Mathematical manipulation (forward dynamics) to calculate power could result in error associated with underestimation of power.[b]
LPT only (or 2-D kinematic analysis[c])	Relatively inexpensive. Reliable measure of velocity if movement is primarily linear (vertical or horizontal only).	Mathematical manipulation (inverse dynamics) can cause magnification of error in calculation, and often, overestimation of power.[a]
Accelerometer	Relatively inexpensive. Reliable measure of jump height during CMJ.	Reliability and bias of velocity and power measures increase minimal difference required when assessing changes in power.[a]

Note: 2-D = two-dimensional; CMJ = countermovement jump; FP = force plate; LPT = linear position transducer.

[a]Measurement of power is based on the velocity of the bar and therefore does not include movements independent of the barbell.

[b]Measurement of power is based on the velocity of the center of mass (system) and therefore does not consider barbell movement.

[c]Two-dimensional kinematic analysis refers to using a marker on the athlete's hip (greater trochanter) to represent the change in the athlete's center of mass.

COMMON POWER TESTS

Some common tests during which power can either be measured or indirectly estimated and that may be of interest to strength and conditioning practitioners will now be discussed in a little more detail than what is summarized in table 2.2 for additional context and considerations.

Standing Broad Jump

The standing broad jump (SBJ), sometimes referred to as the standing long jump, is often used as a proxy for ballistic lower body power rather than a direct measurement, although power can be measured during this test (as later described). The SBJ distance has been shown to be moderately associated (r = 0.335-0.686; $p \leq 0.016$) with P_{peak} attained during a Wingate cycle ergometer test (37) and also moderately associated with P_{peak} and P_{mean} (both r = 0.52; p < 0.01) measured during the SBJ itself (41).

Athletes typically perform the broad jump to a self-selected countermovement depth and with arm swing (25, 41, 69), although sometimes the test has been conducted with the hands remaining on the hips throughout (43). The athlete starts with the toes directly behind a specified start line (usually marked out via a line in the track, court, or pitch or with tape) and is cued to jump as far as possible and to land on both feet (41). The athlete is expected to stick the landing and remain motionless either while in a flexed hip and knee (squatted) position or after standing up following landing. Because there is a requirement to land in a disciplined manner (versus vertical jump assessments), the SBJ may require the completion of additional trials until the required minimum number is achieved. For example, it has been reported that up to 9 attempts of the SBJ are required to provide 3 acceptable trials (69).

The SBJ requires minimal equipment. Typically, only a fiberglass tape measure is used. The horizontal jump distance is measured from the start line to the heel farthest back (i.e., the one closest to the start line). This distance is usually reported to the nearest centimeter (1, 43). The horizonal jump distance is the only variable that can be reported if using a fiberglass tape measure; thus, it is the most often reported, both in practice and research. However, the P_{peak} can be estimated from the SBJ horizontal distance as power (W) = 32.49 × SLJ horizontal distance (cm) + 39.69 × body mass (kg) − 7608, based on a study by Mann and colleagues (41) in which the predictive ability and reliability of this equation were high (r = 0.86; SEE = 488 W; CV% = 9.3%) However, the shared variance between these tests equates to only 74%.

The horizontal jump distance attained during the SBJ can be calculated from force plate data if using a force plate that can concurrently measure both the vertical and anterior–posterior components of the ground reaction force (25, 41). The force plate must be embedded in the ground or securely fixed above the ground to prevent it from slipping when the athlete performs the broad jump. Horizontal jump distance during the SBJ can also be measured via motion capture using two-dimensional cameras if they are placed perpendicular (sagittal plane) to where the SBJ is performed and remain static (e.g., mounted to a tripod) while recording (83). When using a force plate or motion capture to record SBJ performance, it can be deconstructed into various phases, including takeoff, flight, and landing, which may yield more useful information to the practitioner than reporting horizontal jump distance alone.

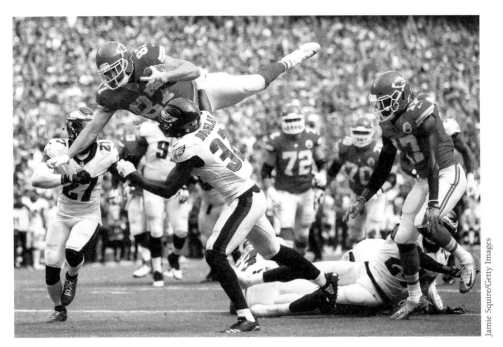

Jamie Squire/Getty Images

Travis Kelce trains power to leap over defenders.

Medicine Ball Chest Pass

The medicine ball chest pass (MBCP), like the SBJ, is used as a field-based proxy for ballistic upper body power, although power can be measured during this test if the medicine ball is instrumented (as later described). The MBCP distance has been shown to be moderately associated ($r = 0.55$; $p \leq 0.001$) with P_{peak} attained during a Wingate test performed on an arm-crank ergometer (38).

A 3 kilogram (6.6 lb) medicine ball is most commonly used for the MBCP test (20, 38), although various medicine ball masses have been reported in the literature, ranging from 9 pounds (0.4 kg) to 13 pounds (5.9 kg) (42). Athletes can perform the MBCP from a seated position or standing position. If seated, the athlete may be positioned with the back oriented vertically against an immovable support, such as a wall (38, 42), with the legs usually positioned straight in front (38, 42, 81). The athlete is instructed to throw the medicine ball from the chest position (like a chest pass in basketball) as far as possible and without flexing the spine (i.e., maintaining the back in a vertical position) (20). The wall or hip position is usually considered the start line (20, 38), and the throw distance is usually measured with a fiberglass tape measure as the horizontal distance from the start line to the point where the medicine ball first contacted the ground. To account for different arm lengths when measuring the horizontal throw distance, Kumar and colleagues (38) had athletes stand with their head, thoracic spine, buttocks, and heels touching the wall; while holding their arms out in front of them (parallel with the floor), the athletes dropped the medicine ball directly onto a tape measure that was extended from the wall. The authors then subtracted this distance from the horizontal throw distance, originally measured from the start line to where the medicine ball first contacted the ground (38).

Aside from measuring the MBCP horizontal throw distance with a fiberglass tape measure, the throw velocity attained during the MBCP can also be measured by using a radar gun (81), three-dimensional motion capture (42), or a medicine ball instrumented with an inertial measurement unit, which has been validated against three-dimensional motion capture for the peak velocity variable (79). In a study in which the load, power, and velocity profile of the MBCP was determined (42), maximal velocity was the only useful measure. This was because power and force estimates were not reliable, but velocity was; thus, the authors suggested that MBCP provides better insight into upper body maximal velocity capabilities than power capabilities (42).

Force–Velocity–Power Profiling

Force–velocity–power profiling is common in strength and conditioning (46). Simple methods of calculating force–velocity–power profiles during a squat jump (65) and a countermovement jump (34) have been proposed, which can be achieved with basic equipment such as a smartphone to videorecord the jumps (18) and then a validated smartphone application to subsequently estimate the associated jump heights using the flight-time method (3).

In addition to estimating jump height from flight time, an estimation of the push-off height during the jump (the assumed displacement of the COM during propulsion) and of body mass (or system mass, if jumps are performed with external load) is also required to construct the force–velocity–power profile (34, 65). The estimation of push-off height during the jump is most commonly not measured during the jump itself but rather separately as the difference in the distance measured between the greater trochanter location and the toes while the athlete lies on the ground with the ankles fully plantar flexed (the assumed COM height at take-off) and the distance between the greater trochanter location and the floor while the athlete adopts a squatted position involving 90 degrees of knee flexion (the assumed COM height at the start of propulsion).

The mean force, mean velocity, and P_{mean} during the jump are then estimated based on the work–energy theorem (see chapter 1 for more information on work and energy). The force–velocity–power profile can be determined if these equations are applied to jumps performed with at least two external loads (21). The efficacy of conducting force–velocity–power profiling of externally loaded countermovement jumps (with either a straight barbell or a hexagonal barbell) has been questioned due to fixed and proportional bias being shown when comparing the simple method, based on jump height from the flight time (34), to the mean force, mean velocity, and P_{mean} measured via a force plate (27). This issue was not noted when using a Smith machine to conduct loaded counter-movement jumps (34). Furthermore, the originators of the method (Samozino and colleagues [66]) attributed discrepancies reported in studies such as that by Hicks and colleagues (27) to sources of error during data collection, and thus, they highlighted the importance of standardizing and controlling for measurement error when applying force–velocity–power equations to derived jump data (66).

Rebound Jump

Rebound jumps performed from a standing position on the ground are conducted by the athlete first completing a maximal-effort countermovement jump followed by a set number of rebound-jump repetitions. Rebound jumps have been performed with 1, 3, 5, 6, and 10 repetitions in the scientific literature (5, 8, 43, 72, 88). Rebound jumps are performed with the athlete attempting to jump with a short ground contact time (i.e., <250 milliseconds) while still aiming to jump as high as possible (19). Therefore, the most frequently reported performance variables following rebound jump testing are jump height, ground contact time, and reactive strength index (RSI) (calculated as the jump height divided by the ground contact time). A plethora of equipment can be used to derive these variables, such as force plates, jump mats, optoelectronic systems, and smartphone applications. The RSI is often considered to be a proxy for how well an athlete can use the stretch-shortening cycle (47).

Although positive ankle joint power (derived by combining motion capture and force plate data) has been described as the most influential factor for the above-mentioned rebound jump performance variables (88), the system P_{peak} and P_{mean} are rarely measured directly. The reason for this, in part, is that numerical integration drift can be an issue when measuring rebound jump tests involving multiple repetitions with a force plate, meaning that the velocity–time record produced from the original force–time record will have accumulated error for the later repetitions performed within the set, and thus, the subsequent power calculations will be incorrect. However, an athlete will have performed the rebound jumps with greater mechanical power if he or she jumped higher (compared with peers or his or her own previous performance) and did so with either the same or a shorter contact time. Therefore, as with the tests discussed earlier, the propulsion P_{mean} can be inferred from various rebound jump tests by measuring jump height (which is dictated by work done during propulsion) and ground contact time, even with minimally expensive equipment.

Squat Jump

The squat jump is often used as a concentric-only (i.e., propulsion) assessment of ballistic lower body power. The squat jump is performed in the same manner as the propulsion phase of the countermovement jump (i.e., aiming to move fast and jump high) but begins from a motionless, squatted position rather than from standing. The depth of the initial squatted position is usually based on the athlete's achieving a knee flexion angle of 90 degrees (typically measured with a goniometer). When commanded to jump, the athlete must immediately extend the hips, knees, and ankles and avoid any initial flexion of these joints (i.e., pre-stretch) before commencing extension. This is important because the purpose of the squat jump is to remove any influence of the stretch-shortening cycle, which is initiated in the countermovement portion of a countermovement jump, or of the braking phase of a rebound jump as the hips, knees, and ankles flex rapidly.

Although it has been shown that a small-amplitude countermovement (SACM) of 0.4 to 1.2 inches (1.0-3.0 cm) performed immediately prior to extending the hips, knees, and ankles during a squat jump did not significantly alter the subsequent jump height based on mean data (26), an SACM has been shown to augment jump height by up to 2.4 inches (6.0 cm) for individual athletes (70). Representative force–time curves for squat jumps performed with and without an SACM are presented in figures 2.4 and 2.5, respectively. Aside from the effect on jump height, performing the squat jump with an initial SACM on a force plate will influence the automated identification of when the jump begins, which, if identified incorrectly, will affect the propulsion phase duration and thus the P_{mean} measurement, among other variables. Indeed, without a force plate or other device with a high sampling rate, it may not be obvious to the strength and conditioning professional that an SACM was performed. For example, when 125 squat jump trials were analyzed, approximately 90% contained an SACM, and of those trials, only approximately 60% were observed in real time by the tester (based on "coach's eye") to have an SACM (70).

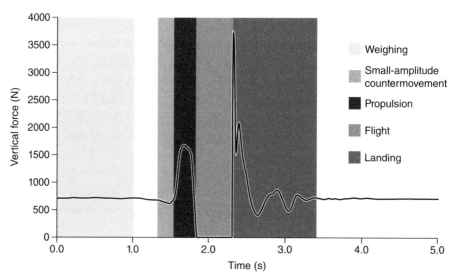

Figure 2.4 A representative unacceptable force–time curve for a squat jump containing a small-amplitude countermovement, which should not occur during this test. The weighing, propulsion, flight, and landing phases of the squat jump are shown for context.

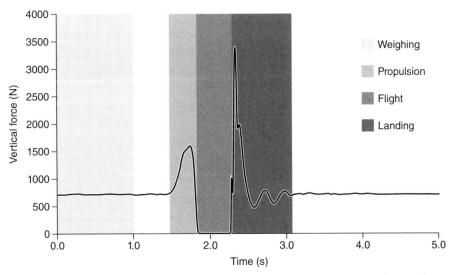

Figure 2.5 A representative acceptable force–time curve for a squat jump. The weighing, propulsion, flight, and landing phases of the squat jump are shown for context.

The main rationale for including the squat jump in an athlete-testing battery is to compare values obtained during it to those attained during the counter-movement jump. The eccentric utilization ratio (EUR) is mainly used as the comparator between the two jump types and has been calculated using both the jump height and the P_{peak} from each jump, although differences between these two variables have been noted when using them in the EUR calculation (48). With the process being the same for the P_{peak}, the EUR equation is shown below with the more commonly used jump height variable included:

EUR = countermovement jump height ÷ squat jump height

The idea behind the EUR is that a value greater than one, which occurs when the countermovement jump height is greater than the squat jump height, indicates that the athlete has benefitted from using the stretch-shortening cycle, which should be experienced only in the countermovement jump because the squat jump should solely involve concentric muscle actions. However, jump height, irrespective of the jump type, tends to increase if the propulsion displacement increases (i.e., the propulsion phase commences from a lower COM position via performing a deeper squat). This is due to the effect of producing force over a greater distance on propulsion net impulse (a larger distance tends to extend time) and work. Thus, if propulsion displacement differs between the countermovement jump and the squat jump, any superior jump heights obtained in the former cannot be attributed to the stretch-shortening cycle alone (74). Researchers have reported a large relationship between the ratio of propulsion displacement (between the countermovement jump and the squat jump) and the EUR (50).

Encouraging athletes to adopt their preferred squat depth during the squat jump rather than with 90 degrees of knee flexion improves test reliability and has been reported to reduce test time (64), although the results of one study highlighted the difficulties in standardizing countermovement depth in the countermovement jump to squat depth in the squat jump (by approximating joint angles, including 90 degrees of knee flexion) in an attempt to enable fairer between-jump comparisons (67). Thus, given that differences in propulsion displacement between the countermovement jump and squat jump will likely be present regardless of test standardization and the fact that many athletes may perform an SACM during the squat jump test, which makes it difficult to analyze some variables accurately when using automated software, practitioners should be aware of these limitations when conducting the squat jump test with athletes solely to calculate the EUR.

Using the information provided, final recommendations can be made to practitioners to ensure they use valid and reliable system-power measurements to assess athletes. However, not all practitioners will have access to the equipment described; therefore, they should use a combination of the most valid and reliable methods possible while understanding the subsequent limitations.

The following is a summary of the overall recommendations for direct measurement of system power during ballistic activities:

▶ Direct measurement of velocity using an LPT—or, most accurately, two LPTs—to remove error caused by horizontal displacement in conjunction with direct force measurement is best practice when assessing the velocity of the bar (10).

▶ A single LPT, either with or without the use of a force plate, can measure the power output of a movement that is primarily linear (vertical). Other movements, such as a clean or snatch, that have as much as 10% of the work done horizontally (22) could result in an inflated velocity and power measure if assessed using only a single LPT.

▶ Caution should be used when using accelerometers to measure system power because of the potentially large errors that may make it difficult to compare between or evaluate changes in power following an intervention (14).

▶ If the system or mechanical power of the COM is of greater interest than the mechanical power of the bar, then a method that uses only a force plate may be the most applicable and may differentiate power improvement based on changes in bar path (technique) from changes in the ability to apply force to the ground (30).

▶ Sampling frequency should be above 200 Hz, particularly if only peak values (e.g., peak power, peak velocity) are of interest. Best practice is a sampling frequency at or above 1,000 Hz when the intention is to assess the rate of force development (54, 73) or more detailed elements of the force–time curve (e.g., by identifying phases). The chosen valid and reliable method should be identical both within and between testing sessions to ensure that results can be compared.

REPORTING POWER RESULTS

When calculating power, the units can be expressed in terms of either an absolute measure (W) or a normalized factor such as body mass (W/kg), which is termed *ratio scaling*. The use of allometric scaling has been proposed as a way to understand a variable independent of body size and has been a topic of great discussion in the literature (13, 15, 33, 56-58). *Allometric scaling* is defined as normalizing data according to dimensionality to remove the effect of body size by normalizing the variable, which is done by dividing it by the body mass (BM) raised to the two-thirds power ($BM^{0.67}$) (56-58). However, before using allometric scaling for normalization, its advantages and disadvantages should be considered. For example, a potential issue with using the proposed exponent ($BM^{0.67}$) is that known variations in body size and composition, particularly the proportion of lean muscle mass, across sexes or different athlete groups (because of body type) can affect the ability of the exponent ($BM^{0.67}$) to correctly remove the effect of body size (57, 58). To handle this potential issue, it is suggested to derive an exponent instead of using the common $BM^{0.67}$ exponent. However, derived exponents lack generalizability because they may be specific to the characteristics of the group used to derive them, such as sex, age, body mass index, and training history (15, 86, 87). This means practitioners may not be able to compare performance data that are normalized using either a proposed or a derived allometric exponent if the athletes' body size characteristics are different, and therefore, simple ratio scaling (dividing by body mass) may be preferable (76). Because data comparison is a common aspect of performance testing, understanding the method of normalization used is critical.

Practitioners should understand both that a bias may exist in ratio scaling (normalizing to body mass) and the potential implications for larger and smaller athletes if ratio scaling is the chosen normalization method. However, when relating results to predictions of performance, ratio scaling has better characterized the relationship between normalized variables and performance than using allometrically scaled variables and performance (15). If it is necessary to eliminate the potential effect of body size to remove confounding factors related to very small or very large athletes, then either derived or proposed allometric scaling can be considered (15). Before applying allometric scaling, practitioners should meet assumptions, understand the implications and use of allometric scaling, and read a variety of resources (6, 58, 82).

PRESENTATION OF TESTING DATA

Beyond data normalization, another important consideration with respect to the presentation of power data is the context of the test performed. As previously mentioned, all movements have a power output. However, the comparison between modes of exercise or loadings may best be evaluated using a standardized score, as is commonly used to compare different aspects of physical performance (e.g., speed and endurance). A standardized score, also termed a *z-score*, calculates how many standard deviations the value is above or below the mean. The z-score can be calculated using the following equation, where x is the score to be standardized, μ is the mean, and ς is the standard deviation:

$$z - score = \frac{x - \mu}{\sigma}$$

CASE STUDY EXAMPLES

The raw data for an athlete are presented in figure 2.6, and two versions of this athlete's standardized data are shown in figure 2.7. Figure 2.6 shows the power profile, or power output, across a range of loadings during the jump squat as commonly assessed in research (17). In addition, these results have been standardized (figure 2.7), allowing a coach to understand how an athlete is improving at each load relative to the team. The difference between figure 2.7*a* and *b* is caused by the means and standard deviations used to calculate the z-score. The team means and standard deviations at each load during pretesting, midtesting, and posttesting, respectively, were used to calculate the z-scores in figure 2.7*a*, while in figure 2.7*b*, only the means and standard deviations at each load during pretesting were used to calculate subsequent z-scores at pretesting, midtesting, and posttesting.

The data in figure 2.6 show a power profile shift upward from pretesting to midtesting and then shifted up further (but not as substantially across all loads) from midtesting to posttesting. In particular, power production in the countermovement jump (load for body mass only) went up vastly. The two blocks of training between pretesting and midtesting were strength-focused blocks and the two blocks of training from midtesting to posttesting were power-focused blocks, explaining the shift in either the whole curve or the higher-velocity, low-load end of the curve (23, 61). Chapter 3 includes a discussion with respect to training the force–velocity curve and the effect on power. This demonstrates how measured power data can be presented to display or determine specific questions about the efficacy of training.

Two professional rugby league players' countermovement jump data obtained on the first day of the preseason period are presented in table 2.4. Player 1 (age, 29 years; height, 181 cm [71.3 in]; body mass, 94 kg [206.8 lb] plays in a back position, and player 2 (age, 30 years; height, 178 cm [70.1 in]; body mass, 97 kg [213.8 lb]) plays in a forward position. Notice that both players jumped 38 centimeters (15 in), but their underpinning power outputs and associated variables were somewhat different, which further highlights the limitations of reporting jump height alone.

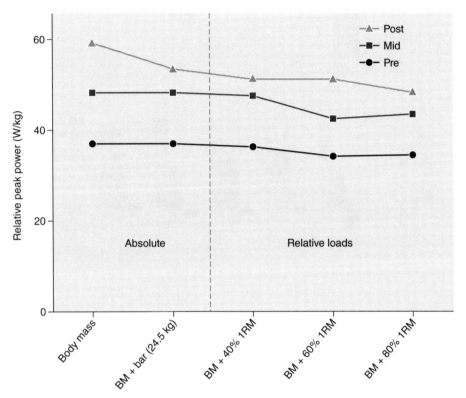

Figure 2.6 Example of a power profile with absolute and relative loads of an athlete at various points in a season (pretesting, midtesting, and posttesting).

For a visual comparison of the players' data, see figure 2.8, which includes both players' z-scores for each variable alongside the squad mean z-scores, which equal zero. Both players performed better than the squad mean when considering each variable (note that the z-scores for propulsion displacement and time have been inverted so that a higher z-score for each variable is achieved by a lower score). The players' P_{peak} values are equivalent, but player 2 produced a larger P_{mean}. This highlights that the P_{peak} and P_{mean} do not tell the same story, because the former represents the maximum power value achieved in just a 0.001 second instant in time (when sampling at 1,000 Hz), whereas the latter represents the average power applied throughout the entire propulsion phase. The larger P_{mean} for player 2 is a consequence of slightly more work being done in a shorter time during the propulsion phase. The slightly greater work done by player 2 occurred

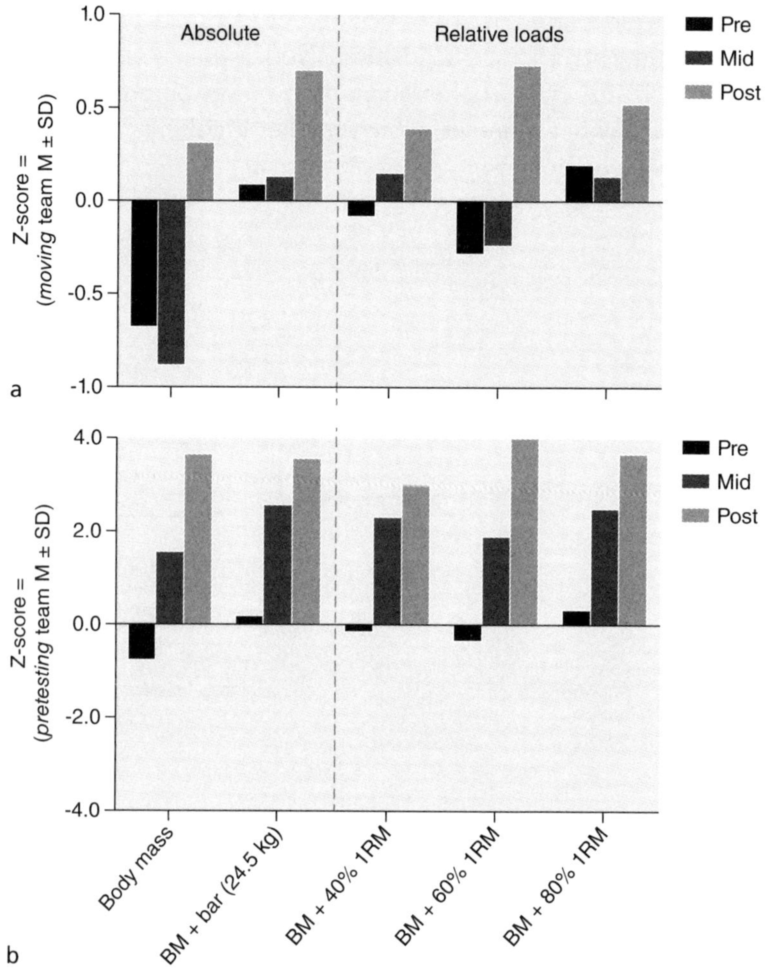

Figure 2.7 Example of standardized scores (z-scores) of an athlete at various absolute and relative loads, calculated with either *(a)* a moving team mean and standard deviation at pretesting, midtesting, and posttesting or *(b)* use of a static team mean and standard deviation at each load from pretesting.

due to greater mean force being applied, because the propulsion displacement was slightly lower compared with player 1.

Based on the countermovement jump results discussed previously, it might be inferred that player 2 performed superiorly to player 1. However, each of the variables shown in table 2.4 and figure 2.8 are based on propulsion or output (jump height). Figure 2.9 shows the full force–, velocity–, displacement–, and power–time curves produced by players 1 and 2. Although the propulsion time was shorter for player 2, the total time to takeoff (i.e., the time from initiating the jump to leaving the ground) was shorter for player 1, meaning that differences occurred in the countermovement portion (i.e., combined unweighting and braking phases) of the jump.

Table 2.4 Two Professional Rugby League Players' Countermovement Jump Data Obtained on the First Day of the Preseason Period

	Peak propulsion power (W)	Mean propulsion power (W)	Mean propulsion force (N)	Propulsion displacement (m)	Propulsion time (s)
#1 Back	5,388	3,011	2,038	0.38	0.232
#2 Forward	5,547	3,292	2,241	0.36	0.208
Squad mean	5,190	3,066	2,057	0.41	0.244
Squad SD	561	331	180	0.04	0.032
	Peak propulsion power (W/kg)	Mean propulsion power (W/kg)	Mean propulsion force (N/kg)	Propulsion work (J)	Jump height (cm) (in)
#1 Back	57.1	31.9	21.6	352	38 (15)
#2 Forward	56.9	33.8	23.0	363	38 (15)
Squad mean	52.7	31.2	20.9	351	36 (14.2)
Squad SD	5.7	3.4	1.8	46	5

Note: SD = standard deviation.

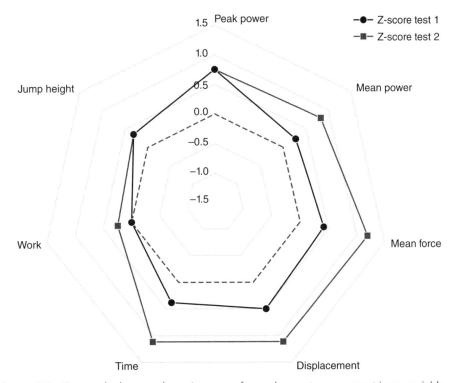

Figure 2.8 Two rugby league players' z-scores for each countermovement jump variable alongside the squad mean z-scores, which equal zero. Player 1's data points are connected by the black line, player 2's data points are denoted by the dark gray line, and the squad mean is represented by the gray dashed line.

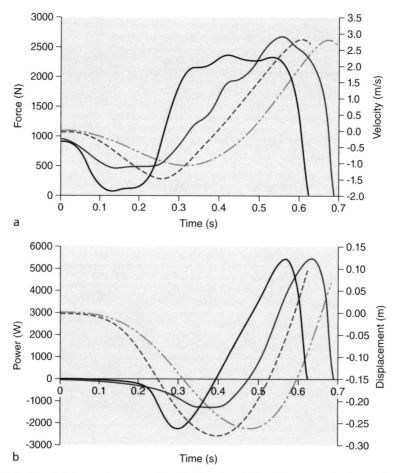

Figure 2.9 The full force–time curve (*a*, solid lines), velocity–time curve (*a*, dotted lines), displacement–time curve (*b*, dotted lines), and power–time curve (*b*, solid lines) produced by player 1 (black lines) and player 2 (gray lines) during the countermovement jump.

Figure 2.10 shows the force–velocity curve for each player. The area underneath the force–velocity curve is equivalent to the total power produced during the jump. The data shown to the left of the vertical axis in figure 2.10 shows that player 1 executed the countermovement portion of the jump with a higher unweighting velocity and a larger mean braking force, which resulted in beginning the propulsion phase with a larger initial force (often termed *force at zero velocity* or *force at minimum displacement*). Despite the more pronounced countermovement portion performed by player 1, the data show that this player gained no additional benefit during the propulsion phase when compared with player 2. Similarly, it is unknown whether player 2 underperformed in the countermovement jump test because the countermovement portion was not used particularly well or whether the propulsion phase would have diminished if the player had unweighted more and then braked harder in the preceding countermovement portion. This scenario illustrates why it is difficult to compare jump strategy variables among athletes within a single testing session but also highlights why monitoring jump strategy variables alongside other metrics, such as power and jump height, can be illuminating in terms of explaining how changes in the latter did or did not occur from a mechanical perspective. Such strategy variables may also provide insight into the physical qualities that the athlete needs to develop during the next phase of training.

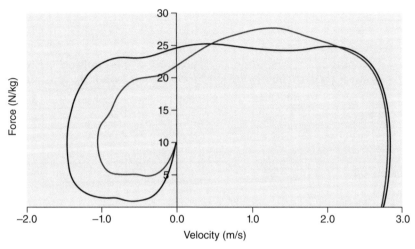

Figure 2.10 The force–velocity curve obtained during the countermovement jump for player 1 (black line) and player 2 (gray line).

Table 2.5 shows player 2's retest scores for the countermovement jump after he completed the initial six weeks of preseason training. When looking at the percentage change values (table 2.5), most variables show a small percentage change that is likely to fall within the associated measurement error of the test. Jump height and the P_{peak} and P_{mean} are, therefore, interpreted as showing no meaningful change from the start of the preseason period.

However, there are some potential interim adaptations worth noting. First, player 2's body mass (total mass only, not specifically muscle mass) increased from 97 to 99 kg (213 to 218 lb). Thus, he can jump the same height despite being 2 kg (4.4 lb) heavier than before, which will be because of a higher propulsive impulse. Second, he went through an 8.6% larger propulsion displacement but in only a 2.6% longer time. He still performed better than his squad for all jump metrics (figure 2.11).

Most interesting of all, player 2 executed the countermovement portion of the jump with a higher unweighting velocity and a larger mean braking force than he did before, resulting in a larger force at the commencement of propulsion (figure 2.12). Although there was no meaningful benefit to the propulsion phase and height of the jump resulting from his use of the countermovement

Table 2.5 Player 2's Retest Scores for the Countermovement Jump After He Completed the Initial Six Weeks of Preseason Training

	Peak propulsion power (W)	Mean propulsion power (W)	Mean propulsion force (N)	Propulsion displacement (cm) (in)	Propulsion time (s)
Pretest	5,388	3,011	2,038	38 (15)	0.232
Posttest	5,513	3,077	2,114	44 (17.3)	0.259
Change (units)	125	65	76	6 (2.3)	0.027
Change (%)	2.3	2.2	3.7	14.5	11.8
	Peak propulsion power (W/kg)	Mean propulsion power (W/kg)	Mean propulsion force (N/kg)	Propulsion work (J)	Jump height (cm) (in)
Pretest	57.1	31.9	21.6	352	38 (15)
Posttest	56.6	31.6	21.7	383	40 (15.7)
Change (units)	−0.4	−0.3	0.1	31	2 (0.7)
Change (%)	−0.7	−0.9	0.6	8.8	5.6

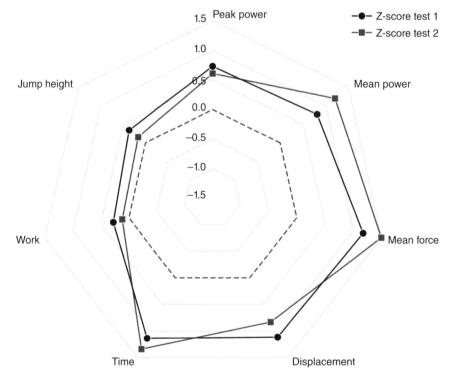

Figure 2.11 Player 2's original test scores (data points connected by the black line) and retest scores (data points connected by the gray line) for the countermovement jump after he completed the initial six weeks of preseason training.

portion to a greater extent that in pretraining, there was also no detriment to these metrics. Thus, these results may reflect interim adaptations to preseason training that would hopefully improve after the completion of more training, particularly with a ballistic focus. Monitoring player 2's countermovement jump performance later in the preseason training period would show whether these desirable adaptations did occur.

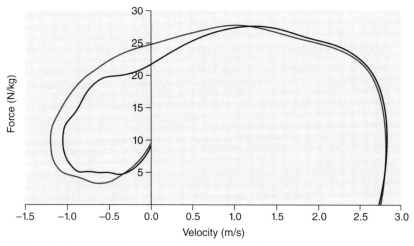

Figure 2.12   The force–velocity curve obtained during the countermovement jump for player 2 before (black line) and after (gray line) he completed the initial six weeks of preseason training.

COMPARING POWER VALUES TO NORMATIVE DATA

In addition to comparing the two rugby league players' power data to the average (mean) obtained by players in their squad, the data may also be compared to published normative data (usually from the population mean and standard deviation reported in relevant studies) provided that a comparable test protocol was adhered to, and this approach would be preferable given that squad descriptive data will likely fluctuate between test occasions due to training-induced adaptations, injury, or seasonal factors. In a published study, percentiles for the countermovement jump P_{mean} and P_{peak} (ratio scaled to body mass) attained by professional male rugby league forwards ($n = 55$) and backs ($n = 49$) were reported (51). Referring to the case study players' countermovement jump results presented in table 2.4, player 1 would be placed in approximately the 75th percentile for relative P_{peak} and the 60th percentile for relative P_{mean}, whereas player 2 would be placed in approximately the 85th percentile for relative P_{peak} and the 90th percentile for relative P_{mean} (51). It is worth noting that the 50th percentile is equal to a z-score of zero. After completing six weeks of preseason training, player

2's P$_{peak}$ dropped to approximately the 80th percentile and his P$_{mean}$ remained at approximately the 90th percentile. As mentioned earlier, player 2's body mass increased by 2 kg (4.4 lb) and thus influenced the ratio scaled power outputs. Both before and after preseason training, player 2's relative P$_{peak}$ and P$_{mean}$ were in the top quartile for a professional rugby league forward. His jump height of 38 centimeters (15 in) is also in the top quartile, based on a study by McMahon and colleagues (51); however, player 1's jump height equals approximately the 65th percentile, due to backs jumping higher than forwards on average.

The different position-specific countermovement jump attainment by players 1 and 2 highlight the benefit of comparing individual athletes' data to position-specific normative data where possible; however, this is often difficult to achieve when published research involving athletes generally involves small sample sizes and may have included protocols or equipment different from what is used by individual strength and conditioning professionals. Additionally, the guidance is that 30 or more athletes should be included when z-scores are calculated from the associated mean and standard deviation values and the data are normally distributed (80). Thus, when strength and conditioning professionals compare their athletes' data to published normative data, they are encouraged to read the *subject information* section to check that the sample size is at least 30; read the *protocols* section to check whether the equipment used, the verbal cues given, and the methods of analyzing the data match their own (or have been validated against their own); read the *statistical analysis* section of the manuscript to check that the data were assessed for normal distribution; and read the *results* section (including associated tables) to check that the mean and standard deviation values for the data of interest are presented. Once these checks are completed, strength and conditioning professionals can be reasonably confident in the normative data to which they are comparing their own athletes' data.

In a similar study, McMahon and colleagues (52) provided some normative countermovement jump data for 121 professional rugby league players, but power was not included. However, a process of compiling benchmarks from countermovement jump test data was presented, which can be applied to any other performance test data. The process involved the calculation of t-scores (80), which can be directly calculated or calculated from the more familiar z-score via the following equation:

$$t = (z\text{-score} \times 10) + 50$$

The t-score involves a scale from 0 to 100 that is equal to a z-score range from −5 to 5. Another standardized score that may be of interest is the standard ten (STEN) score, which scales data from 0 to 10 (78). The STEN score can also be calculated directly from the z-score as follows:

$$STEN = (2 \times z\text{-score}) + 5.5$$

Table 2.6 illustrates how z-scores, t-scores, and STEN scores compare to each other and the ratio-scaled relative P_{peak} values to which they each would equate based on normally distributed mean and standard deviation values of 50.6 ± 7.4 W/kg derived from a sample size of 30 or greater. Thus, the above equations can be used to calculate strength and conditioning professionals' preferred standardized score both for their own athletes' data and from normative data when the data pass the above-mentioned quality assurance checks. When used in conjunction with the corresponding qualitative descriptions outlined by McMahon and colleagues (51), also shown in table 2.6, the strength and conditioning professional can easily interpret the magnitude of a given performance test variable (in this case, P_{peak}) and feed this information back to athletes and coaches, in addition to setting benchmarks for the athletes to aspire to after completing a predetermined period of training.

Table 2.6 Comparison of Z-Scores, T-Scores, and STEN Scores and the Corresponding Ratio-Scaled Relative Peak Power

Description	T-score	Z-score	STEN	Peak power (W/kg)
Excellent	≥80	≥3.0	≥10.0	≥72.8
Very good	70	2.0	9.5	65.4
Good	60	1.0	7.5	58.0
Above average	55	0.5	6.5	54.3
Average	50	0.0	5.5	50.6
Below average	45	−0.5	4.5	46.9
Poor	40	−1.0	2.5	43.2
Very poor	30	−2.0	0.5	35.8
Extremely poor	≤20	≤−3.0	0.0	≤28.4

Note: STEN = standard ten.

It is important that practitioners understand the different information that methods of data presentation convey. If the purpose of the testing data is to show the development of an athlete over time, independent of team changes, then either presentation of the raw data as previously described (figure 2.6) or keeping a constant (e.g., pretesting) mean and standard deviation is advised (figure 2.7*b*), which could also be based on published normative data. If the purpose is to understand how an athlete is developing in comparison to the team over time, then a moving team mean and standard deviation at each time of testing should be used (e.g., pretesting, midtesting, and posttesting) (figure 2.7*a*). Figure 2.7*a* provides an example of how a constantly changing mean and standard deviation, or the "goalpost of comparison," can affect the interpretation of an individual athlete's improvement. For example, in figure 2.6, it is clear that at both absolute loads and relative loads, the athlete improved at pretesting, midtesting, and posttesting points. However, when evaluating this athlete relative to the improvements of the team (figure 2.7*a*), this athlete performed below or near the team mean until the final testing, when the performance improved vastly, not only compared to the athlete's own scores (as indicated in figure 2.6) but also in comparison to the team (figure 2.7*a*), as indicated by the high z-scores at each load. Comparing the change score for the individual athlete to the change score for the team as a whole at each time point would also illustrate this pattern. The presentation of data in figure 2.7*a* is quite different from that in figure 2.7*b*, which indicates that in comparison to the team mean at pretesting, the athlete far exceeded this baseline level at midtesting and posttesting sessions despite starting near the team mean at pretesting.

Different ways of presenting data have been discussed. Understanding the purpose of testing and the question to be answered by using those data will help when choosing the appropriate data presentation. This concept is critical for gathering data that aid rather than detract from the ability to make decisions on training and athlete improvement. Furthermore, the normalized power output of an athlete can be compared to the ranges that are commonly produced under the same loads or modes of exercise, as discussed in chapter 3.

ADVANTAGES AND DRAWBACKS OF POWER ASSESSMENT

It is common to compare the power output of various ballistic movements and loading paradigms in an effort to understand the power profile of an athlete, as previously presented in figure 2.6. These power profiles are regularly used to discuss various loads that maximize power (12, 17, 84). However, the drawback of this approach is a potential overemphasis on finding the load that maximizes power. Instead, a mixed-methods approach to effectively train this proposed power spectrum is recommended (7, 23, 59).

Impulse could be considered directly to understand the determinants of an athlete's performance, but this provides the same information as the eventual jump height (if body mass remains constant). However, time—an aspect of impulse that may provide insight—can be evaluated, as in figure 2.13. Specifically, understanding time with respect to performance can be described using different ratio variables, such as the reactive strength index (either jump height or flight time divided by contact time) during plyometric jumps or the modified reactive strength index (jump height divided by time to takeoff) or flight time to contraction time (FT:CT) ratio (which is technically the same as time to takeoff) during ballistic jumps. Although athlete 1 in figure 2.13 has a higher jump performance, it may be hypothesized through investigation of other variables that this athlete may strive to improve the rate of force development (RFD) or should be assessed using shorter stretch-shortening cycle (SSC) activity to see whether the athlete still has the capacity to perform when time is restricted or limited, such as with a rebound jump. In sport, time limitation is an important consideration with respect to performance. For example, if two people have the same capacity for jump height but one can jump the same height with less force production time, that individual may have an advantage in seeing the angle a ball will bounce during a rebound or when diving to prevent a goal. This is because the individual who can jump within less time can move with the same capacity but more quickly. The data that may be used to draw such conclusions can come from both inspection of the displacement–time curve and direct analysis of ratio variables such as the FT:CT, which in the previous example demonstrated a 28% difference between the two athletes, while their actual performance (jump height) only differed by 10% (figure 2.13). However, it was the inspection of many variables that characterize performance beyond just power that helped to draw such conclusions. Therefore, power has a great capacity to describe the combination of force and velocity within a single simple

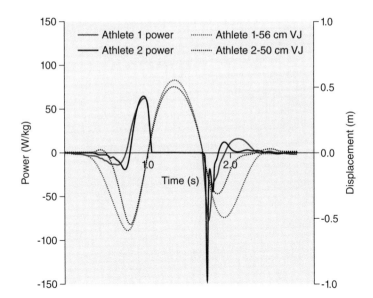

	Peak velocity	Relative peak force	Relative peak power	Force at peak power	Velocity at peak power	Ratio of flight time to contraction time
Athlete 1	2.93	62.63	21.07	21.57	2.90	0.64
Athlete 2	2.75	64.78	21.34	24.29	2.67	0.85
% Difference	6%	-3%	-1%	-12%	9%	-28%

Figure 2.13 Comparison of two athletes with identical power outputs normalized to their body mass. Observe the differences in the displacement and power curves as well as the percentage difference of various chosen variables. This provides an example of how power as a standalone variable can be misleading in the comparison of athletes and should be accompanied with a comprehensive understanding of how the athlete develops his or her power.

metric, but deeper analysis is required to understand underlying determinants of athlete performance. For this reason, power, as a variable, should never be used exclusively, and the presentation of results using force–velocity or evaluation of different metrics beyond power is justified.

CONCLUSION

Although power is a highly discussed and measured variable, its usefulness is determined partially by the methodology chosen and partially by the intent or question to be answered with the measurement of power (see figure 2.3 for an overview of considerations for the development of a test battery). Valid and reliable methodologies are used to accurately assess the P_{peak} and P_{mean} during a variety of tasks. Practitioners who cannot directly measure power can choose indirect power assessments while understanding their limitations. Furthermore, the best method to present results that provide meaningful information about the physical characteristics of the athlete must be considered. Understanding the limitations of the equipment and methods used to measure power, the best methods to express the data collected, and the underpinning information variables, such as force and velocity, will give practitioners direct insight into the mechanism by which athletes produce their performance.

Periodization and Programming for Maximizing Power

G. Gregory Haff

Periodization is a widely accepted theoretical and practical paradigm for guiding the preparation of athletes (10, 41, 43, 47, 93, 114, 117). Although periodization is both widely accepted and considered an essential tool for guiding training, coaches and sport scientists often misunderstand it and misapply it. While this confusion has many causes, the most important appears to be centered on what periodization is and how it differs from programming and planning (9, 41, 43, 117). *Planning* is the process of organizing and arranging training structures into phases to achieve a targeted goal. *Programming* is the application of training modes and methods into this structure. Periodization, on the other hand, contains elements of both planning and programming in that it defines the training structure, modes, and methods used within the global training plan. Based on this construct, the manipulation of sets, repetitions, and training loads would be considered programming, not periodization, as it is sometimes incorrectly termed in the literature (16, 30, 31, 77). Periodization is an inclusive theoretical and practical construct that allows for the management of the workloads of all training factors (e.g., physical, tactical, and technical training) to direct adaptation and elevate performance at appropriate times through the integrative and sequential manipulation of programmatic structures (40, 41, 47, 102, 104, 121).

The ability to manipulate training factors in a structured fashion allows periodized training plans to target several distinct goals. These include the optimization of the athlete's performance capacity at predetermined times or the maintenance of performances across a season, targeting the development of specific physiological and performance outcomes with precise training interventions, reducing overtraining potential through the appropriate management of training stressors, and facilitating long-term athlete development (37, 40-43, 47, 114). The multidimensional application of training interventions in an integrative and sequential manner largely affects the ability of periodized training models to accomplish these goals. While a central component of an appropriately designed periodized training plan is training variation, one should avoid random or excessive variation, because this results in what is referred to as the *blender effect*, where performance gains can be muted (41) and there is an increased risk of injury (103). Training variation should be logical and systematic so that the training responses are modulated while accounting for fatigue and elevating performance at appropriate times (41, 43, 47).

To apply these principles to maximize power development, one must consider several key aspects of periodization, planning, and programming. This chapter discusses the general principles of periodization and the hierarchical structure of periodization cycles and is designed to help improve coaches' understanding of the periodization process, approaches to planning used in periodization, models of periodization, fundamentals of power development, and planning training and power development.

GENERAL PRINCIPLES OF PERIODIZATION

The ability to develop specific physiological adaptations and translate those adaptations into performance outcomes is largely dictated by the ability to sequence and structure the periodized training plan to manage both recovery and adaptive processes (22, 41, 87, 104). Because it is well documented that peak performance can only be maintained for a relatively short period of time (8-14 days) (6, 14, 69, 94-96, 134), the sequential structure of the training plan becomes a critical consideration for periodization (11-13, 104, 120, 140). Ultimately, the average intensity contained in the training plan is inversely related to the magnitude of the performance peak and the duration with which that peak can be maintained (27, 41, 55, 120). Three basic mechanistic theories can be used to understand how periodized training programs can manage the recovery and adaptive processes: the general adaptive syndrome (25, 40, 41, 43, 47, 111, 120, 147), the stimulus-fatigue-fitness-adaptation theory (25, 40, 41, 43, 47, 120, 147), and the fitness–fatigue paradigm (25, 40, 41, 43, 47, 120, 147).

General Adaptive Syndrome

One of the foundational theories that underpins the periodization of training is Hans Selye's *general adaptive syndrome* (GAS) (25, 43, 120, 147). The GAS describes the body's specific responses to stress, either physiological or emotional (111). While the GAS offers a potential model that explains how the body adapts to training stimuli, it does not explain all the responses to stress that occur (figure 3.1) (120).

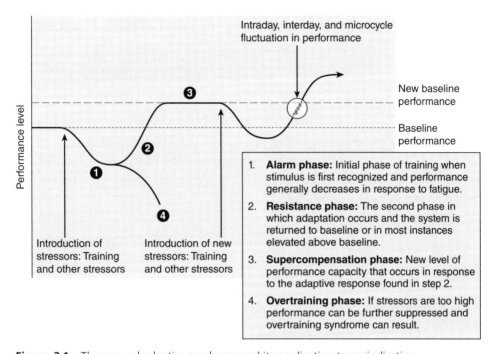

Figure 3.1 The general adaptive syndrome and its application to periodization.

Reprinted by permission from G.G. Haff and E.E. Haff, "Training Integration and Periodization," in *NSCA's Guide to Program Design*, edited for the National Strength and Conditioning Association by J. Hoffman (Champaign, IL: Human Kinetics, 2012), 215.

When applying GAS to training theory, it is important to note that the body appears to respond in a similar fashion regardless of the type of stressor that is applied (41, 43, 47). If new training stimuli (e.g., stress) are introduced to the athlete, the initial response, or *alarm phase*, results in a reduction in the athlete's performance capacity as a result of the accumulation of fatigue, stiffness, soreness, and reductions in available energy stores (41, 43, 47). The *alarm phase* initiates the adaptive processes that lead into the *resistance phase*. If training is programmed correctly, the athlete's overall performance capacity will be maintained or elevated (i.e., supercompensation) as a result of being able to adapt to the applied training stimuli. Conversely, if the training stimuli are excessive or randomly applied, the athlete will be unable to adapt to the training stress. As a consequence, performance capacity will continue to decline, initially resulting in a state of nonfunctional overreaching, which can eventually lead to the occurrence of *overtraining* (34). An additional consideration is that the athlete's ability to adapt and respond to training stimuli can be affected by other stressors (e.g., interpersonal relationships, nutrition, or career pressures), because all stressors are additive.

Stimulus-Fatigue-Recovery-Adaptation Theory

Whenever a training stimulus is applied, a general response occurs, which can be explained by the stimulus-fatigue-fitness-adaptation theory (figure 3.2). When the training stimulus is applied, fatigue ensues, resulting in a reduction in both preparedness and performance in proportion to the magnitude and duration of the workload (41, 43, 47). As the recovery process begins and the accumulated fatigue dissipates, both preparedness and performance increase. If, after the recovery process is complete, no new training stimulus is encountered, both preparedness and performance will progressively decline, and a state of *involution* (i.e., loss of training effect, or detraining) will occur.

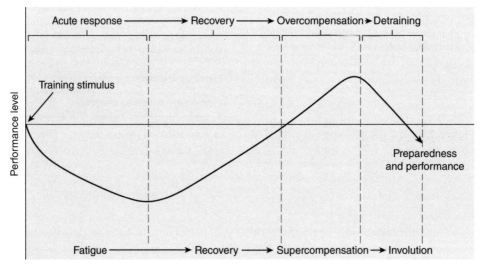

Figure 3.2　The stimulus-fatigue-recovery-adaptation theory.

Reprinted by permission from G.G. Haff and E.E. Haff, "Training Integration and Periodization," in *NSCA's Guide to Program Design*, edited for the National Strength and Conditioning Association by J. Hoffman (Champaign, IL: Human Kinetics, 2012), 216. Adapted from Yakovlev (110); Verkishansky (104); Rowbottom (81); and Stone et al. (94).

Careful inspection of the base concept reveals that the magnitude of the training stimulus affects the length of the recovery–adaptation portion of the process (41, 43, 47). For example, a large training load will cause a large amount of fatigue, which will require more recovery time before the recovery–adaptation process can occur (107, 120). Conversely, if the training load is light, the athlete will experience less accumulated fatigue, and the recovery–adaptation process will proceed more rapidly. In the training literature, this response is often referred to as a delayed or residual training effect (41, 43, 47, 107, 120). One can modulate delayed training effects by manipulating the training program to ensure that preparedness and performance are supercompensated at key time increments (42). Central to the ability to modulate residual training effects is how one integrates and sequences the workloads in the periodized training program.

While the stimulus-fatigue-recovery-adaptation theory is often considered in a global context, this general response pattern occurs as a result of a single exercise, training session, microcycle, mesocycle, and macrocycle (25, 41, 43, 47). Additionally, complete recovery is not required before encountering another training stimulus (98). In fact, it is recommended that coaches modulate the volume load of training (i.e., heavy and light training days) to facilitate recovery and maximize adaptive potential (15, 32) and to further develop fitness (41, 43, 47). The ability to maximize adaptive responses to training relies on the ability to take advantage of the recovery–adaptation process by manipulating training factors (e.g., intensity, volume load, and number of exercises) within the programmatic structure that are used in the context of the periodized training plan. This concept is a foundation from which several sequential periodization models presented in the literature have been developed (107, 137-139).

Fatigue–Fitness Paradigm

The interrelationship between fitness, fatigue, and preparedness are partially explained by what Zatsiorsky (146) termed the *fatigue–fitness paradigm*. This paradigm gives a more complete picture of the athlete's response to the training stimulus (17). Central to the understanding of the paradigm are the two aftereffects of fitness and fatigue, which summate to dictate the athlete's overall preparedness (17, 62, 146). Classically, these aftereffects are presented as one fatigue–fitness curve (figure 3.3) (17, 146). However, it is more realistic that multiple independent fitness and fatigue aftereffects occur in response to training and exert a cumulative effect on the preparedness curve (figure 3.4) (17, 41, 43, 47, 62).

The existence of multiple fatigue and fitness aftereffects may partially explain the individual responses to variations in training stimuli (41, 43, 47). Stone and colleagues (120) suggest that different training targets have different aftereffects and that targeted training interventions modulate which aftereffects occur and how an athlete can progress in preparedness throughout the training plan. These training-induced aftereffects are also referred to as residual training effects and serve as the foundation for the theories that underpin sequential training (64, 117, 137, 140). Sequential training theory suggests that the rate of decay of a residual training effect can be maintained by a minimal training stimulus or through the periodic dosing of the training stimuli to modulate the athlete's preparedness. The rate of decay of a given residual training effect can be modulated by manipulating the training stimulus. In sequential modeling, it appears that residual training effects can be magnified if specific training stimuli are sequenced and integrated correctly, resulting in a delayed training effect or a phase-potentiation effect (28, 41, 43, 47, 64, 67, 117).

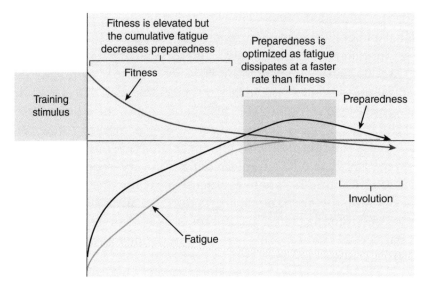

Figure 3.3 The fitness–fatigue paradigm.

Reprinted by permission from G.G. Haff and E.E. Haff, "Training Integration and Periodization," in *NSCA's Guide to Program Design*, edited for the National Strength and Conditioning Association by J. Hoffman (Champaign, IL: Human Kinetics, 2012), 219. Adapted from Stone et al. (94); Zatsiorsky (115).

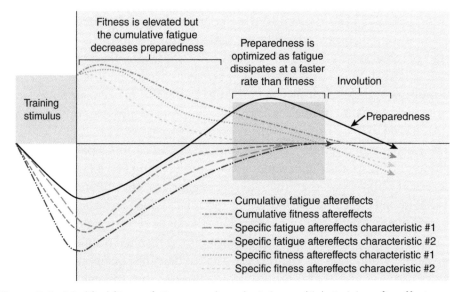

Figure 3.4 Modified fitness–fatigue paradigm depicting multiple training aftereffects.

Reprinted by permission from G.G. Haff and E.E. Haff, "Training Integration and Periodization," in *NSCA's Guide to Program Design*, edited for the National Strength and Conditioning Association by J. Hoffman (Champaign, IL: Human Kinetics, 2012), 209-254. Adapted from Stone et al. (94) and Chiu and Barnes (18).

When the GAS, stimulus-fatigue-fitness-adaptation theory, and fitness–fatigue paradigm are used collectively to examine periodization models, it is clear that the modulation of the adaptive responses is accomplished through careful planning. The training plan must be designed to develop various fitness characteristics while managing fatigue to maximize the performance capacity of the athlete (41, 43, 47). The ability to control the athlete's level of preparedness centers on the ability to manage training loads in order to modulate both fatigue and fitness aftereffects (41, 104). When designing the training plan, it is essential to consider the training interventions, the actual sequential pattern, and the integration of the training interventions to maximize the performance capacity and fitness aftereffects while minimizing accumulated fatigue.

While the structure of the training program is one of the major factors affecting preparedness and performance, it is important to note that all stressors affect the athlete's ability to recover from training stress. As a good example of the individual nature of recovery, emerging data suggest that psychoemotional stress can increase the fatigue response, extend the time frame of recovery, and delay elevations in preparedness (122). Ultimately, the time course of recovery is highly individualized and can be affected by the athlete's current training state, psychoemotional stress, and other modifiable factors, such as diet and sleep (41).

HIERARCHICAL STRUCTURE OF PERIODIZATION CYCLES

The periodization of training is facilitated by a hierarchical structure that allows for several distinct, interrelated levels that can be used in the planning process (table 3.1). Each level of the periodization process should be based on the training goals established for the athlete or team. Conceptually, these levels of organization start with a global context and then progress into smaller, more defined structures. Seven hierarchical structures are typically used in the periodization of training.

The highest level of the hierarchical structure is the multiyear plan, which is most typically built around the Olympic quadrennial cycle (10, 40, 41, 43, 70, 98, 102, 120, 147). This cycle presents the athlete's longer-term training goals and contains multiple annual training plans. The next hierarchical level is the annual training plan, which contains the training structures within an individual training year (10, 22, 40, 41, 43, 87, 102, 107). Annual plans can contain one or more macrocycles, depending on how many competitive seasons are contained in the annual training plan (10, 22, 68). Each macrocycle is then subdivided into three periods: preparation, competition, and transition (40, 41, 46). The preparation period is divided into the general preparation and specific preparation phases. The general preparation phase develops a general physical base and is marked by high volumes of training, lower training intensities, and a large variety of training means (65, 87). The specific preparation phase targets sport-specific motor and technical abilities, which are built on the foundation of the general preparation phase (40, 41, 46). The competition period is structured

Table 3.1   Hierarchical Structure of Periodized Training Plans

Level	Name	Duration	Description
1	Multiyear training plan	2-4 years	This plan lays out the long-term goals for the athlete. The most common multiyear plan is the 4-year quadrennial plan.
2	Annual training plan	1 year	This plan outlines the entire year of training. It can contain 1-3 macrocycles, depending on the number of competitive seasons contained in the training year.
3	Macrocycle	Several months to a year	Some authors refer to this as an annual plan. It contains preparatory, competitive, and transitional periods of training.
4	Mesocycle	2-6 weeks	This medium-sized cycle is often referred to as a block of training. The most typical duration for the mesocycle is 4 weeks. Regardless of length, the cycle consists of linked microcycles.
5	Microcycle	Several days to 2 weeks	This smaller training cycle consists of several training days and typically lasts 7 days.
6	Training day	1 day	A training day is designed in the context of the microcycle goals and defines when training sessions are performed within the microcycle.
7	Training session	Minutes to hours	A training session contains all the scheduled training units. It can be performed individually or within a group. If the training session contains >30 min of rest between training units, then multiple sessions are performed.
8	Training unit	Several minutes to hours	A training unit is a focused training activity. Warm-up, agility, resistance training, and technical drills are examples of training units. Several training units can be strung together to create a training session.

Adapted from G.G. Haff, "Periodization and Power Integration," in *Developing Power* edited by M. McGuigan (Champaign, IL: Human Kinetics, 2017), 39. Adapted from Bompa and Haff (2009); Haff (2019); Haff (2021); Haff and Haff (2012); Issurin (2010); and Stone et al. (2007).

to slightly improve or maintain the physiological and sport-specific skills established in the preparation period (41). This period is typically subdivided into the precompetition and main competition phases. Conceptually, the precompetition phase is a link between the preparation period and the main competition phase (38, 41). Finally, the transition phase is the most important linking phase and can bridge either multiple macrocycles or annual training plans (38, 40, 41, 43).

The next hierarchical structure, the mesocycle, is sometimes referred to as a medium-duration training cycle (41, 64, 65, 81, 102, 147). It is often referred to as a block of training and is a central training cycle in the block-periodization model (38, 40, 41, 43, 68). Mesocycles typically contain two to six microcycles, which are next in the hierarchy (38, 40, 41, 43). Each microcycle is made up of both training days and sessions, which contain the individual training units.

These last components of the hierarchy form the foundation for the whole training system and outline the main training factors delivered (41, 65, 66).

UNDERSTANDING THE PERIODIZATION PROCESS

The overall periodization process must be considered in the context of three basic levels: periodization, planning, and programming (figure 3.5).

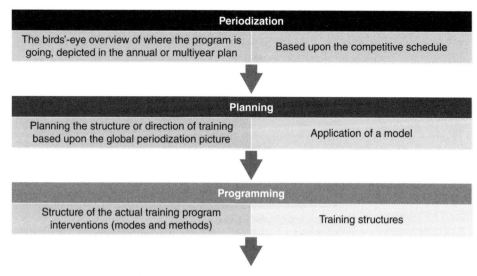

Periodization	
The birds'-eye overview of where the program is going, depicted in the annual or multiyear plan	Based upon the competitive schedule

Planning	
Planning the structure or direction of training based upon the global periodization picture	Application of a model

Programming	
Structure of the actual training program interventions (modes and methods)	Training structures

Figure 3.5 Interrelationship of periodization, planning, and programming.

The first level is periodization, which dictates the long-term development of the athlete across the multiyear or annual training plan. This level includes the overall breakdown of the preparation, competition, and transition periods. It may also include the travel and testing schedule. The second level is planning, which forms the foundation for choosing the training model used to design the training structures. This can include parallel, sequential, block, or emphasis training models. The third level, programming, contains the basic training structures, such as the modes and methods used. This level contains the training loads (i.e., intensity and volume) as well as the structures (e.g., complexes, cluster sets) and exercises used to construct the training interventions.

APPROACHES TO PLANNING USED IN PERIODIZATION

When examining the periodization process, and in particular, the planning of training, numerous models can be used in accordance with the overall periodized plan. These include parallel, sequential, and emphasis approaches to designing training interventions (9, 41, 43, 71, 97).

Parallel Approach

Coaches use the parallel approach to train multiple biomotor abilities simultaneously and to train all targets across the annual training plan (figure 3.6). Using this approach, all targeted biomotor abilities may be trained within one training session, training day, series of training days, or microcycle. Sometimes this approach is called a concurrent or complex parallel approach (9, 41). While this approach may work well for novices or those who are in the early stages of their long-term athlete development plan, it is generally not recommended for intermediate to advanced athletes (41).

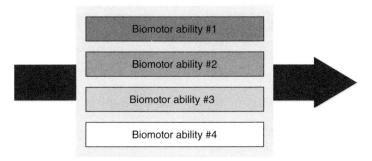

Figure 3.6 Parallel training approach.

One issue with the parallel approach is that to continue the improvement of any specific biomotor ability, a greater training volume or load is required, resulting in a cumulative increase in overall training load. Because athletes have a limited training tolerance, the increases in volume or load required to further induce changes in performance capacity eventually exceed an athlete's ability to tolerate training (68) and ultimately may lead to a state of nonfunctional overreaching or overtraining. This approach to training may work well for novice and youth athletes (41) but may not be as beneficial for intermediate to elite athletes, because these athletes require greater training stimuli to further develop key biomotor abilities (9, 97, 104). Therefore, other approaches to training may be warranted for more advanced strength and power athletes (68).

Sequential Approach

The sequential approach arranges training for biomotor abilities or training targets to occur one after another in a logical pattern (figure 3.7) (9, 41).

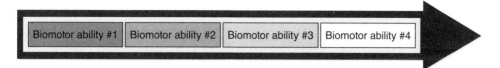

Figure 3.7 Sequential training approach.

By working specific targets sequentially, the athlete is able to undertake higher training loads and intensities to target a given training attribute. Strong scientific evidence supports this approach when targeting power development (56, 58, 60, 91, 123, 145). Specifically, Zamparo and colleagues (145) and Minetti (91) suggest that the optimization of power development is achieved through a sequential pattern that develops a muscle's cross-sectional area, improves force production capacity, and increases movement speed, resulting in increased power production capacity. Additionally, Harris and colleagues (56) demonstrated that training football players with a sequential training approach resulted in significantly greater increases in both power and strength measures when compared to a parallel training approach. The sequential approach to planning training serves as the foundation for the *block model of periodization* (64, 68, 117). While the sequential approach is a useful planning paradigm, it is possible that as the athlete moves through the sequence, detraining effects for the attributes not being trained will occur (90). The longer the sequence of training stimuli, the greater the chance for a detraining effect. Depending on the sport, it may be beneficial to use an approach that modulates training responses within the sequential structure.

Emphasis Approach

The emphasis, or pendulum, approach lies between the two extremes of the parallel and sequential approaches in that it incorporates aspects of both models (9, 41, 43). As noted by Zatsiorsky and colleagues (147) and Munroe and Haff (97), this approach allows for the sequential training of various biomotor abilities with frequent intermittent changes in training emphasis. In this approach, the athlete may train several biomotor abilities (i.e., parallel approach) with varying degrees of emphasis, which change over time (i.e., sequential approach). For example, the athlete may target the development of strength while maintaining the ability to express power (figure 3.8).

Zatsiorsky and colleagues (147) recommend changing the targeted biomotor ability every two weeks to optimize performance capacity. This approach seems to be particularly beneficial when attempting to maximize strength, power, and the rate of force development (97, 147) and appears to be a good choice for intermediate to advanced athletes who have congested competition schedules or are

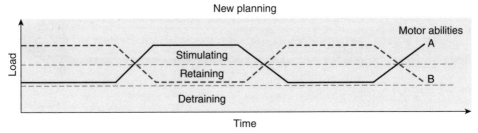

Figure 3.8 Sample emphasis approach.

Reprinted by permission from V.M. Zatsiorsky, *Science and Practice of Strength Training* (Champaign, IL: Human Kinetics, 1995), 126.

competing in a team sport (41, 43). Emphasis models have been implemented in individual sports such as track cycling (97), sprinting (33), and mixed martial arts (23). The most noted example of this model is the vertical integration model for sprinting presented by Francis (33). This application targets the simultaneous development (parallel model) of six training factors that are trained with varying degrees of emphasis (sequential model) to better align with a sprinter's targeted training goals. Fundamentally, this approach allows all training factors to be trained with varying degrees of emphasis so that some training factors are developed while others are maintained.

MODELS OF PLANNING USED IN PERIODIZATION

Coaches can choose from several models to construct a periodized training plan. These models can be broken into parallel, sequential, and emphasis models.

Parallel Model

The parallel model is a complex system that involves the parallel development of biomotor abilities (22, 41, 43, 113, 137). This model tends to use training structures that contain relatively limited variations in training methods and means (104, 117, 120), constructed to create gradual wavelike increases in workload (87, 117). These increases are sequenced into predetermined training structures (22, 41). The load progressions are depicted as a ratio of the volume to the intensity of training (87). Early in the periodized training plan, the workload is primarily increased as a result of increased volumes of work and marginal increases in intensity (22, 41). As training progresses, the volume of training decreases while the intensity of training increases. These fluctuations in intensity and volume are depicted in the figure presented by Matveyev (87). This figure was, however, only meant to be a graphic illustration of the central concepts of the periodization model (figure 3.9) and was not intended to be rigidly applied to the training practices of all athletes.

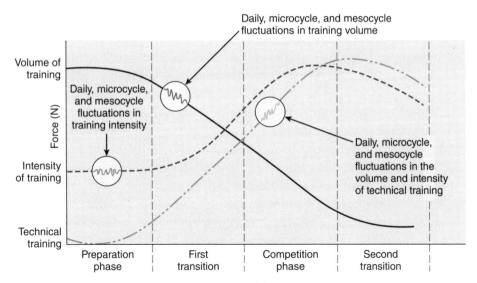

Figure 3.9 Matveyev's classic periodization model.

Reprinted by permission from G.G. Haff and E.E. Haff, "Training and Integration and Periodization," in *Strength and Conditioning Program Design*, edited by J. Hoffman (Champaign, IL: Human Kinetics, 2012), 219. Originally adapted by permission from M.H. Stone and H. S. O'Bryant, *Weight Training: A Scientific Approach*, 2nd ed. copyright © 1987 by Burgess International Publishing. Adapted by permission of Pearson Learning Solutions, A Pearson Education Company.

A gross misinterpretation of this model is the source of the term *linear periodization* (7, 26, 31, 73, 78, 105), which, based on the major tenets of periodization, is not possible because central to the periodization concept is the removal of linearity (87). Careful inspection of Matveyev's seminal text (87) reveals that the model is in fact nonlinear and is marked by variation at several levels of the periodization hierarchy (e.g., training session, training day, microcycle, mesocycle, and macrocycle).

A key aspect of the traditional model is that it uses a complex parallel approach that attempts to develop multiple biomotor abilities necessary for a variety of sports simultaneously (22, 113, 136). Most of the research that supports the use of this model is somewhat dated and was collected from beginner athletes (22, 113, 136). As such, this model may not adequately address the needs of intermediate and advanced athletes (41, 43, 136).

Sequential Model

Central to the sequential model is the idea that training needs to be prioritized and sequenced to allow the athlete to better manage training stressors through a more focused training approach. Strong scientific evidence supports the use of sequential periodization models for the development of muscular strength and maximal capacity for power generation (8, 35, 41, 43, 56, 63, 117). One of the early pioneers in the development of the sequential model system was Dr. Anatoliy Bondarchuk, who devised a system that used three specialized mesocycle blocks for the development of throwers (12, 67, 68). These included developmental, competitive, and restoration blocks. Developmental blocks were used to increase working capacity toward the maximal level, while competitive blocks were focused on elevation of competitive performance. Restoration blocks were used to prepare the athlete for the next developmental block and served as transitions periods. The sequence of these blocks was predicated by the competition schedule and the athlete's responses to the training stressors (12). Issurin (67, 68) proposed a model that used three basic blocks similar to those proposed by Bondarchuk (12). This model used accumulation blocks to develop basic abilities (e.g., strength, endurance, or movement technique), transmutation blocks to develop more specific abilities (e.g., aerobic–anaerobic or anaerobic endurance, specialized muscular endurance, power, or event-specific technique), and realization blocks to maximize performance. In its purest form, the block model uses minimal training targets in each training block and takes advantage of delayed training effects and training residuals (figure 3.10).

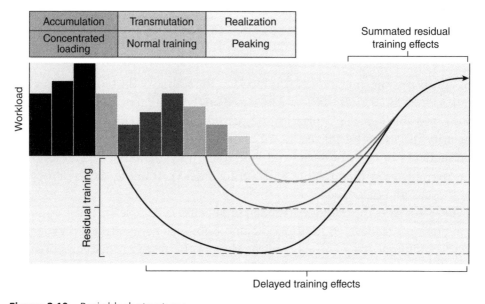

Figure 3.10 Basic block structures.

Emphasis Approach

The emphasis approach, as outlined by Zatsiorsky and colleagues (147), trains several targets simultaneously with various degrees of focus, then shifts to sequential training according to the demands of the periodized training plan. Similarly, Verkhoshansky and Siff (137) give examples of integrating primary, secondary, and tertiary training emphases for a training block in their conjugated sequencing model. In this model, each block of training is vertically integrated, meaning complementary training targets are trained to varying degrees of emphasis (emphasis approach) and horizontally sequenced (sequential approach). Horizontal sequencing then capitalizes on the training residuals and delayed training effects established in the previous block. Zatsiorsky and colleagues (147) suggest that this model maybe ideal for the development of maximal strength, rate of force, and power in athletes in several power sports. Verkhoshansky and Siff (137) give examples of how this approach can be used with athletes who are targeting the development of explosive strength or power output (figure 3.11).

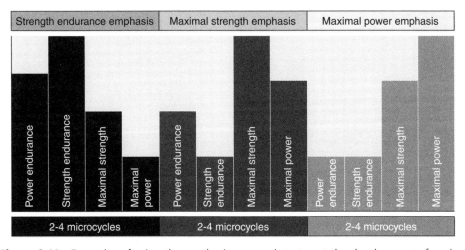

Figure 3.11 Examples of using the emphasis approach to target the development of explosive strength or power output.

FUNDAMENTALS OF POWER DEVELOPMENT

The ability to generate high power outputs is facilitated by the ability to generate high levels of force rapidly and express high contraction velocities (74). Examination of the relationship between force and velocity reveals that they are inversely related, as indicated by the force–velocity curve (figure 3.12). See chapter 1 for additional detail regarding the fundamentals of power development.

When examining the force–velocity curve, it is apparent that as the velocity of movement increases, the force that the muscle can produce during the concentric contraction will decrease. Because of the relationship between force and velocity, it is clear that the expression of maximal power outputs occurs at compromised levels of maximal force and velocity (figure 3.13).

When targeting the optimization of power output in a training program, three key elements should be considered. First, *maximal strength* must be increased, because it has a direct relationship with the ability to express high rates of force development and power output (2, 4, 20, 50, 85, 91, 126, 145). Second, a high

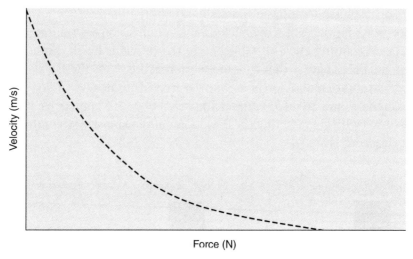

Figure 3.12 Basic force–velocity relationship.

Reprinted by permission from G.G. Haff and S. Nimphius, "Training Principles for Power," *Strength and Conditioning Journal* 34, no. 6 (2012): 2-12.

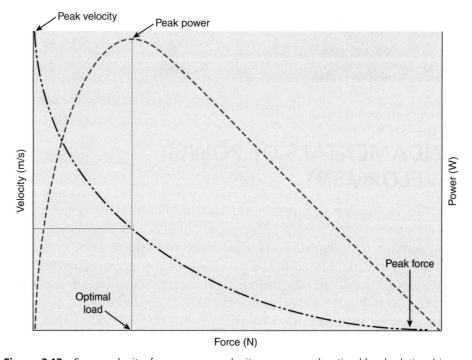

Figure 3.13 Force–velocity, force–power, velocity–power, and optimal load relationships.

Reprinted by permission from G.G. Haff and S. Nimphius, "Training Principles for Power," *Strength and Conditioning Journal* 34, no. 6 (2012): 2-12.

rate of force development (RFD) must be achieved; this is the ability to express high forces in short periods of time and is central to the ability to express high power outputs (20, 52, 53, 88, 148), because impulse (force × time) relative to the object's mass determines velocity (see chapter 1). Finally, it is important to develop the ability to express high forces as the velocity of shortening increases (50). The interplay among these elements is strong, and the athlete's overall strength serves as the main factor dictating the ability to express higher power outputs (50, 74). Within the scientific literature is evidence of the interrelationship between maximal strength, RFD, and the ability to express maximal power output (45, 52). Based on these interactions, any periodized training plan designed to optimize power must consider the development of each of these key interrelated attributes.

Maximal Strength and Power

As noted previously, one of the foundational elements in the development of power is the athlete's maximal strength (4, 50, 91, 126, 145). Clearly, stronger athletes demonstrate a greater potential to develop higher power outputs and often express higher power outputs when compared to their weaker counterparts (4, 118, 126). Haff and Nimphius (50) suggest that stronger people are able to generate higher forces at a higher rate when compared to weaker people (3, 4, 19, 79). Support for this contention can be seen in the research literature, which reports that weaker athletes who undertake resistance training targeting the development of maximal strength experience significant increases in muscular power (4, 19), which translates into improvements in athletic performance (19, 118). Once athletes have established adequate strength levels, they are then able to better capitalize on the benefits of specific power development exercises, such as plyometrics, ballistic exercises, complexes, or contrast training methods (50). In fact, stronger athletes exhibit a greater overall responsiveness to power-based training methods (19, 50).

Based on the literature, it is clear that maximization of strength levels is a prerequisite for the development of higher power outputs. However, it is often difficult to determine what an adequate level of strength is for a given athlete or group of athletes. Based on the contemporary body of knowledge, athletes who can squat more than 2.0 × body mass express higher power outputs than their weaker counterparts (1.7 or 1.4 × body mass) (7, 118). Research suggests that athletes between the ages of 16 and 19 years who compete in strength and power sports or team sports should be able to back squat a minimum of 2.0 × body mass (75). Additionally, when using strength–power potentiation complexes or plyometric exercises, it appears that athletes who are able to squat double their body weight are able to optimize the effectiveness of these exercises (108, 109, 128). Maximal lower body strength is also related to the degree of difficulty or intensity of plyometric exercises that maximize performance adaptations, with a minimum back squat of 2.0 × body mass being a prerequisite for maximizing the benefits of higher-level plyometrics, such as depth and drop jumps performed from moderate to high heights (i.e., more than 30 cm [11.8 in]). Based on this literature, Haff and Nimphius (50) suggest that a minimum back squat of 2.0 × body mass is a requirement for undertaking specialized training to optimize lower body power output. Specifically, higher-level plyometric activities, such as depth and drop jumps and loaded ballistic exercises (e.g., squat jump with 40% of the 1-repetition maximum [1RM]), should be reserved for athletes who can back squat a minimum of 2.0 × body mass, because this level of strength allows the athlete to better tolerate these activities and achieve greater training benefits (127, 128). Importantly, this does not mean that athletes who back squat less than 2.0 × body mass should not perform plyometric training. Weaker athletes should perform lower-level plyometric activities (e.g., pogo jumps, repeated countermovement jumps, and hops) as part of their training program, but they should only engage in higher-level plyometrics once their 1RM back squat is a minimum of 2.0 × body mass (128).

Maximal strength levels also seem to be an important prerequisite for the development of higher upper body power outputs (24), with stronger athletes being able to display significantly higher power outputs (4). While high levels of strength are an important factor underpinning the ability to express higher upper body power outputs, there is currently no consensus in the contemporary body of knowledge on the minimal level of upper body strength required when seeking to maximize upper body power development (126). There is, however, an emerging body of evidence suggesting that a bench press of at least 1.35 × body mass may be a minimum requirement for undertaking upper body strength–power potentiation complexes or plyometric exercises (21, 110). As such, until further research is conducted examining the effect of upper body strength on power development, a minimum bench press of at least 1.35 × body mass may be a minimum requirement for specialized training to optimize upper body power output.

Rate of Force Development

The rate at which force is expressed during sporting movement is often referred to as the RFD, or explosive muscular strength (1, 85). In its most simplistic form, the RFD is determined from the slope of an isometric force–time curve (39, 50, 142) (figure 3.14). One can calculate the RFD in a variety of ways, including the peak value in a predetermined sampling window and in specific time bands, such as the slope of 0 to 200 m/s (39, 51). Typically, contraction times of 50 to 250 m/s are associated with jumping, sprinting, and change-of-direction movements. With short contraction times, it is unlikely that maximal forces can be developed, and it has been reported that it may take more than 300 m/s to generate maximal forces (1, 129, 131). With this in mind, several authors recommend ballistic exercises performed with light loads as a method to optimize RFD, and subsequently, the overall power output (20, 50, 53).

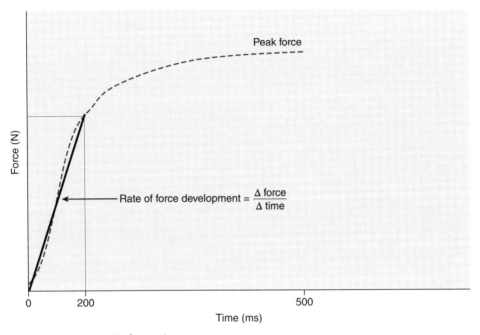

Figure 3.14   Isometric force–time curve.

Reprinted by permission from G.G. Haff and S. Nimphius, "Training Principles for Power," *Strength and Conditioning Journal* 34, no. 6 (2012): 2-12.

When examining the scientific literature, it is clear that performing resistance training exercises with heavy loads results in an increase in maximal strength (20, 101, 125) and RFD in weaker or untrained people (84). While training with heavy loads increases most athletes' strength reserve and can positively affect their RFD, it is likely that explosive or ballistic exercises may be necessary to optimize the RFD in stronger, more experienced athletes (20, 50, 53). Based on this phenomenon, Haff and Nimphius (50) suggest that varying the training foci has the potential to affect various parts of the force–time curve (figure 3.15) and force–velocity curve (figure 3.16).

Heavy resistance training and explosive or ballistic resistance training have the potential to increase an untrained athlete's maximal strength and RFD (figure 3.15). Conversely, ballistic training does not increase maximal strength but results in a greater increase in the RFD when compared to heavy resistance training in stronger athletes. When examining the force–velocity relationship, it is clear that heavy resistance training results in increases in the velocity

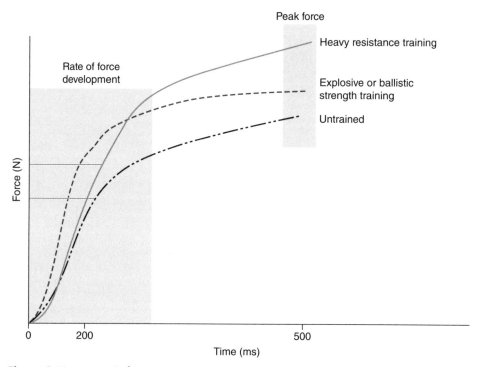

Figure 3.15 Isometric force–time curve depicting force–time curve responses to training.

Reprinted by permission from G.G. Haff and S. Nimphius, "Training Principles for Power," *Strength and Conditioning Journal* 34, no. 6 (2012): 2-12.

of movement at the high-force end of the force–velocity curve (figure 3.16b), while ballistic movements result in increases in the velocity of movement at the low-force end of the force–velocity curve (figure 3.16c). It is clear that mixed methods that target high-velocity and high-force movements are necessary to exert a more global effect on the force–velocity relationship (figure 3.16a and d) and ultimately increase RFD and power output (50).

PLANNING TRAINING AND POWER DEVELOPMENT

The periodization literature offers several planning models to target the maximization of power. The first is the traditional approach, in which the athlete attempts to develop all key biomotor abilities in a parallel manner (figure 3.17).

In this approach, equal attention is given to each of the key attributes across the entire annual training plan. As noted earlier, this approach may work for novice or youth athletes but is probably not ideal for more advanced athletes, who may require more advanced planning models to fully maximize the development of power.

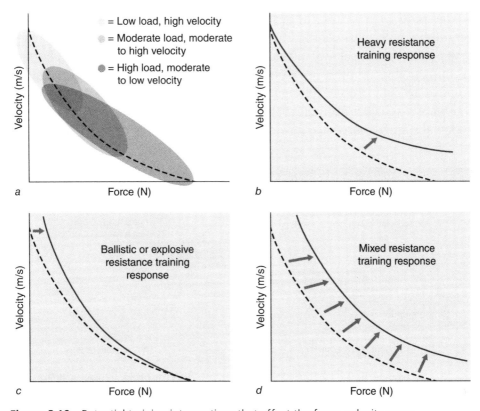

Figure 3.16 Potential training interventions that affect the force–velocity curve.

Reprinted by permission from G.G. Haff and S. Nimphius, "Training Principles for Power," *Strength and Conditioning Journal* 34, no. 6 (2012): 2-12.

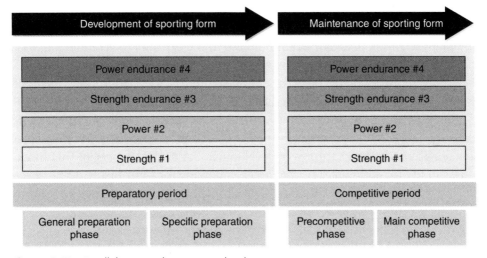

Figure 3.17 Parallel approach to power development.

The second approach to the development of power is the sequential model of periodization. Strong scientific support demonstrates that by dedicating specific time periods to a target, key attributes can be developed in a sequential fashion, resulting in the optimization of power-generating capacity. Based on the model proposed by Zamparo and colleagues (145), Minetti (91), and Stone and colleagues (117), a coach could use an approach that sequentially targets muscle hypertrophy, maximal strength, strength–power, and then power development (figure 3.18).

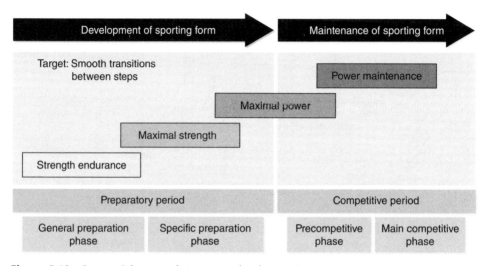

Figure 3.18 Sequential approach to power development.

This model is similar to the approach presented by Stone and colleagues (119) in their seminal paper on periodization for resistance training. In this model, distinctive training targets were sequentially developed across a 12-week training plan, resulting in a significant increase in the capacity to generate maximal power. This approach appears to work well for intermediate to advanced athletes.

A third model of planning is the emphasis approach. In this model, the main training factors are vertically integrated and horizontally sequenced (figure 3.19).

Complementary training factors are trained at various levels of emphasis and then sequenced across a series of mesocycle blocks to optimize the transfer of key adaptive responses to power development. A central aspect of this model is the ability to modulate training targets, allowing for some factors to be developed while others are maintained (97). Ultimately, by modulating the training emphasis, training stimuli are supplied to minimize the detraining effects that may occur in sequential models while reducing the potential for workload issues such as the blender effect (41). As with the sequential model, this approach works well for intermediate to advanced athletes and may be ideally suited for team sport athletes, athletes with dense competitive schedules, and tactical athletes who maintain a variety of capacities to perform at a high level (41).

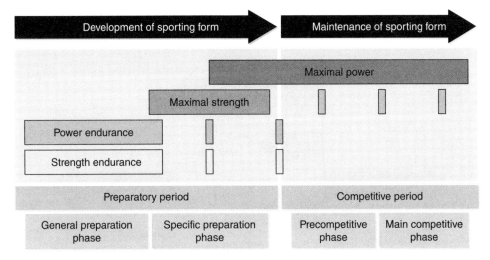

Figure 3.19 Emphasis approach to power development.

PROGRAMMING AND POWER DEVELOPMENT

Once the overall periodization plan and the training model are established, a training program can be developed. Essential to programming is establishing the intensity of training, the set structures and types of exercises used, and the exercise order.

Intensity of Training

Much research has been conducted to determine the *optimal load* for power development when performing resistance training. There is no one optimal load for power, because different exercises have different loading ranges that have been shown to optimize power output (figure 3.20) (83, 115, 116). For example, loads ≥70% of the 1RM have been associated with the optimal load during the power clean or hang power clean, while the optimal load for the jump squat or bench throw is generally ≤30% of the 1RM (115, 116). As such, it has been proposed that there are three exercise-specific optimal loading zones for optimizing power output—low (≤30% of the 1RM), moderate (30%-70% of the 1RM), and high (≥70%) loads—which can be used to target power development (115, 116). Several authors have suggested that using the optimal load is an effective method for improving power output (72, 74, 89, 92, 115, 116, 132, 133). However, the results of few studies actually support this contention (72, 83, 89, 92, 143), and based on several studies, it has been suggested that training with heavy loads (19, 57) or mixed loads (19, 57, 132, 133) produces superior enhancements in power output.

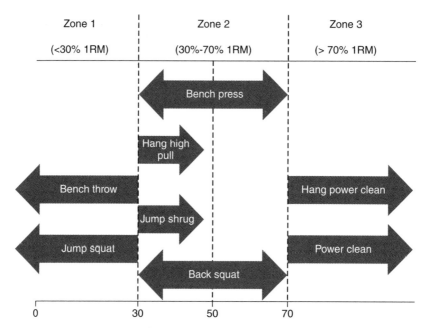

Figure 3.20 Example exercises for optimal power load zones.

Based on data from Suchomel and Sole (2017). Power-Time Curve Comparison between Weightlifting Derivatives. *Journal of Sports Science and Medicine* 16: 407-413; Soriano, et al. (2017). The Optimal Load for Maximal Power Production During Upper-Body Resistance Exercises: A Meta-Analysis. *Sports Medicine* 47(4): 757-768. Soriano, et al. (2015). The Optimal Load for Maximal Power Production During Lower-Body Resistance Exercises: A Meta-Analysis. *Sports Med* 45(8): 1191-1205.

Training at the optimal load, while conceptually sound, appears to be flawed because the current body of knowledge indicates that many athletes require the ability to express high power outputs under loaded conditions (4, 5). In fact, in sports such as rugby league, a critical differentiator of performance is the athlete's overall strength level and ability to express high power outputs under loaded conditions (4, 5). For these types of athletes, consistently training at the optimal load to develop power will result in a muted ability to improve strength levels (19, 57, 89, 132, 133), which is detrimental to these athletes. Therefore, it may be warranted to use training loads in excess of the optimal load to improve the ability to express high power outputs under loaded conditions. In support of this contention, Moss and colleagues (92) report that training with heavier loads (90% of the 1RM) enhances power development under loaded conditions (>60% of the 1RM) when compared to training with low to moderate training loads (15%-35% of the 1RM). When working with athletes who must express high power outputs in loaded conditions (e.g., rugby league, rugby union, and American football), it is critical that strength development be a central component of training.

Many athletes must produce force against external sources of resistance and therefore need to train at a variety of training loads to develop power more globally in a variety of conditions. This becomes important when athletes must develop power in unloaded conditions, such as sprinting, and are often required to make large changes of direction, which magnify the load that the athlete must resist or move against (50). Additionally, athletes must also produce force against external resistance in activities such as tackling or rowing, where high forces are met continually during performance. Because athletes encounter a continuum of loads in sport, it is imperative to expose them to a variety of loads in training (50). Therefore, to optimize the continuum of power needed in sport, the strength and conditioning professional should adopt a mixed-methods model of training that develops the athlete's ability to generate power across the entire range of the force–velocity profile (50, 74).

One strategy for using a mixed-methods approach is to use a variety of training loads when constructing the training program (50). For example, higher loads (>75% of the 1RM) are typically used with the back squat to develop lower body strength. However, this exercise can also be performed as a speed squat with lighter loads (e.g., 30%-70% of the 1RM) to develop power (figure 3.21) (61). When the speed squat is used, approximately 45% of the final range of motion during the exercise is used for deceleration, and the overall velocity of movement achieved during this exercise is less than what is achieved during the jump squat (76, 80).

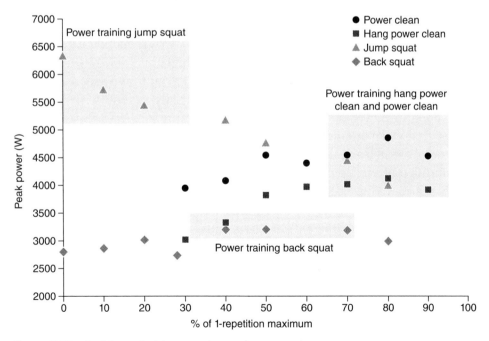

Figure 3.21 Resistance training exercises and power zones.

Reprinted by permission from G.G. Haff and S. Nimphius, "Training Principles for Power," *Strength and Conditioning Journal* 34, no. 6 (2012): 2-12.

An additional consideration in power-based training is the use of the warm-up set as a key contributor to performing training at various parts of the force–velocity relationship (50). For example, if an athlete were using the back squat to develop lower body strength with loads of 80% to 85% of the 1RM, he or she would perform a series of lower-loaded warm-up sets, and if these were performed explosively, they could be used to develop power (76). Lifting submaximal and maximal loads as quickly as possible in an explosive manner provides a greater potential for developing power across a range of training loads even when using exercises that are traditionally reserved for strength development (50, 76).

Set Structures

When examining the ability to develop power within a given exercise, the structure of the set can play an integral role. Traditional set structures, in which repetitions are performed continuously without rest between them, reduce the power output achieved in each repetition in the set (48, 82, 135). For example, Lawton and colleagues (82) reported that during the bench press, there was a nearly linear reduction in peak power output across a series of 6 repetitions performed at the 6RM. Similarly, Hardee and colleagues (54) reported that across a set of 6 repetitions in the power clean, there was a 15.7% reduction in power output from repetitions 1 to 6. Additionally, Gorostiage and colleagues (36) reported a 7% to 20% reduction in average peak power during the leg press when traditional sets of 5 were used and a 35% to 45% reduction when sets of 10 repetitions were performed. Interestingly, the higher-volume sets resulted in a greater reduction in adenosine triphosphate (ATP) and phosphocreatine and a greater increase in lactate (36), which may partially explain why there was a reduction in power output across the set structure. Collectively, these data suggest that when attempting to maximize power output using traditional set structures, sets of fewer than 6 repetitions are needed. To maximize power outputs during training, other resistance training set strategies, such as cluster sets, may be warranted, especially if higher-volume work is targeted (48, 99, 100).

The *cluster set*, as defined by Haff and colleagues (44, 49), is a set structure that applies a short rest interval (15-45 seconds) between individual repetitions or small groupings of repetitions to induce partial recovery and maximize the velocity and power of the movement (figure 3.22).

Hardee and colleagues (54) noted that performing power cleans with 80% of the 1RM using cluster sets with 20 seconds of rest between repetitions resulted in only a 5.5% reduction in power output across 6 repetitions. They compared this to a traditional set that demonstrated a 15.7% decrease. When the rest interval used in the cluster set was extended to 40 seconds, the reduction in power output was only 3.3%. The increased power output that occurs by extending

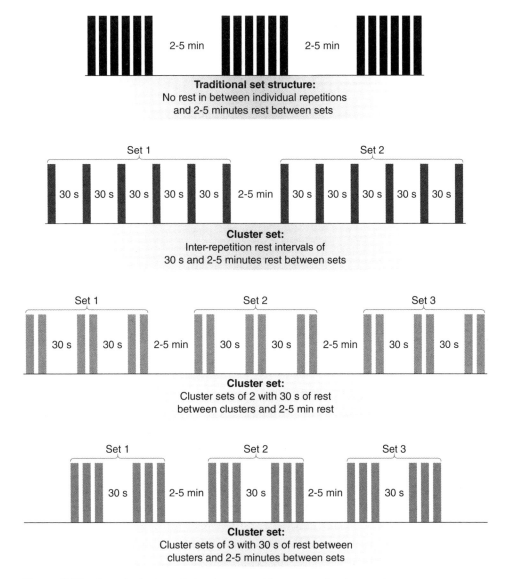

Figure 3.22 Sample cluster set structures used for power development.

the interrepetition rest interval to 30 to 40 seconds appears to capitalize on the ability to partially replenish phosphocreatine and ATP during these recovery periods (44, 49).

When structuring cluster sets, Haff and Harden (48) suggest that five basic variants can be used: standard, undulating, wave-loaded, ascending cluster, and descending (table 3.2).

The standard cluster set uses a loading scheme in which every repetition is performed with the exact same load and only the interrepetition rest interval is manipulated. An alternative approach is to use a wave-loaded, undulating, or

Table 3.2 Sample Cluster Set Structures for the Power Clean

Type of cluster	Sets	Reps	Average intensity, % 1RM	Sample structures for cluster set repetition loading (weight [kg] / rep)					Inter-rep rest interval (s)
Standard	1-3	5/1	85	106/1	106/1	106/1	106/1	106/1	30
	1-3	6/2	85	106/2	106/2	106/2	-	-	30
	1-3	6/3	85	106/3	106/3	-	-	-	30
Wave	1-3	5/1	85	103/1	110/1	103/1	110/1	103/1	30
	1-3	8/2	85	103/2	110/2	103/2	110/2	-	30
Undulating	1-3	5/1	85	103/1	106/1	113/1	106/1	103/1	30
	1-3	6/2	85	104/2	110/2	104/2	-	-	30
Ascending	1-3	5/1	85	98/1	103/1	105/1	110/1	113/1	30
	1-3	6/2	85	100/2	106/2	113/2	-	-	30
Descending	1-3	5/1	85	113/1	110/1	105/1	103/1	98/1	30
	1-3	6/2	85	113/2	106/2	100/2	-	-	30

Note: 5/1 = 5 total repetitions broken into 5 clusters of 1, 6/2 = 6 total repetitions broken into 3 clusters of 2, etc.; 1RM = 1-repetition maximum. All weights are based on a maximum power clean of 125 kg (276 lb) (106 kg [234 lb] = 85% of the 1RM).

ascending cluster set, manipulating the repetition load and the interrepetition rest interval. In the wave-loaded cluster set structure, the load is alternated between each repetition to create a load contrast, while in the undulating set, the load increases in a pyramid fashion. During the ascending cluster set, the load of each repetition performed in the set increases, while in the descending cluster set, the load decreases with each repetition. A cluster set could also be modified by manipulating the number of repetitions performed. For example, a cluster set of 6 repetitions could be performed with rest between individual repetitions (6/1), between pairs of repetitions (6/2), or between groups of 3 repetitions (6/3), with varying rest intervals. By varying the repetitions and the rest intervals between repetitions or clusters of repetitions, different aspects of power may be developed. Regardless of the cluster set structures used, the rest interval between sets is typically 2 to 5 minutes when attempting to maximize power (48).

When contextualized to the periodized training plan, cluster sets seem to be the most beneficial as a tool for optimizing power development during the specific preparatory, precompetition, and competition phases of the annual training plan (48, 106). For example, Roll and Omer (106) recommend using cluster sets with the clean and bench press exercises during the specific preparatory phase (e.g., strength–power phase) of the annual training plan when working with American football players. Similarly, Haff and colleagues (44, 49) suggest that cluster sets are ideally suited for the specific preparatory phase when maximizing power development is a central training target. Haff and Harden (48) recommend integrating standard, wave-loaded, ascending, and undulating cluster sets into the precompetition and main competition phases of the annual training plan, because these structures allow for both strength and power to be developed.

Types of Exercises Used

When developing a resistance training program that is in line with the periodization and planning goals, the actual training exercises selected play a key role in effectively developing power. Haff and Nimphius (50) suggest that a mixed-methods approach is essential when attempting to develop various parts of the force–velocity curve. Training exercises can be broken into several distinct categories, including shock- or reactive-strength, speed–strength, strength–speed, maximal strength, and supramaximal strength methods. Each of these methods develops different aspects of the force–velocity curve and therefore affects power development in different ways. For example, shock- or reactive-strength training maximizes the engagement of the stretch-shortening cycle and generally requires the athlete to couple an eccentric with a concentric muscle action in an explosive manner. The best example of a reactive-strength activity is high-level plyometrics, such as a drop or depth jump from a box, requiring the athlete to rapidly jump vertically after contacting the ground (chapter 6). Speed–strength resistance training enhances the RFD and in general has a high power output (124). On the other hand, strength–speed training targets the development of the RFD but tends to use heavier loads, although not as heavy as those used to develop maximal or supramaximal strength. Some of these methods are introduced here but will also be discussed in more detail in chapter 8.

As examples, ballistic methods could use plyometric activities, which target the low-load, high-velocity portion of the force–time curve (50). Strength–speed methods could use moderate loads of 70% to 95% of the 1RM with exercises such as the clean pull or power clean to develop power across a wide range of the force–velocity curve (18). Maximal-strength methods would use loads >85% of the 1RM and a variety of exercises, such as the back squat, to develop loaded power output at the high-force end of the force–velocity curve. Each exercise has a different power profile and can be used in different ways, depending on loading, to affect the development of specific strength and power attributes according to how it is used in the training program.

When examining the power profile of a variety of exercises, it is apparent that each exercise has a different power profile (see figure 3.23). For example, weightlifting movements (e.g., snatch, clean, and jerk) and their derivatives (e.g., clean pull, snatch pull, and push press) offer the ability to develop large amounts of power across a wide range of the force–velocity relationship (18) (see chapter 7).

Conversely, powerlifting exercises (i.e., squat, bench press, and deadlift) produce very little power, due to the low movement velocity. Therefore, they affect the high-force portion of the force–velocity curve.

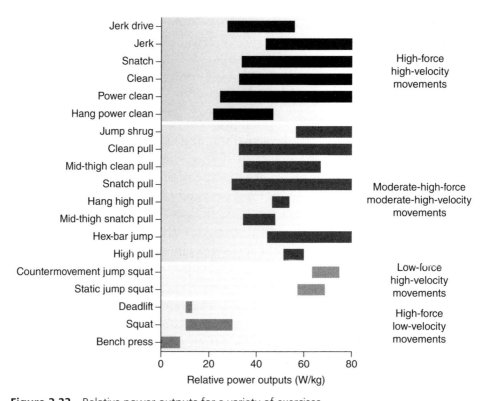

Figure 3.23 Relative power outputs for a variety of exercises.

Reprinted by permission from G.G. Haff and S. Nimphius, "Training Principles for Power," *Strength and Conditioning Journal* 34, no. 6 (2012): 2-12.

Exercise Order

When constructing a training program, most guidelines for the order of exercises suggest that power exercises be performed before core and assistance exercises (46). This order is effective because power exercises often require more effort, skill, and focus than multijoint core exercises and single-joint assistance exercises and thus should be performed when fresh. While this strategy is excellent, it may not be the best approach for stronger, more developed athletes, because they may need more advanced training structures to maximize performance gains. As such, several alternative strategies for sequencing training exercises within a training session have been proposed and are often classified as complex training (21, 86). Complex training involves implementing a specific exercise order in which movement velocity or load is systematically manipulated to improve the athlete's slow and fast force production and, ultimately, ability to express high power outputs (table 3.3). Generally, four categories of complex training, including contrast, ascending, and descending methods and the French contrast method, are discussed within the scientific literature (21).

Table 3.3 General Training Recommendations for Complex Training Targeting Power Development

Complex type	Sequence	Intensity	Recovery interval	Examples
Contrast	Exercises are alternated between high-load (high force) and low-load (high velocity) exercises in a set-by-set fashion within the same session	• Conditioning activity: 0%-85% 1RM • Subsequent task: BM to 60% 1RM	• Intracontrast rest: stronger athletes, 3-7 min (individualize); weaker athletes, >7 min • Interset rest: 3-4 min	1. Quarter back squat from pins—85% 1RM 2. Box jump 3. Quarter back squat from pins—85% 1RM 4. Box jump
Ascending	Several sets of high-velocity exercises are completed before several sets of high-load exercises within the same session	• Light load: BM to 60% 1RM • High load: ≥85% 1RM	• Interset rest: 3-4 min	1. Jump squat—30% 1RM 2. Jump squat—30% 1RM 3. Back squat—90% 1RM 4. Back squat—90% 1RM
Descending	Several sets of high-load exercises are completed before performing several sets of low-load, higher-velocity exercises within the same session	• High load: ≥85% 1RM • Light load: BM to 60% 1RM	• Interset rest: 3-4 min	1. Bench press—85% 1RM 2. Bench press—85% 1RM 3. Bench throw—30% 1RM 4. Bench throw—30% 1RM
French contrast method	In this complex method, a series of exercises is performed in a predetermined sequence: heavy compound exercise→plyometric exercise→light-to-moderate compound exercise to maximize power→plyometric exercise	• Heavy compound: 80%-90% 1RM • Plyometric exercise: BM • Light-to-moderate compound: 30%-40% 1RM • Plyometric exercise: BM, or can be assisted (−30% to 40% BM)	• Intracontrast rest: 20 s between exercises • Interseries rest: 4-5 min	1. Back squat—85% 1RM 2. Depth jump 3. Jump squat—30% 1RM 4. Assisted CMJ (−30% BM)

Note: 1RM = 1-repetition maximum; BM = body mass; CMJ = countermovement jump.

Adapted by permission from P Cormier, T.T, Freitas, I. Loturco, et al., "Within Session Exercise Sequencing During Programming for Complex Training: Historical Perspectives, Terminology, and Training Considerations," *Sports Medicine* 52 (2002), Springer Nature.

The first way to organize a training program is to implement contrast training methods where high-load (i.e., high-force) and low-load (i.e., high-velocity) exercises are alternated on a set-by-set basis. With this programming strategy, the high-load activity is used to stimulate a postactivation performance enhancement (PAPE; see page 257 for more details), which is expressed as an increase in power output or movement velocity during the low-load activity (21).

Another way to organize a training program is through ascending or descending workouts (21, 130). Ascending workouts generally require the athlete to perform several sets of exercises that use low-load, high-velocity movements followed by several sets of high-load, low-velocity exercises (21). For example, a session could start with shock- or reactive-strength exercises (i.e., plyometric tasks), followed by ballistic, strength–speed, and heavy-load strength exercises (table 3.4) (130). Ascending workouts increase force application and reduce the velocity of movement across training sessions.

Table 3.4 Sample Ascending Workout

Exercise	Sets × reps	Load (% 1RM)	Focus
Depth jump	3 × 5	0	Shock or reactive strength
Jump squat	3 × 5	0-30	Ballistic
Power clean	3 × 5	75-85	Strength–speed
Back squat	3 × 5	80-85	Strength

Conversely, descending workouts reverse this order, starting with heavy load strength exercises and ending with shock or ballistic exercises (table 3.5). By reversing the order of the session, the athlete progresses from higher- to lower-load activities while increasing movement velocity.

Table 3.5 Sample Descending Workout

Exercise	Sets × reps	Load (% 1RM)	Focus
Back squat	3 × 5	80-85	Strength
Power clean	3 × 5	75-85	Strength–speed
Jump squat	3 × 5	0-30	Ballistic
Depth jump	3 × 5	0	Shock or reactive strength

Another method of organizing training that has gained in popularity is the French contrast method, in which exercises are sequenced to target maximum strength, speed–strength, strength–speed, and maximum speed with approximately 20 seconds of rest between exercises and 4 to 5 minutes of interseries rest (table 3.6) (21, 29, 59). By sequencing the order of the training session in this manner, it is believed that a PAPE will be elicited while targeting four different components of the force–velocity relationship (21).

Table 3.6 French Contrast Workout

Exercise	SERIES #1 Reps	SERIES #2 Reps	SERIES #3 Reps	Load	Intracontrast rest	Focus
Front squat	5	5	5	85% 1RM		Maximal strength
					20 s	
Countermovement jump	3	3	3	Body weight		Speed–strength
					20 s	
Clean grip jump shrug	5	5	5	35% 1RM		Strength–speed
					20 s	
Band-assisted countermovement jump	3	3	3	–20% Body weight		Maximal speed
Interseries rest	4 min	4 min	4 min			

Ultimately, the various complex methods allow development of various portions of the force–velocity curve and can affect power development across a variety of loading structures.

General Programming Recommendations

While programming for the development of strength and power is a highly individualized process, some basic recommendations can be made (table 3.7). When targeting power development, it is generally recommended that 3 to 5 sets, with 1 to 5 repetitions per set, are performed with a focus on maximizing the quality of exercise (46, 112). The intensity used will depend on the exercise (115, 116). For example, for weightlifting movements such as the power clean, loads of ≥70% of the 1RM should be programmed when targeting power development. Conversely, when implementing jump squats and bench throws, loads ≤30% of the 1RM are typically used. Although these loads give a programmatic starting point, variation in loading should be programmed to maximize various aspects of the force–velocity curve, which can enhance the development of power. Finally, a key aspect of training for power development is providing adequate recovery (i.e., 2-5 minutes of rest) between sets and exercises targeting power development.

Table 3.7 General Programming Guidelines

Sets	Single-effort event	3-5	Example exercises		
	Multiple-effort event	3-5			
Reps	Single-effort event	1-2			
	Multiple-effort event	3-5			
Intensity	Optimal load zone 1 exercises	≤30% 1RM	Plyometric exercises		
			Bench throw		
			Jump squat		
			Hex-bar jump squat		
	Optimal load zone 2 exercises	30%-70% 1RM	Jump shrug		
			High hang pull		
			Back squat		
			Leg press		
			Bench press		
			Mid-thigh pull		
	Optimal load zone 3 exercises	≥70% 1RM	Power clean		
			Hang power clean		
			Snatch		
			Clean		
			Power snatch		
			Jerk		
Rest interval		2 to 5 min			

CONCLUSION

Based on the contemporary body of scientific knowledge, periodized training plans are an essential component of the development of athletic performance. Once a multiyear or annual training plan is established, the organization of the training structures can be planned and the training methods to include in the program can be determined for developing maximal strength and power. A parallel planning structure may be an adequate tool for guiding the training process of novice athletes. However, for intermediate to advanced athletes, sequential or emphasis models may provide a superior training stimulus for maximizing both strength and power. Regardless of the planning structure used, it is essential for the strength and conditioning professional to understand that strength is the foundation from which power is built and that the development of strength should always be part of the training process. When targeting strength and power development, a mixed-training-model approach is necessary. Training structures, such as cluster sets and complexes, can be useful when constructing training interventions. Additionally, contrast, ascending, descending, and French contrast methods can be useful components of a training plan to maximize power development.

CHAPTER 4

Adapting Power Training to Special Populations

Robert C. Linkul
Rhodri S. Lloyd

Many strength and conditioning professionals and personal trainers work with a range of ages and abilities among their clientele. This chapter presents power training guidelines for populations that have distinctive characteristics and may require modification of standard training protocols to maximize training effects and minimize risk of injury. When designing programs to improve power, it is important to understand power training in the context of both young, developing athletes and older people who may have a variety of complicating factors in their medical history.

TRAINING YOUTH POPULATIONS

Alongside physical fitness qualities such as motor skills, strength, and speed, power is recognized as one of the key components of athleticism for children and adolescents (51). Leading consensus indicates that enhancing levels of athleticism over time to improve health, fitness, and physical performance and reduce injury risk are the hallmarks of long-term athletic development for youths (51). The capacity to produce high quantities of neuromuscular power is a requirement for dynamic sporting performance (32, 35) and can differentiate between playing levels in young athletes (45, 67). Neuromuscular power is also an important physical attribute for deceleration and reacceleration when rapidly

The authors would like to acknowledge the significant contribution of N. Travis Triplett to this chapter.

changing direction or dealing with unanticipated movements (84). Therefore, both children and adolescents should engage in training methods that promote the development of neuromuscular power to enhance performance and reduce injury risk.

The most common training modality for developing neuromuscular power in youths is some form of resistance training (5, 26, 31, 46), a specialized method of training whereby a person works against a wide range of resistive loads applied through the use of body weight, weight machines, free weights (barbells and dumbbells), elastic bands, and medicine balls (53). Despite previous concerns regarding its safety, resistance training is now recognized as a safe and effective vehicle for developing muscular strength and power in children and adolescents and should serve as an essential component of physical activity for all youths (53). Strength and conditioning professionals and personal trainers who plan, deliver, and guide athletic development programs for youths should possess a sound understanding of pediatric exercise science, a recognized professional certification credential, a background in pedagogy (i.e., the method and practice of teaching), and an ability to communicate with youths of different ages and abilities (55).

Natural Development of Neuromuscular Power in Youths

The natural development of neuromuscular power mirrors that of muscular strength, which is unsurprising given the close association between the two physical qualities (101) (see chapter 1 regarding the relationship between strength and power). Indeed, much like muscular strength, natural increases in neuromuscular power (as measured by performance in the standing long jump, with jump distance as a proxy for power) have been shown to occur in prepubertal children between the ages of 5 and 10 years (9). Maturation of the central nervous system is typically responsible for the adaptations seen in neuromuscular power during childhood. Specifically, the ability to activate and coordinate motor units and the increased neural myelination improve neural drive through this stage of development (25, 26). A secondary natural "spurt" in neuromuscular power then appears to commence approximately 18 months before peak height velocity (PHV), with peak gains typically occurring 6 to 12 months after PHV (7). Peak height velocity refers to the maximum rate of growth during the adolescent growth spurt and occurs at approximately 11.5 years for girls and 13.5 years for boys. In addition to the continuing maturation of the nervous system, adolescence is associated with structural and architectural changes in contractile tissue, which ultimately increase the capacity to generate force (88). Proliferations in hormonal concentrations (including testosterone, growth hormone, and insulin-like growth factor) mediate changes in muscle size, muscle pennation angle, and further motor unit differentiation (102). One study indicated that school-aged boys who achieved large, worthwhile changes in sprint speed (80% of the sample) and jump height (50% of the sample) also achieved large changes in vastus lateralis and physiological muscle thickness over an 18-month period (87).

The ability to produce high levels of muscular power depends on the type of muscular action involved, and research has demonstrated that when a muscle uses a stretch-shortening cycle (SSC), it can produce greater power outputs than an isolated concentric muscle action (42). Owing to the dynamics of sport and physical activity, rarely is a concentric action used in isolation; therefore, it is important to consider how the regulation of SSC function changes as children mature. Researchers have shown that the development of the SSC is nonlinear, with periods of accelerated adaptation for a range of measures of SSC function reported for age ranges indicative of before and after PHV (59). Research examining the way the neural regulation of SSC function changes in children of different maturity groups showed that as children become older and more mature, they become more reliant on feed-forward mechanisms (pre-activation) to regulate cyclical high-speed activities that produce a high rate of force, such as submaximal or maximal rebounding in place (57). Feed-forward activity reflects involuntary anticipatory muscle activity prior to the observation of any spinal or supraspinal reflexive activity. Previously, researchers showed that from a sample of 127 school-aged children, post-PHV boys achieved greater measures of reactive strength index (RSI) during a maximal five-rebound jump test than their pre-PHV peers, likely underpinned by the larger relative net impulses driving higher jump heights in the more mature group (86). Similarly, drop jump data from a sample of 341 young male athletes (aged approximately 10-16 years) showed that moderate increases in RSI from before to after PHV were underpinned by large changes in jump height (attributable to very large increases in relative net impulse) in the absence of any changes in ground contact time (44).

The increase in SSC function reported in boys does not necessarily follow the same trajectory in girls. For example, drop jump data from 1,013 girls in middle and high school showed that RSI and its constituent variables, jump height and ground contact time, remained unchanged between prepubertal, pubertal, and postpubertal groups (75). Therefore, there appear to be potential sex-specific differences in SSC function that likely emerge during adolescence, which can be attributed to the divergent development of neuromuscular properties in males and females during adolescence (26). However, data from young female gymnasts indicate that squat jump, countermovement jump, and drop jump heights increased from early prepuberty to puberty among girls (65). Considering the training practices of gymnasts, this demonstrates that appropriate training can enhance SSC function despite the sex-related differences in neuromuscular power that may manifest during adolescence.

Trainability of Neuromuscular Power in Youths

Researchers have shown that muscular power increases in a nonlinear fashion throughout childhood and adolescence, with both boys and girls of all ages and maturity levels able to show improvement as a result of growth and maturation alone (8). This is an important factor for researchers, strength and conditioning professionals, and personal trainers to consider as they plan and deliver training programs, because growth and maturity-related increases in neuromuscular power may be misinterpreted as training-induced adaptations. Consequently, to confidently determine meaningful changes in performance associated with training, these professionals should understand the typical increases in performance expected because of growth and maturation in addition to the measurement error associated with the testing equipment used.

Researchers have shown that traditional resistance training, ballistic exercises, plyometrics, and weightlifting are the most commonly used forms of resistance training to develop neuromuscular power (13). While the interaction between growth, maturation, and the trainability of neuromuscular power requires further research, the results of several studies show that both children and adolescents are able to increase this physical quality following exposure to appropriate resistance-based training interventions (47, 54, 76, 99). Within the pediatric literature, researchers have shown that traditional resistance training (52, 62, 66), plyometrics (58, 76), weightlifting (11), explosive resistance training (30), and combined training (107) are all safe and effective means of enhancing various indices of neuromuscular power. Resistance training, as part of an integrative neuromuscular training program, has also been shown to reduce the relative risk of injury, with exposure at earlier stages of development proving to offer more protective benefits (71). Resistance training has also been shown to increase insulin sensitivity in youths who have obesity, because the training mode can increase both the size and recruitment of fast-twitch muscle fibers (95).

Because there is little evidence of hypertrophic adaptations in children, resistance training–induced increases in neuromuscular power during childhood are likely determined by changes in the nervous system (6). Conversely, training-induced gains in neuromuscular power during adolescence typically reflect not only adaptations to the nervous system but also structural and architectural properties (26, 63). Researchers have indicated that maturity status, in addition to baseline fitness, is a key predictor of training responsiveness in measures of strength and power (52). More research is required to examine the specific mechanisms that mediate training-induced gains in neuromuscular power in youths, especially mechanisms that underpin long-term adaptations across different stages of maturation. Previously, researchers have shown that a training prescription can be manipulated to mirror the training stimulus with naturally occurring adaptations to augment the training response, a concept referred to as *synergistic adaptation* (50). Specifically, a six-week, school-based, resistance training intervention showed that pre-PHV boys responded more favorably to plyometric training compared to post-PHV peers, who experienced a greater training response to traditional resistance training (50). Plyometrics are likely to stimulate neural adaptations, which also undergo marked natural development from growth and maturation, whereas resistance training will drive neural and structural adaptations and are likely to mirror the ongoing neural and structural changes that are stimulated by adolescence. While synergistic adaptation is in its relative infancy in the research, there is some supporting evidence that it influences the development of strength and power (6) and sprint speed (69). Additionally, meta-analytical data from 75 studies and >5,000 participants show that the plyometric training response is heightened in pre-PHV boys, whereas youths who are approaching or have reached PHV appear to respond more favorably to traditional resistance training (76).

There is a fundamental relationship between muscular strength and neuromuscular power (see chapter 1). Evidence indicates that people with higher strength levels have a greater capacity to produce power (13). Given its multiple health and performance benefits and its ability to reduce the risk of injury, resistance training should form an integral part of any youth-based strength and conditioning program (53). Strength and conditioning professionals and personal trainers should ensure that all children and adolescents are provided with developmentally appropriate training strategies to develop sound movement mechanics while simultaneously increasing muscular strength levels (53). In combination, movement competency and muscular strength will serve as the foundations for a robust system through which high levels of muscular power can be produced and attenuated during whole-body dynamic activities. Researchers have demonstrated the interplay between muscle strength and movement competency, with data showing that relatively weaker school-aged boys (as determined from relative peak force in the isometric mid-thigh pull [IMTP]) were about 8 times more likely to be classified as lower competency (assessed via the Resistance Training Skills Battery) than relatively stronger boys (80). Similar data have emerged from adolescent females, with relatively stronger girls (as measured via IMTP peak force) demonstrating fewer technical deficits in both the back squat assessment and the drop jump (100). The emphasis on muscular strength and movement competency is especially prudent considering the negative trends in muscular strength levels and motor fitness of modern-day youths (12, 91). Because of the increased sedentariness of children (103) and the fact that they are less capable of maximally recruiting their high-threshold type II motor units (18), it is highly probable that in most cases, simply focusing on increasing their movement competency and muscular strength capacities will indirectly increase neuromuscular power.

Researchers have examined the effects of a two-year resistance training program on strength performance in youth soccer players and have shown that the magnitude of strength gains increases with age (41). Long-term exposure to periodized resistance training resulted in relative strength levels being 0.7 × body weight in 11- to 12-year-olds, 1.5 × body weight in 13- to 15-year-olds, and 2.0 × body weight in 16- to 19-year-olds (41). In a separate study, the same group of researchers showed that after two years of resistance training, 13-, 15-, and 17-year-old soccer players simultaneously improved 1-repetition maximum (1RM) squat strength by 100% to 300% and sprinting speed by 3% to 5%, which was used as a surrogate measure of power (92). Collectively, these studies underline the meaningful improvements that children and adolescents can make in response to resistance training, especially over long-term training durations.

Not all youths wish to engage in competitive sports; therefore, strength and conditioning professionals and personal trainers should not base strength and power training programming on data from homogeneous populations (e.g., elite youth soccer players). Researchers have examined the effectiveness of integrative neuromuscular training interventions on the health- and skill-related measures of fitness in seven-year-old children (23). They showed that children were able to make significant gains in curl-up and push-up performance (increased muscular strength and endurance) and in standing long jump and single-leg hop performance (increased neuromuscular power) by following an eight-week training program of 15-minute sessions twice a week (23). A follow-up study showed that after an eight-week detraining period, training-induced gains in curl-up and single-leg hop performance (muscular strength and endurance) were maintained, while those for long-jump performance (neuromuscular power) significantly decreased (24). This might suggest that muscular strength is easier to maintain in children, while neuromuscular power capacities require more frequent stimuli to prevent detraining.

Improvements in muscular power have also been shown in school-aged youths who followed a four-week plyometric training program (58). Results showed that 12- and 15-year-old boys were able to significantly improve SSC function, while nine-year-olds were also able to show improvements, albeit not significantly. This may highlight an age-dependent response to plyometric training and may indicate that younger children possibly require a different amount of training to elicit gains similar to those their more mature peers experience. Conversely, it could simply suggest that training-induced adaptation takes longer to materialize in younger children, which supports the notion of a long-term approach to training for athletic development in youths. Moeskops and colleagues (66) showed that prepubertal female gymnasts who completed a 10-month training program made significant improvements in a range of isometric and dynamic kinetics, standing long jump, sprint speed, and vaulting vertical takeoff velocity and that these changes were not evident in the "gymnastics only" group or the "nongymnastics" control group. The results of this study also highlighted that the adaptations realized in the program followed a sequence aligned with classic block periodization theory. Notably, strength-related improvements were

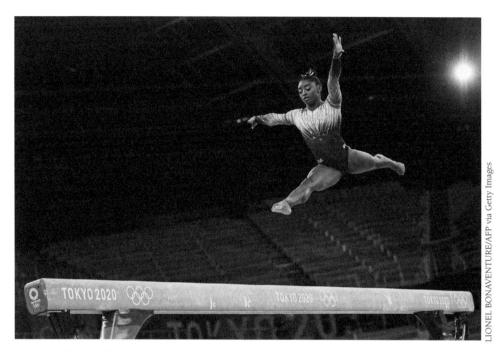

Simone Biles utilizes muscular power to achieve incredible jump heights.

noted at four months, further strength gains and "power" adaptations were noted at seven months, and improvements in sprint speed, spring-like behavior, and vaulting takeoff velocity were determined at 10 months. Collectively, these findings emphasize that even prepubertal children can make meaningful improvements in strength and power but also that a periodized, long-term approach to programming is highly effective.

Cumulatively, the results of existing studies within the literature base show that both children and adolescents can make resistance training gains in neuromuscular power, that youths can make improvements in neuromuscular power as a result of increasing their muscular strength capacities, and that training-induced gains in neuromuscular power may diminish at a faster rate than muscular strength in youths.

Translating the Science into Program Design

When designing training programs for children or adolescents, progression should be based primarily on their technical competency. Strength and conditioning professionals and personal trainers should also consider the training age of the child or adolescent (72), which reflects their relative experience (e.g., number of years) of formalized training and, potentially, the type of training to which they have been exposed. Coaches should also be aware of the biological maturation of the person, because stages of development are characterized by unique physiological adaptations that may influence the training response (56). Because of the inherent variations in the timing, tempo, and magnitude of maturation, chronological age should not determine training prescriptions for youths. Psychosocial maturity should also be taken into account when designing a program to meet their individual needs (53). For example, an inexperienced and introverted child lacking confidence may need simpler exercises, more conservative progressions, and a greater degree of patience than an experienced, confident, and extroverted adolescent. The following case studies demonstrate how training prescription is altered in accordance with the individual needs of children or adolescents with varying degrees of experience and technical competency.

Case Study 1: Child With No Training Experience and Low Technical Competency

When young children are first exposed to a formalized strength and conditioning program, it is not uncommon that they will be unable to demonstrate competency in a range of motor skills. Consequently, the initial focus should be directed toward developing a diverse range of motor skills alongside basic strength development, which, combined, will positively influence power and overall athleticism (figure 4.1).

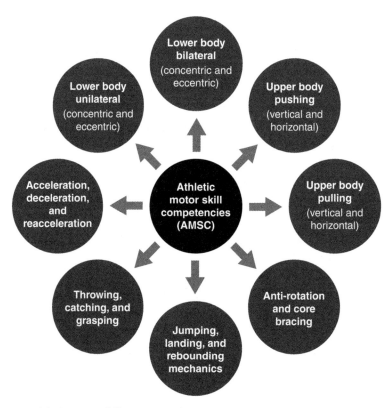

Figure 4.1 Athletic motor skill competencies.

From J.A. Moody, F. Naclerio, P. Green, and R.S. Lloyd, 2013, Motor skill development in youths. In *Strength and conditioning for young athletes: Science and application*, edited by R.S. Lloyd and J.L. Oliver (Oxon: Routledge), 53.

Before trying to develop muscular power, coaches should first look to increase muscular strength levels, because untrained children with low technical competency will likely be a considerable distance from their ceiling potential of force-producing capacities. Therefore, in addition to training motor skills, base levels of muscular strength should also be trained during the early stages of the training program to enable the expression of higher levels of neuromuscular power. This approach should also develop a robust and highly coordinated neuromuscular system that youths can use to withstand the reactive and unpredictable forces typically experienced within free play, sports, or recreational physical activity. A sample training session for an inexperienced child with low technical competency is provided in table 4.1.

Children with low technical competency should also be exposed to a range of activities that enable the simultaneous development of other fitness qualities, such as coordination, speed, power, agility, and flexibility (54). This is because of the heightened neural plasticity associated with childhood and the accompanying trainability of neuromuscular qualities (6). While the development of neuromuscular power is critical for sport performance, recreational physical activity, and general health and well-being, taking a broader approach to athletic development in youths is important because of the inherent trainability of all fitness components at all stages of development (54). Consequently, strength and conditioning professionals should not focus on one or two measures of fitness but should rather provide complementary training activities that develop a wide range of fitness components in a holistic program.

Additionally, a varied and holistic approach to athletic development is necessary from a pedagogical perspective to keep training sessions fun, interesting, and motivating for young children (51). Strength and conditioning professionals and personal trainers should remember that many activities children engage in on the playground (e.g., hopscotch) present opportunities for power training and that child-friendly activities that might not reflect the traditional training modes (e.g., advanced plyometrics or weightlifting) can still be effective in developing neuromuscular power.

In terms of developing neuromuscular power, childhood can be viewed as an opportune time to lay the foundation for general athleticism that will enable youths to participate in more advanced training strategies as they become more experienced. For example, a major goal for a child with low technical competency might be to develop the ability to jump and land effectively. This should be viewed as a critical athletic motor skill that is required for a range of activities—for example, plyometric training. Over time, and as technical competency and muscular strength increase, the child can challenge this movement pattern through a higher plyometric training stimulus that provides greater eccentric stress (e.g., drop jumps or bounding). Another example could be in the development of weightlifting ability, whereby childhood should be viewed as an opportunity to

Table 4.1 Sample Training Session for a Child With No Training Experience and Low Technical Competency

Phase	Exercise	Description	Volume (sets × reps)	Intensity	Rest (s)
Fun warm-up	Animal shapes warm-up games	The child moves around and on the floor in multiple directions, mimicking various animal shapes (e.g., bear, crab, or seal).	4 × 30 s	Body weight	30
Bodyweight management	Deadbug	The child lays on his or her back with the arms extended toward the ceiling and the hips, knees, and ankles at 90 degrees. The child extends one leg and one arm asynchronously, then returns them to center.	2 × 10 (each side)	Body weight	30
	Inchworm	The child places the hands in front of the feet, then walks the hands out as far as possible while maintaining torso control. The child then walks the feet into the hands.	2 × 8	Body weight	30
	Dish-to-arch roll	The child rolls from a dish position to an arch and back to a dish position without the feet, hands, or head touching the floor.	2 × 8 each side	Body weight	30
	Front support (plank) walk	The child adopts a front support (plank) position, while a partner supports his or her ankles and shins. The first child then moves around the floor in multiple directions and maintains torso control.	2 × 10 m	Body weight	45
Main	12 in. (30.5 cm) box jump	See the regressions for the double-leg snap down (chapter 6, page 141).	3 × 4	Body weight	45
	Resistance band overhead squat	See the chain- or band-resisted back squat* (chapter 6, page 172).	3 × 6	Body weight plus band tension	60
	Push-up	See the band push-up (page 132), but exlude the band.	3 × 6	Body weight	45
	Band standing row	(chapter 5, page 134).	3 × 6	Body weight plus band tension	45

*This is a similar, but not identical, version of the recommended exercise that includes a bar; the resistance band overhead squat does not include a bar and has the child holding a resistance band in an overhead (shoulder press) position while doing a squat.

develop basic motor skills that will help in the execution of full weightlifting movements and their derivatives as technical competency improves (70).

Case Study 2: Technically Competent Adolescent With Six Years of Training Experience

When a child has engaged with formalized training during childhood, adolescence can serve as an ideal opportunity to build on existing levels of neuromuscular fitness. Developmentally appropriate training can be prescribed to work synergistically with the heightened hormonal concentrations that result from puberty. This enables adolescents to achieve greater neural, structural, and architectural adaptations. Consequently, technically competent adolescents with a sound training age should be able to generate greater force outputs at higher velocities, thus enhancing their ability to produce high levels of neuromuscular power. As part of their athletic development program, technically competent adolescents of an appropriate training age should incorporate a variety of resistance training modes to develop neuromuscular power, using higher intensities (e.g., greater external loads or movement velocities), more sophisticated training strategies (e.g., complex training or cluster training), more advanced technical demands (e.g., accentuated plyometric training, weightlifting derivatives), or a

Table 4.2 Sample Training Session for a Technically Competent Adolescent With Six Years of Training Experience

Phase	Exercise	Description	Volume (sets × reps)	Intensity (% 1RM)	Rest (min)
Physical Preparation	Foam rolling	The adolescent gently rolls specific body parts over the top of the foam roller, paying particular focus to areas of muscle tightness or soreness.	2 × 10 (each side)	N/A	1
	Mini-band walk	The adolescent steps laterally with a mini band positioned just above the knees or around the ankles.	2 × 10 (each side)	N/A	1
	Glute bridge	Lying on his or her back with the knees raised and the feet in contact with the floor, the adolescent squeezes his or her glutes to extend the hips toward the ceiling.	2 × 10 (each side)	N/A	1
	Single-leg hop and hold	See the progresssions and regressions for the single-leg snap down (chapter 6, page 143).	2 × 4 (each leg)	N/A	1
Main	12 in. (30.5 cm) depth drop	(See chapter 6, page 144).	4 × 3	Body weight	1-2
	Power clean	See the power clean–related progressions (chapter 8, page 215).	4 × 2	85	2-3
	Back squat	(See chapter 6, page 170).	4 × 5	85	2-3
	Jump squat	See the chain- or band-resisted back squat variations (chapter 6, page 173).	4 × 4	30	2-3

combination of these variables. Regardless of an adolescent's training history, his or her motor skill competency should be regularly revisited to prevent technical deficiencies over time stemming from sudden growth spurts, muscle imbalances, or injury. A sample training session for an experienced and technically competent adolescent is provided in table 4.2.

One Size Does Not Fit All: The Need for Flexible Programming

Table 4.2 outlines an approach to develop neuromuscular power in an adolescent who has engaged in formalized training during childhood. However, this plan may not be appropriate for adolescents with no experience in athletic development, irrespective of their maturity status. In this situation, the program should still focus on mastering technical competency; however, the pedagogy involved in coaching more basic training methods (e.g., to improve fundamental motor skills) in older youths will likely differ from those used for younger children. Additionally, while possibly possessing greater levels of muscular strength, untrained adolescents will typically lack flexibility or may present with muscle imbalances that should be addressed in the early stages of the program before attempting to specifically develop neuromuscular power. Conversely, when coaching a naturally gifted and highly athletic child, they should be allowed to progress to more advanced training strategies or increased intensities while being careful not to sacrifice technical competency. These scenarios underscore the need to take a flexible and individualized approach to training youths and coach what is seen.

TRAINING OLDER ADULTS

The ability of older adults (aged ≥65 years) to produce power is thought to be vital for retaining neuromuscular function as they age. Eccentric strength and power production in multiple different planes is key in preventing falls, which can lead to increased morbidity and mortality (3, 29, 98). Retaining neuromuscular function is important for a variety of reasons, including the ability to perform the activities of daily living and preserve muscle mass, which is essential for maintaining a healthy body composition and weight (61, 74, 89). Older adults best develop neuromuscular power through tempo-based resistance training, with heavily loaded compound movements. A good portion of their exercises should include heavily loaded movements (2, 38, 49) in addition to a specific emphasis on explosive or ballistic movements that are age- and ability-appropriate, such as tempo lifting, certain plyometric exercises, and implement release exercises (e.g., throws) (15).

Older adults should keep physical limitations in mind and perform power-based movements only after developing a base level of strength (82). Therefore, strength and conditioning professionals and personal trainers who choose to incorporate power training into resistance exercise programs for older adults should conduct a thorough assessment, needs analysis, and medical history to truly understand any physical limitations and/or altered ability levels their client might have, because this information is vital to the program design process (33). These professionals should also hold a recognized strength and conditioning qualification, ideally one specific to the older population, and understand the expected physiological and biomechanical responses and adaptations in older adults.

Neuromuscular Decline With Aging

To understand the potential training adaptations to a strength and power training program in the older population, it is necessary to first be familiar with typical decline in physiological functioning of the muscular, neural, and skeletal systems. One of the most evident changes in the aging body is *sarcopenia*, a condition that causes long-term muscular atrophy and loss of function (3). Sarcopenia is commonly associated with the involuntary loss of skeletal muscle mass and strength, and it affects as much as 25% to 45% of the older adult population (19, 20, 48, 83). Much of this total muscle mass loss is caused by disproportionate losses of the faster-contracting type II muscle fibers (48, 97), likely the result of a reduction in high-force and rapid, "explosive" activities (19). In conjunction with the atrophy of type II muscle fibers, the related motor neurons also decline in function, firing at a lower rate in their range (105, 106). In addition, the motor unit (a group of muscle fibers and the motor neuron that controls them) remodels, resulting in denervation of the type II muscle fibers and reinnervation by the neurons associated with the slower-contracting type I muscle fibers (105, 106). Other changes brought on with age include decreased amounts of myelin covering the motor neuron and reduced transmission of the neural signal to the muscle cells (37, 40, 106). Combined, these alterations reduce force production and contraction speed, thereby reducing power production in aging muscle.

Connective tissue that forms the joints and other connections between the muscles and bones loses some elasticity and increases in stiffness beyond what is optimal for the translation of force from the muscle to the tendon (1). The ability of a tendon to absorb muscle force and store it as potential energy is critical to the functioning of the SSC. Therefore, reduced storage of elastic energy results in a reduction in force and power production (1). Between the ages of 30 and 50 years, strength and power decline gradually. The greatest decline in strength and power occurs after the age of 60. Starting the sixth decade of life, older adults will experience a 3.6% loss in muscle strength and a 3% loss in muscular power each year, on average (96). This is a staggering amount of strength and power loss and is one of the primary reasons why fall risks are projected to increase from 63% of older adults experiencing falls in 2014 to 66% by the year 2030 (33, 96).

Trainability of Power in the Older Population

Numerous researchers have used a variety of power training modalities and programming in older populations (39, 104). The most common modalities have been hydraulic or pneumatic resistance exercise machines, release exercises (e.g., throws), and traditional free weights (17, 28, 74, 79). The most common way to test for power involves a countermovement jump or exercises performed with the intent to move rapidly (e.g., double-leg press in a pneumatic or hydraulic machine) (10, 61). Because of the previously mentioned neural decline with aging, machine exercises may be easier for novice individuals to learn because the movements are less complex and are generally restricted to one plane of movement, which should improve safety. In addition, hydraulic or pneumatic resistance is accommodating and adjusts to the individual's level of effort. Release exercises (e.g., throws) are more advanced and therefore are typically performed on a Smith machine (i.e., a guided bar) or with a sandbag, Jam-Ball (also called a slam ball; i.e., a nonreactive medicine ball), medicine ball, or sand-filled kettlebell type of implement that can be safely thrown without damaging the equipment or the facility (15, 38).

Across any age, the relationship between muscular strength and neuromuscular power is the same, and stronger people have greater capacity to produce power (13). Thus, the benefits of power training in older populations are better realized after establishing a strength base. The other primary component of power—movement speed—can be addressed successfully in a power training program for older adults (21, 28, 64, 94). While the magnitude of improvement in power is more modest than in a young person, positive functional adaptations are nonetheless possible, and studies of power training in older adults have shown varying levels of success (36, 64, 77, 79, 90, 93).

Power training can be approached in two ways. The most common method is to perform high-speed, "explosive" movements (34, 73, 81), while the other method is to perform movements with a specific emphasis placed on lifting the tempo with the intent to move quickly (4, 61), which may or may not be possible based on the load. Each approach has pros and cons. Performing exercises "explosively" commonly requires applying braking force (i.e., a net force less than the system mass to permit deceleration via gravitational forces) to slow the movement before reaching the end of the range of motion. This approach is more commonly used for novice to intermediate clients. Because of the previously mentioned losses in muscle mass, motor neuron function, and elasticity in the connective tissues, older individuals are more affected by the higher forces seen in explosive power exercises. This has implications for higher risk of injury, so the emphasis must first be on developing consistent and flawless technique and ensuring that an eight-week adaptation phase focused on improving strength is implemented and successfully achieved.

Pneumatic or Hydraulic Training

Pneumatic or hydraulic machine exercises have the advantage that movements can be performed with the intent to move fast but without the ballistic characteristics at the end of a joint's range of motion. A drawback to pneumatic or hydraulic training is that many of these exercises take place in a fixed plane of movement and are less likely to mimic daily life movements. Research using eccentric training with a pneumatic training machine or open fly wheel device has shown promise in improving clients' power production with minimal wear and tear on their body and joints (43). Eccentric-focused training with a consistent load, an accommodating load, or a fly wheel resistance have shown to improve balance, stability, strength, and power in older adults while producing less stress and wear and tear on their joints (43). Pneumatic, hydraulic, and fly-wheel eccentric and power-based training is a successful way to develop strength and power with older adults; however, this style or tempo of lifting does take time to master and requires a solid foundation of strength as a prerequisite to minimize risk of injury and maximize potential for success.

Free Weight Training

Researchers have reported that free weight training with loads between 40% and 80% of the 1RM (or a 4-8 on the rate of perceived exertion scale) is ideal for older adults to maximize their power production in all modalities of power training (60). Low to moderate loads (40%-80% of the 1RM) moved in a concentric phase of less than 1 second followed by a 1- to 2-second controlled eccentric phase allows the individual to move a low to moderate load quickly. This will improve power (via the concentric phase) and increase strength (via the eccentric phase) by maximizing the potential of the controlled eccentric contraction, change of direction, and reacceleration of the load during a completed repetition (60, 96). Performing 3 to 4 sets of 6 to 10 repetitions with this low to moderate load should allow the individual to move concentrically with high velocity and eccentrically with smooth low velocity even when fatigued (22). Building power and strength in the same exercise is a very efficient and effective way to train. However, it can be very exhausting and may require longer bouts of recovery between sets and training days (96).

Release Exercises

Power can be developed using free weights, by performing plyometrics, or by performing release (e.g., throwing) exercises. Free-weight training works well for older adults and has a relatively low injury rate; however, performing plyometrics (bounds, leaps, skips, jumps, etc.) can be rather risky for the aging body that is undertrained or untrained. Plyometric and ballistic (i.e., jump training) exercises, using only body weight, can result in impact forces on landing that easily exceed three times the participant's body weight (if not more), putting overload stress on the joints and skeleton. This dynamic plyometric load can be too much for an aging body to manage (if not already well trained), because simply manipulating their own body weight at a slow and controlled speed can be a challenge for older individuals.

Release exercises are an alternative to maximize the older adult's ability to produce power. Low loads (30%-50% of the 1RM for release exercises and 5%-30% of the 1RM for throwing exercises) can be effectively stabilized and accelerated during these exercises to allow for power production to be safely obtained (15, 49). Free-weight and machine-based power training has been researched and reported on for decades, showcasing that it does work efficiently, but does it truly allow for "maximal" power production? Free-weight and machine-based movements must be controlled through the entire range of motion with specific emphasis on the end range of motion, commonly known as the follow-through phase. An exercise such as a hang power clean must be pulled from the knees to the shoulders (acceleration or concentric phase), where the weight has to be stopped (or caught at the follow-through phase) and then returned (preparation or eccentric phase) to the starting position to be repeated. Due to the deceleration and catch of the follow-through phase, novice- to intermediate-level clients do not typically possess the ability to truly perform the movement with 100% maximal effort, because they must keep control of the load being lifted. If clients could simply let go of the implement they are accelerating (i.e., in the vertical sandbag toss), they would be able to maximize all their power-production abilities. This is where release exercises such as a throw can be beneficial.

Release exercises (e.g., using a Smith machine to do the bench press, overhead press, or high pull) and throwing exercises (e.g., using a sandbag, sand bell, or medicine ball to do a slam, vertical toss, or lateral toss) are all movements suitable for the aging body to safely and appropriately train for power without having to control or catch weight; clients can simply let go at the top of the acceleration phase (15). They will still experience the follow-through phase; however, the load will no longer be present. During release exercises, the lifting implement (the platform of the leg press or the bar in the Smith machine) will have to be caught gently and shifted into the preparation phase by eccentrically decelerating the load, changing direction, and then reaccelerating the load to perform the next repetition (2, 15).

Regarding throwing exercises, strength and conditioning professionals and personal trainers need to educate their clients on three criteria and practice them regularly to ensure the safety and maximum performance of the client's experience. When throwing an implement, the following three rules should be observed:

1. Never take the eyes off the implement. Even if receiving instructions from a coach or workout partner, the person *must* stay focused on the implement, or serious injury can occur.

2. Never attempt to catch the implement in flight. Thrown implements have massive momentum and rotational spin and are made of shifting or sand-based materials that make catching them very dangerous.

3. Never turn away from someone throwing an implement. It is the responsibility of those around the individual throwing to get out of the way of the implement being thrown. Some throwing movements, such as a between-the-legs vertical toss, are performed with the participant's back to the landing area, and the throwing participant cannot see individuals walking into the landing area. Thus, it is the responsibility of the non-throwing participants to be aware of their surroundings and not get hit by a thrown implement.

Translating the Science Into Program Design

The key concept when designing resistance training programs that include power exercises or a phase of power development for older adults is the needs analysis. Individual differences in training and medical histories will heavily influence not only progressions in exercise selection (shown from left to right in table 4.3) but also the programming and periodization of the training volume (table 4.4) and other activities and additional stressors. Older adults should be cleared by a physician for participation in an exercise program and should not have serious orthopedic or cardiorespiratory conditions or be on medications that may interfere with their ability to exert themselves physically (78). A secondary concept when designing resistance training programs for older populations is the amount of recovery, which is generally suggested to be longer regardless of whether the primary program goal is hypertrophy, strength, or power. Research reviewing 11 studies specific to power- and resistance-training recovery protocols for older adults found that resistance training could be safely used by older populations without concern for impaired recovery (27, 33). The traditional guideline suggestion of 48 to 72 hours of recovery between training sessions (for the same muscle group) is ideal. To break that down even further, the novice older adult client (six months of experience or less) could benefit from a full 72 hours of true recovery between similar training sessions, whereas the advanced older adult client (one year or more of experience) may benefit from 48 hours of active recovery between similar training sessions (2).

After the assessment of the older adult has been completed and, where necessary, a medical clearance has been provided, exercises can be selected. For power training, the most common and effective explosive exercises involve multiple joints and muscles and include machine exercises, free weights, and release or throwing exercises such as the bench press release and the vertical throw. Strength and conditioning professionals and personal trainers need to keep in mind that developing a strength base for each of these exercises is

Table 4.3 Exercise Selection Progression Guide for Training the Older Adult

Movement or position	Exercise 1	Exercise 2	Exercise 3	Exercise 4	Exercise 5	Exercise 6
Hinge or squat	Bridge	Stiff-leg deadlift	Sit to stand	Goblet squat	Deadlift	Swing
Row or pull	Chest pull	Seated row	Pullover	High pull	Pulldown	Single-arm row
Push or press	Chest press	Decline press	Overhead press	Bench press	Incline press	Push press
Split stance	Sled push	Step-up	Split squat	Lunge	Drop-step lunge	Dynamic step-up or split squat
Loaded carry	Farmer carry	Suitcase carry	Goblet carry	Hex or trap bar carry	Waiter carry	Overhead carry
Complexes	Hinge and high pull	Slam	Jerk	Clean	Snatch	Throw

Note: Reading the rows from left to right, the exercises progress in relative difficulty, complexity, or challenge from exercise 1 to exercise 6.

Table 4.4 Volume Guide for Training the Older Adult

Reps	Sets	Load	Tempo	Recovery
6-15	2-4 per exercise	40%-80% 1RM; 4-8 RPE	2:1 Standard 3:1 Eccentric 4:1 Eccentric	30-60 s

Note: 1RM = 1-repetition maximum; RPE = rate of perceived exertion.

necessary before attempting to perform them in a ballistic or explosive fashion. Due to the risk of injury, older adult clients should participate in and complete an 8- to 12-week adaptation-based traditional resistance training program (table 4.5) prior to the introduction of power-based movements (2).

Incorporating a variety of exercises into a periodized program is beneficial for well-rounded physical development. Training the aging body comes with some additional considerations of which strength and conditioning professionals and personal trainers should be aware. Older adults may need more time to learn each exercise thoroughly (neuromuscular adaptation) and be able to perform each with proper technique because of the motor-unit recruitment changes that occur with aging (105, 106). The common limitations that accompany aging (i.e., arthritis, joint impingement or inflammation, and general muscle soreness and tightness) may dictate a slower learning curve. Therefore, it may be best not to introduce new exercises too frequently within the program, especially for a novice client.

Table 4.5 Adaptation Phase Training Program (Beginning Older Adults)

Exercise	Week 1	Week 2	Week 3	Week 4	Week 5	Week 6	Week 7	Week 8
Focus and lifting tempo	Adaptation 2:2	Adaptation 2:2	Adaptation 2:2	Eccentric 3:1	Adaptation 2:2	Adaptation 2:2	Adaptation 2:2	Eccentric 4:1
DB sit to stand	2 × 12 (40%)	2 × 10 (45%)	2 × 8 (50%)	2 × 8 (40%)	3 × 12 (50%)	3 × 10 (55%)	3 × 8 (60%)	3 × 8 (50%)
DB bench press	2 × 12 (40%)	2 × 10 (45%)	2 × 8 (50%)	2 × 8 (40%)	3 × 12 (50%)	3 × 10 (55%)	3 × 8 (60%)	3 × 8 (50%)
KB stiff-leg deadlift or RDL	2 × 12 (40%)	2 × 10 (45%)	2 × 8 (50%)	2 × 8 (40%)	3 × 12 (50%)	3 × 10 (55%)	3 × 8 (60%)	3 × 8 (50%)
Pulley seated row	2 × 12 (40%)	2 × 10 (45%)	2 × 8 (50%)	2 × 8 (40%)	3 × 12 (50%)	3 × 10 (55%)	3 × 8 (60%)	3 × 8 (50%)
DB suitcase split squat or step-up	2 × 12 (40%)	2 × 10 (45%)	2 × 8 (50%)	2 × 8 (40%)	3 × 12 (50%)	3 × 10 (55%)	3 × 8 (60%)	3 × 8 (50%)
Sled push	—	—	—	—	2 × 30 s (40%)	2 × 35 s (45%)	2 × 35 s (45%)	2 × 40 s (50%)
Sled drag	—	—	—	—	2 × 30 s (40%)	2 × 35 s (45%)	2 × 35 s (45%)	2 × 40 s (50%)

Note: For novice and intermediate older adults, some of the loads and repetitions usually associated with training athletic populations may be too ambitious and are therefore modified slightly here. The emphasis should be to create progressive overload through increasing volume (i.e., hypertrophy), load (i.e., strength), or movement velocity (i.e., power and speed) to target the desired adaptations. The percentages in parentheses indicate the load; see table 4.4 for more detail. DB = dumbbell; KB = kettlebell; RDL = Romanian deadlift.

Once the exercises have been chosen, incorporating them into a periodized program is the next step (see chapter 3). Some exercises may not be performed in a particular program phase because they are not the best choice for the set, repetition, and load scheme (volume) in that phase or simply due to the complexity of the movement pattern. It is important to think through which exercises will be performed during each primary training phase based on the training outcome or goal (e.g., hypertrophy, strength, power). For the novice older client, the focus of each phase is more singular. Strength development should be the initial focus, followed by muscular development (hypertrophy) and then by power development (tables 4.6 and 4.7). The novice client should not hurry through any phases of their training program, because neuromuscular development of movement patterns and the development of foundational strength-binding sites are necessary for the progression of more muscular growth (hypertrophy) or for power development (moving a load quickly) (2, 38). A more highly trained older adult may spend more or less time on a particular training phase due to their training outcomes or goals (tables 4.8 and 4.9).

Table 4.6 Novice Older Adults: Workout 1 (Monday)

Exercise	Week 1	Week 2	Week 3	Week 4	Week 5	Week 6	Week 7	Week 8	Week 9	Week 10	Week 11	Week 12
Focus and lifting tempo	Adaptation 2:2	Adaptation 2:2	Speed 2:1	Eccentric 3:1	Hypertrophy 2:1	Hypertrophy 2:2	Speed 2:1	Eccentric 3:1	Hypertrophy 2:1	Hypertrophy 2:2	Speed 2:1	Eccentric 3:1
DB single-arm clean and press	2 × 12 (40%)	2 × 10 (45%)	2 × 8 (50%)	2 × 6 (60%)	3 × 12 (50%)	3 × 10 (55%)	3 × 8 (60%)	3 × 6 (65%)	3 × 12 (60%)	3 × 10 (65%)	3 × 8 (70%)	3 × 6 (75%)
Hex bar deadlift*	2 × 12 (50%-55%)	2 × 10 (60%-65%)	2 × 8 (70%-75%)	2 × 6 (75%)	3 × 12 (60%)	3 × 10 (65%)	3 × 8 (70%)	3 × 6 (75%)	3 × 12 (65%)	3 × 10 (70%)	3 × 8 (75%)	3 × 6 (80%)
DB bench press	2 × 12 (50%-55%)	2 × 10 (60%-65%)	2 × 8 (70%-75%)	2 × 6 (75%)	3 × 12 (60%)	3 × 10 (65%)	3 × 8 (70%)	3 × 6 (75%)	3 × 12 (65%)	3 × 10 (70%)	3 × 8 (75%)	3 × 6 (80%)
DB suitcase drop step lunge	2 × 12 (40%)	2 × 10 (45%)	2 × 8 (50%)	2 × 6 (60%)	3 × 12 (50%)	3 × 10 (55%)	3 × 8 (60%)	3 × 6 (65%)	3 × 12 (60%)	3 × 10 (65%)	3 × 8 (70%)	3 × 6 (75%)
DB three-point single-arm row	2 × 12 (50%-55%)	2 × 10 (60%-65%)	2 × 8 (70%-75%)	2 × 6 (75%)	3 × 12 (60%)	3 × 10 (65%)	3 × 8 (70%)	3 × 6 (75%)	3 × 12 (65%)	3 × 10 (70%)	3 × 8 (75%)	3 × 6 (80%)
BALLISTIC WORK												
Sled push	—	—	—	—	30 s (50%)	35 s (60%)	40 s (65%)	45 s (70%)	30 s (55%)	35 s (60%)	40 s (65%)	45 s (70%)
Medicine ball lateral toss	—	—	—	—	2 × 12 (60%)	2 × 10 (65%)	2 × 8 (70%)	2 × 6 (75%)	2 × 12 (60%)	2 × 10 (65%)	2 × 8 (70%)	2 × 6 (75%)

Note: For novice and intermediate older adults, some of the loads and repetitions usually associated with training athletic populations may be too ambitious and are therefore modified slightly here. The emphasis should be to create progressive overload through increasing volume (i.e., hypertrophy), load (i.e., strength), or movement velocity (i.e., power and speed) to target the desired adaptations. The percentages in parentheses indicate the load; see table 4.4 for more detail. DB = dumbbell.

*Clients can use the loaded sit-to-stand squat or leg press if they are unable to perform this exercise.

Table 4.7 Novice Older Adults: Workout 2 (Thursday)

Exercise	Week 1	Week 2	Week 3	Week 4	Week 5	Week 6	Week 7	Week 8	Week 9	Week 10	Week 11	Week 12
Focus and lifting tempo	Adaptation 2:2	Adaptation 2:2	Speed 2:1	Eccentric 3:1	Hypertrophy 2:1	Hypertrophy 2:2	Speed 2:1	Eccentric 3:1	Hypertrophy 2:1	Hypertrophy 2:2	Speed 2:1	Eccentric 3:1
DB single-arm snatch	2 × 12 (40%)	2 × 10 (45%)	2 × 8 (50%)	2 × 6 (60%)	3 × 12 (50%)	3 × 10 (55%)	3 × 8 (60%)	3 × 6 (65%)	3 × 12 (60%)	3 × 10 (65%)	3 × 8 (70%)	3 × 6 (75%)
Kettlebell or DB goblet squat*	2 × 12 (50%-55%)	2 × 10 (60%-65%)	2 × 8 (70%-75%)	2 × 6 (75%)	3 × 12 (60%)	3 × 10 (65%)	3 × 8 (70%)	3 × 6 (75%)	3 × 12 (65%)	3 × 10 (70%)	3 × 8 (75%)	3 × 6 (80%)
Band or pulley single-arm chest press	2 × 12 (50%-55%)	2 × 10 (60%-65%)	2 × 8 (70%-75%)	2 × 6 (75%)	3 × 12 (60%)	3 × 10 (65%)	3 × 8 (70%)	3 × 6 (75%)	3 × 12 (65%)	3 × 10 (70%)	3 × 8 (75%)	3 × 6 (80%)
DB suitcase single-leg step-up	2 × 12 (40%)	2 × 10 (45%)	2 × 8 (50%)	2 × 6 (60%)	3 × 12 (50%)	3 × 10 (55%)	3 × 8 (60%)	3 × 6 (65%)	3 × 12 (60%)	3 × 10 (65%)	3 × 8 (70%)	3 × 6 (75%)
Band or pulley seated row	2 × 12 (50%-55%)	2 × 10 (60%-65%)	2 × 8 (70%-75%)	2 × 6 (75%)	3 × 12 (60%)	3 × 10 (65%)	3 × 8 (70%)	3 × 6 (75%)	3 × 12 (65%)	3 × 10 (70%)	3 × 8 (75%)	3 × 6 (80%)
BALLISTIC WORK												
Sled pull	—	—	—	—	30 s (50%)	35 s (60%)	40 s (65%)	45 s (70%)	30 s (50%)	35 s (60%)	40 s (65%)	45 s (70%)
Medicine ball scoop toss	—	—	—	—	2 × 12 (60%)	2 × 10 (65%)	2 × 8 (70%)	2 × 6 (75%)	2 × 12 (60%)	2 × 10 (65%)	2 × 8 (70%)	2 × 6 (75%)

Note: For novice and intermediate older adults, some of the loads and repetitions may be too ambitious and are therefore modified slightly here. The emphasis should be to create progressive overload through increasing volume (i.e., hypertrophy), load (i.e., strength), or movement velocity (i.e., power and speed) to target the desired adaptations. The percentages in parentheses indicate the load; see table 4.4 for more detail. DB = dumbbell.

*Clients can use the loaded sit-to-stand squat or leg press if they are unable to perform this exercise.

Table 4.8 Advanced Older Adults: Workout 1 (Monday)

Exercise	Week 1	Week 2	Week 3	Week 4	Week 5	Week 6	Week 7	Week 8	Week 9	Week 10	Week 11	Week 12
Focus and lifting tempo	Hypertrophy 2:1	Hypertrophy 2:2	Speed 1:1	Eccentric 5:1	Hypertrophy 2:1	Hypertrophy 2:2	Speed 1:1	Eccentric 4:1	Hypertrophy 2:1	Hypertrophy 2:2	Speed 1:1	Eccentric 3:1
DB single-arm clean and press	3 × 12 (50%)	3 × 10 (55%)	3 × 8[b] (60%)	3 × 6 (65%)	4 × 12 (55%)	4 × 10 (60%)	4 × 8[b] (65%)	4 × 6 (70%)	4 × 12 (60%)	4 × 10 (65%)	4 × 8[a] (70%)	4 × 6 (75%)
Hex bar deadlift[a]	3 × 12 (50%-55%)	3 × 10 (60%-65%)	3 × 8[b] (70%-75%)	3 × 6 (75%)	3 × 12 (60%)	4 × 10 (65%)	4 × 8[b] (70%)	4 × 6 (75%)	3 × 12 (65%)	4 × 10 (70%)	4 × 8[a] (75%)	4 × 6 (80%)
DB bench press	3 × 12 (50%-55%)	3 × 10 (60%-65%)	3 × 8[b] (70%-75%)	3 × 6 (75%)	4 × 10 (65%)	4 × 10 (65%)	4 × 8[b] (70%)	4 × 6 (75%)	3 × 12 (65%)	4 × 10 (70%)	4 × 8[a] (75%)	4 × 6 (80%)
DB suitcase drop step lunge	3 × 12 (40%)	3 × 10 (45%)	3 × 8 (50%)	3 × 6 (60%)	3 × 10 (55%)	3 × 10 (55%)	3 × 8 (60%)	3 × 6 (65%)	3 × 12 (60%)	3 × 10 (65%)	3 × 8 (70%)	3 × 6 (75%)
DB three-point single-arm row	3 × 12 (50%-55%)	3 × 10 (60%-65%)	3 × 8 (70%-75%)	3 × 6 (75%)	3 × 10 (65%)	3 × 10 (65%)	3 × 8 (70%)	3 × 6 (75%)	3 × 12 (65%)	3 × 10 (70%)	3 × 8 (75%)	3 × 6 (80%)
BALLISTIC WORK												
Sled push	—	—	—	—	2 × 30 s (50%)	2 × 35 s (60%)	3 × 40 s (65%)	3 × 45 s (70%)	3 × 30 s (50%)	3 × 35 s (60%)	3 × 40 s (65%)	3 × 45 s (70%)
Medicine ball lateral toss	—	—	—	—	2 × 12 (60%)	2 × 10 (65%)	3 × 8 (70%)	3 × 6 (75%)	3 × 12 (60%)	3 × 10 (65%)	3 × 8 (70%)	3 × 6 (75%)

Note: For novice and intermediate older adults, some of the loads and repetitions usually associated with training athletic populations may be too ambitious and are therefore modified slightly here. The emphasis should be to create progressive overload through increasing volume (i.e., hypertrophy), load (i.e., strength), or movement velocity (i.e., power and speed) to target the desired adaptations. The percentages in parentheses indicate the load; see table 4.4 for more detail. DB = dumbbell.

[a]Clients can use the loaded sit-to-stand squat or leg press if they are unable to perform this exercise.

[b]Emphasize a power-based lifting tempo.

Table 4.9 Advanced Older Adults: Workout 2 (Thursday)

Exercise	Week 1	Week 2	Week 3	Week 4	Week 5	Week 6	Week 7	Week 8	Week 9	Week 10	Week 11	Week 12
Focus and lifting tempo	Hypertrophy 2:1	Hypertrophy 2:2	Speed 1:1	Eccentric 5:1	Hypertrophy 2:1	Hypertrophy 2:2	Speed 1:1	Eccentric 4:1	Hypertrophy 2:1	Hypertrophy 2:2	Speed 1:1	Eccentric 3:1
DB single-arm snatch[a]	3 × 12 (50%)	3 × 10 (55%)	3 × 8[b] (60%)	3 × 6 (65%)	4 × 12 (55%)	4 × 10 (60%)	4 × 8[b] (65%)	4 × 6 (70%)	4 × 12 (60%)	4 × 10 (65%)	4 × 8[a] (70%)	4 × 6 (75%)
Kettlebell or DB goblet squat[a]	3 × 12 (50%-55%)	3 × 10 (60%-65%)	3 × 8[b] (70%-75%)	3 × 6 (75%)	3 × 12 (60%)	4 × 10 (65%)	4 × 8[b] (70%)	4 × 6 (75%)	3 × 12 (65%)	4 × 10 (70%)	4 × 8[a] (75%)	4 × 6 (80%)
Band or pulley single-arm chest press	3 × 12 (50%-55%)	3 × 10 (60%-65%)	3 × 8[b] (70%-75%)	3 × 6 (75%)	4 × 10 (65%)	4 × 10 (65%)	4 × 8[b] (70%)	4 × 6 (75%)	3 × 12 (65%)	4 × 10 (70%)	4 × 8[a] (75%)	4 × 6 (80%)
DB suitcase single-leg step-up	3 × 12 (40%)	3 × 10 (45%)	3 × 8 (50%)	3 × 6 (60%)	3 × 12 (50%)	3 × 10 (55%)	3 × 8 (60%)	3 × 6 (65%)	3 × 12 (60%)	3 × 10 (65%)	3 × 8 (70%)	3 × 6 (75%)
Band or pulley seated rows	3 × 12 (50%-55%)	3 × 10 (60%-65%)	3 × 8 (70%-75%)	3 × 6 (75%)	3 × 12 (60%)	3 × 10 (65%)	3 × 8 (70%)	3 × 6 (75%)	3 × 12 (65%)	3 × 10 (70%)	3 × 8 (75%)	3 × 6 (80%)
BALLISTIC WORK												
Sled pull	—	—	—	—	2 × 30 s (50%)	2 × 35 s (60%)	3 × 40 s (65%)	3 × 45 s (70%)	3 × 30 s (50%)	3 × 35 s (60%)	3 × 40 s (65%)	3 × 45 s (70%)
Medicine ball scoop toss	—	—	—	—	2 × 12 (60%)	2 × 10 (65%)	3 × 8 (70%)	3 × 6 (75%)	3 × 12 (60%)	3 × 10 (65%)	3 × 8 (70%)	3 × 6 (75%)

Note: For novice and intermediate older adults, some of the loads and repetitions usually associated with training athletic populations may be too ambitious and are therefore modified slightly here. The emphasis should be to create progressive overload through increasing volume (i.e., hypertrophy), load (i.e., strength), or movement velocity (i.e., power and speed) to target the desired adaptations. The percentages in parentheses indicate the load; see table 4.4 for more detail. DB = dumbbell.

[a]Clients can use the loaded sit-to-stand squat or leg press if they are unable to perform this exercise.

[b]Emphasize a power-based lifting tempo.

Selecting Specific Exercises for Training the Aging Body

The program design workouts found in tables 4.3 and 4.4 feature exercises selected specifically for the aging body. It is the belief of this chapter's first contributor that bilateral lifting of one implement (i.e., barbells) can be more uncomfortable for older clients who have physical limitations more commonly found in the aging body (shoulder impingements, arthritis, medial or lateral epicondylitis, etc.). Training with two individual implements that can move independently of each other (dumbbells, fatbells or center-mass bells, kettlebells, etc.) can provide a more comfortable lifting experience for the aging body with physical limitations (108). For example, the pronated barbell bench press, pronated barbell back squats, the pronated barbell overhead press, and pronated barbell prone bench rows can stress physical limitations commonly associated with aging. Using implements that allow for independent range of motion and movement, such as dumbbells, kettlebells, or fatbells, allows clients to control or advance their varying degrees of freedom via range of motion and the angle in which they hold and maneuver the implement throughout the repetitions (108).

Along the same line of thinking, the trap bar or hex bar deadlift can provide a more comfortable and safe lifting experience for the older and aging body, because clients are placed inside the load as opposed to countering the load in front of them. The neutral grip position of the trap bar or hex bar deadlift and the extra height (1-3 inches [2.5-7.6 cm]) of the handles make this deadlift a more anatomically comfortable lift with regard to the wrists, elbows, shoulders, hips, and knees and their alignment in the neutral starting position. For an older adult, the kettlebell deadlift (with a pulling height of 12 inches [30.5 cm]) can produce an effect similar to the trap bar or hex bar deadlift, because clients can place themselves directly over the top of the load and properly pull it from the floor into a stable standing position, keeping the weight pulled as close to their body as possible to reduce low back stress or pressure. Most older adults lack the mobility and flexibility to address and grab a barbell (with a pulling height of 8 inches [20.3 cm]) in a deeply flexed and pronated grip position with their hands addressing the bar outside their knees; however, opening the stance (a wide or sumo stance) and properly addressing a kettlebell with their hands between their feet allows for a greater range of motion (depth), resulting in a comfortable, safe, and effective movement.

One aspect with which strength and conditioning professionals may struggle is how best to load the exercise when training for power with older adults. Though research has been collected on this topic, the specifics of what load is ideal for ultimate power production are still unclear. Currently, research supports using a load ranging from 40% to 80% of the 1RM (16, 17, 28, 90). However, the results of some studies showed ideal power development for both upper and lower body exercises using 40% to 60% of the 1RM across the board (87, 100). This is supported anecdotally by the first contributor of this chapter, because he has used the 40% to 60% load and repetition scheme with his clients successfully for over a decade.

Ideally, a variety of loads will be used, but load determination is influenced by both the exercise selection and the goal of training (see chapter 3). Some researchers have shown that balance and gait speed are more positively affected by loads in the lower end of the training range (body weight to about 40% of maximum), while getting up out of a chair or climbing steps is more positively affected by loads of 50% to 80% of maximum (14, 90). Phases of a program that use these varying loads can also vary in length. In more highly trained older adults, a short phase (two weeks) may effectively be used, while a frailer novice client may need eight weeks to make significant improvements.

How to Select the Proper Load for Older Adults: Criteria for Success and Reduced Risk of Injury

Although the following three questions are quite simple, they are often overlooked or simply ignored in the general scheme of program design for any client, let alone the older adult. By addressing these three criteria, the strength and conditioning professional or personal trainer should be able to select loads safely and efficiently for their participants on a regular basis (49).

1. Can the client perform the number of repetitions set as the goal?
2. Can the client perform the number of repetitions and the exercise with the proper technique throughout the entire set?
3. Can the client perform the number of repetitions with the proper technique at the lifting tempo that is required?

Criteria one and two are typically achieved; however, criterion three is what most participants fail to maintain. The tempo will switch as fatigue sets in with a load that is too heavy and a proper lifting tempo is no longer possible. For example, a deadlift tempo of 3 seconds eccentric to 1 second concentric (i.e., 3:1) is maintained for 5 of the desired 10 repetitions, but at repetition 6, the tempo changes to 2 seconds eccentric and 2 seconds concentric (2:2) as the client begins to struggle, and by repetition 8, the tempo has flipped to 1 second eccentric and 3 seconds concentric (1:3) because the load is now obviously too heavy for the client and he or she is struggling to perform any more repetitions.

Addressing these three criteria will reduce risk of injury due to overload and will work toward pushing the client's limits without exceeding them. Great success, strength, and power gains can be achieved by enforcing these three lifting criteria (49).

Otherwise, a program design for older adults is not that dissimilar to a design for a younger adult, except for a slower overall progression. Loads are relative to the person's own strength levels, and programming should be goal driven, with variety and adequate recovery (figure 4.2).

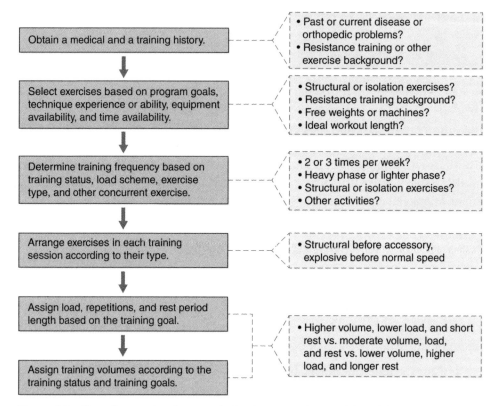

Figure 4.2 Steps for constructing a periodized program for an older adult.

CONCLUSION

When developing neuromuscular power in youths, recognize and follow these key points:

▶ In children and adolescents, neuromuscular power will naturally increase as a result of growth and maturation.

▶ All youths can make worthwhile gains in neuromuscular power when exposed to developmentally appropriate training programs.

▶ While enhancing neuromuscular power might be the ultimate aim of a youth-based strength and conditioning program, strength and conditioning professionals and personal trainers should first look to develop motor skill competency and requisite levels of muscular strength.

▶ Irrespective of whether the training program attempts to develop motor skills, muscular strength, or neuromuscular power, progression should be based on a combination of technical competency, training age, and biological and psychosocial maturation.

▶ Allow flexibility when designing and following a program to ensure that the training prescribed meets an individual's needs.

When a primary training goal is to develop neuromuscular power in an older adult, take note of and follow these guidelines:

▶ Neuromuscular power is a function of both peak strength levels and the ability to perform a movement rapidly.

▶ All older adults have the capacity to improve their neuromuscular power somewhat with well-designed and well-implemented training programs, using traditional resistance training, high-tempo or eccentric resistance training, and release and throwing exercises. The range of their success will depend on their individual work ethic, physical limitations, and medical history.

▶ Training for neuromuscular power should be performed only after an older adult has completed an eight-week adaptation-phase training program and can perform movements with proper technique for the desired number of sets and repetitions, both under load and at high or low lifting tempos.

Upper Body Power Exercises

Disa L. Hatfield

Upper body power is critical in sports involving overhand or underhand throwing, hitting, combat, or upper body propulsion. The physiology and physics of power development of the upper body are the same as those of the lower body. However, upper body power training presents unique training considerations. Variance in recommendations for training intensity based on sex, experience, and sport can make programming for developing upper body power challenging. In addition, the research literature has not adequately addressed many commonly debated issues, such as the role of rotational exercises in improving transfer of momentum and the use of variable resistance devices as training aids. The purpose of this chapter is to address performance aids, training devices, and testing devices that are specific to upper body power training and to provide techniques, instructions, and exercise variations for upper body power exercises.

SPECIAL AIDS FOR UPPER BODY POWER TRAINING

Coaches, strength and conditioning professionals, and athletes are always seeking training devices or aids that will promote athletic performance. Aside from dietary and supplemental ergogenic aids, a variety of products can enhance power training and performance.

Power Training Aids

A key component of power training implements is the ability to train for ballistic movements, allowing the athlete to accelerate throughout the entire concentric range of motion and resulting in greater power output (35, 36). For this to occur, athletes must release any weight or resistance they are holding. Thus, medicine balls are the most common aids used in upper body power training and have continued to evolve since they were first noted in modern literature in the late 19th century. Although medicine balls are often described within the scope of plyometric exercises, many medicine ball exercises exceed 250 milliseconds of movement time associated with plyometric tasks and are, in most cases, ballistic. Medicine ball variations include those with handles, ropes, and rebounding and nonrebounding capabilities (soft toss balls) and those that come with additional rebounding components, such as vertical trampolines. Medicine balls come in a variety of sizes and weights, are widely available at retail stores and through fitness equipment manufacturers, and are cost-effective compared to other resistance training modalities. Many of the exercises described in this chapter use a medicine ball, which should be considered the minimum equipment required for upper body power training.

A second ballistic training variation is a bench press throw. While the bench press throw exercise has been shown to improve upper body power in the literature, it is a high-risk exercise (3, 5). A Smith machine allows an athlete to catch a barbell more easily on the descent and also allows for a greater eccentric preload. Most Smith machines come with adjustable stops that can be set to stop the bar before impact in case of a missed catch. Some Smith machines are equipped with a magnetic braking system to catch the bar, but a braking system requires more time to reset between repetitions and negates the stretch-shortening cycle between repetitions. Overall, a Smith machine is an added cost, takes up a great amount of space, and still involves risks. Because of this, the popularity of variable-resistance training aids that require increased concentric force through the range of motion has increased.

Special aids, such as resistance bands and chains, were first used by powerlifters in their bench press training to increase the rate of force development. While both aids increase resistance through the concentric range of motion, resistance bands enhance the eccentric loading of a free-weight exercise, leading to maximized power output during the concentric phase (7, 21, 27). In addition, proponents of these training aids suggest they may be beneficial in decelerating bar speed (20, 27). However, research concerning the effectiveness of using bands to increase strength is conflicting and fraught with potential validity issues (7, 10, 26, 27, 44). Some evidence suggests that short-term training (seven weeks) with elastic bands in addition to a free-weight barbell improves upper and lower body strength and lower body power (1). In one study that measured upper body power after training with bands, the authors reported no significant differences between the results of using resistance bands in conjunction with free-weight bench press training compared to seven weeks of free-weight bench press training (21). In another study, large effect sizes for the variable-resistance group (i.e., the group using bands) were reported, but these differences were not statistically significant (39). The authors speculated that this result was due to a small sample size and short duration of training (e.g., six weeks.) One potential drawback to using resistance bands during traditional free-weight training is that the intensity of the load is not easily characterized because of individual differences in bar path trajectory and length with and without bands. This means that intensity can only be prescribed as a repetition range (RM) and that the quantifying volume-load cannot be compared across individual athletes. Researchers have noted that bands contribute 20% to 32% of an individual's 1RM to the training load (1, 27), but measuring this requires additional equipment during practical application. The available literature is too sparse to recommend the addition of resistance band training as a necessary component of upper body power training, but it can be considered a novel addition to training, with both potential benefits and limitations. This modality is discussed in more detail in chapter 9.

Acute Performance Aids

Only a small body of literature addresses specialized aids to improve upper body power production in an acute setting, such as an individual training session. Compression garments are the most popular acute training aid.

How compression garments work to aid acute athletic performance is not fully understood. Compression garments enhance the early concentric phase of an exercise through stored elastic energy from the eccentric phase and subsequent increased velocity following the amortization phase (47). Some evidence suggests that compression garments may aid in recovery after a strenuous resistance training session, but sport-specific performance information is limited (22, 24, 30) and suggests some markers of sport performance (i.e., throwing or swinging accuracy) may be acutely improved but that velocity and power are not affected (37).

Despite little research in this area, compression garments for upper body athletic performance are popular in certain athletic populations, particularly powerlifters. This has led to the development of commercially available devices, such as the Sling Shot, for recreational powerlifters. The Sling Shot is an elastic band worn across the chest while bench pressing. Researchers suggest that the Sling Shot and similar devices, such as graduated compression sleeves, lead to acute increases in 1RM and bar velocity during submaximal repetitions (16, 32). However, despite a higher absolute load in the Sling Shot condition, a decrease in muscle activation during both a 3RM (at 87.5% of the 1RM) and an 8RM (at 70% of the 1RM) in the triceps brachii and pectoralis major, as measured by electromyograph, was observed due to the higher average 1RM load, suggesting that muscular adaptations from chronic training might be negatively affected (16,

47). Compression garments may be useful in acute training to enhance power and accuracy, but chronic training performance and physiological outcomes have not been reported.

Bar Speed and Power Measuring Devices to Monitor Training Progress

Independent of athletic performance, a variety of methods are available for monitoring the progress of upper body power training. Commonly used field tests include a simple medicine ball throw, such as a chest pass, for distance (see chapter 2). While this test is certainly inexpensive and easy to administer, few normative data are available that can be used for comparing athletes to the sporting population (19).

Several commercially available devices, such as linear position transducers, accelerometers, and laser devices, can determine power and velocity during bar, medicine ball, and bodyweight exercises. These devices use either tensiometry (to approximate bar speed from time displacement) or accelerometry (to calculate velocity). The reported validity and reliability of these devices are good in experimental conditions; however, measurement error in the field may be quite high. To maintain good reliability within individual facilities, strength and conditioning professionals should be trained in the setup and placement of these devices so that within- and between-tester measurement conditions are consistent. In addition, only a few devices have been validated for accuracy across a wide range of loads (45).

Wearable inertial devices have been found to have good validity and reliability to determine upper body power, but the results have not been documented with a variety of training loads (38, 42). In addition, as with field tests, normative data do not exist for a wide variety of populations (13, 19), although this does not affect the use of these devices for longitudinal monitoring as long as the testing procedures are standardized. Aside from testing, anecdotal evidence suggests that some of these devices are used during training to monitor power and velocity in acute sessions. Athletes typically try to remain within a certain percentage of their maximum velocity or power output at a given load and thus receive instant feedback that motivates them to maintain a high-power output on each repetition or throw. However, more research is needed to fully understand where velocity-loss thresholds should be set, especially for upper body power training. A velocity-loss threshold set at 10% to 30% is potentially within the measurement error of some devices. While kinematic software analysis has been shown to be effective in teaching complex movements, programming based on power output and barbell or ball velocity has not been well studied in upper body power training (40). The use of velocity-based training is discussed in more detail in chapter 9.

UPPER BODY POWER TRAINING CONSIDERATIONS

There are multiple factors to consider when training to enhance upper body power. For instance, production of upper body power rarely happens without concomitant movement from the lower body. Optimizing the transfer of force and power production from lower body movements can enhance upper body power output (referred to as transfer of momentum). In addition, the prescription of acute resistance program variables, such as intensity, when training for power are not as well defined in evidence-based research as other performance outcomes such as strength.

Transfer of Momentum

Ballistic exercises, in which deceleration of the bar or person is negated, are necessary in upper body power training. Deceleration is needed in exercises such as the bench press, because the bar must slow at the end of a bench press motion so it does not leave the athlete's hands (34). Thus, the agonist muscle is not concentrically active through the whole range of motion (ROM) (36). Momentum is the tendency of an object to continue moving and is defined as mass multiplied by velocity. In a traditional bench press exercise, the point of deceleration (sometimes referred to as the *sticking point*) theoretically depends on training status, load, kinematics of muscle activation (such as in a concentric-only versus an eccentric–concentric bench press,) and mechanical advantage of the agonist muscles (31, 41, 46). To overcome the deceleration phenomenon (e.g., ≤45% of the range of motion during a bench press, depending on load) (36), it is necessary to either transfer the momentum to another object or continue to accelerate and allow the bar to leave the athlete's hands, such as in a bench press throw (37). Resistance bands decrease the need for eccentric deceleration by increasing the external resistance through the concentric ROM and allow the muscle to continue to work concentrically through a greater ROM (21, 27).

The results of multiple studies suggest that upper body power has a meaningful relationship with lower body power, similar to its relationship with dynamic core strength (9, 11, 12). In an acute setting, throwing distance, velocity, and peak power output of the upper body are all significantly increased when lower limbs are used in the movement (9, 11, 12). Motions such as throwing a shot put, shooting a basketball, or throwing a punch require a sequence of activation from the ground up, in which momentum passes from the lower body to the torso, the torso to the shoulder, the shoulder to the elbow, the elbow to the wrist and fingers, and finally to the implement (37). Thus, lower body and torso power movements and exercises that transfer momentum through the upper body should be included in acute training sessions and longer-term training programs.

Intensity

Researchers have indicated that the intensity of upper body power training may depend on sex, sport, arm length, and training experience (2, 3, 6). For instance, researchers have reported that trained athletes produce maximal power at a lower percentage of their 1RM in comparison to untrained individuals (3). This training adaptation is important because it indicates the ability of trained athletes to synchronously recruit motor units and shift the force–velocity curve up. In basic terms, trained athletes are more explosive and require less initial resistance to recruit fast-twitch fibers.

Researchers have reported that maximal power outputs during a bench press throw in various athletic populations lie between 15% and 60% of the 1RM (2, 4, 8, 33, 37). Athletes should strive to perform weighted upper body power exercises at an intensity that produces the highest power. Bar speed measuring devices, as described earlier in this chapter, allow for easy monitoring of power during an exercise such as a bench press throw. If these devices are not available, choose loads of 30% to 60%. One study found that while upper body peak power occurred at 30% of the 1RM in the sample population, there were no significant differences between power at 30%, 40%, or 50% of the 1RM (8). In addition, the relative load that produced peak power in the upper body was different from the relative load that produced peak power in the lower body. Additionally, training power at a specific load tends to result in enhanced performance at that load; therefore, training power across a spectrum of loads may be most beneficial (14, 23). Because of the many factors that influence the load at which peak power occurs, monitoring power during training may be essential for an individualized training prescription.

Regardless, few field-friendly methods exist for monitoring velocity and power while performing upper body power exercises such as medicine ball throws and plyometric drills. Despite a lack of peer-reviewed recommendations of loading intensity for medicine ball drills, plyometric and medicine ball training both have been shown to improve athletic performance parameters such as throwing and hitting velocity (11, 19). As such, plyometric and medicine ball training should be thought of as essential to upper body power training, because both work to enhance the stretch-shortening cycle (SSC), thus increasing explosive ability and power over time.

Rotator Cuff Mechanics

The muscles of the shoulder joint serve several purposes during power movements, including dynamic stabilization of the joint, force generation, and eccentric deceleration toward the end of the full ROM (25, 28, 37). Unlike other joints, the glenohumeral joint is largely unstable, because only a small portion of it articulates with the glenoid fossa; subsequently, the purpose of the surrounding musculature is mainly to provide stabilization, not to produce power. The unique functions of these muscles and the anatomy of the shoulder joint result in a high rate of strain, impingement, and tendinitis in the surrounding structures (25). Muscular imbalance caused by repetitive motion and overuse is a factor in these injuries (28). However, despite the incidence of shoulder injury, little research has been conducted concerning exercise volume, technique, and adaptations in strength and conditioning programming, which may help reduce the risk of injury in athletes (28). The research that does exist is highly specialized and often uses clinical equipment that is not widely available, such as isokinetic machines (19). Probably the most common generalized advice for training rotator cuff mechanics is to address muscular imbalances that may lead to injury (15, 28).

For the purposes of this chapter, coaches, strength and conditioning professionals, and athletes should consider the following:

▶ Despite the lower load of many power exercises, upper body power exercises that contain an enhanced eccentric portion should be classified as high intensity. Partner-assisted loading, rebounding, and resistance-band exercises will increase the eccentric loading of the shoulder joint and should be performed in lower volumes. While resistance bands increase the resistance at the top end of an exercise to aid in decelerating the movement, they also increase the eccentric force, which may increase injury potential. The effects of acute and chronic training with these devices on shoulder mechanics and movement have not been addressed.

▶ Release exercises such as the bench press throw and medicine ball exercises can reduce but do not fully negate the need for deceleration.

▶ No power exercises exist for the rhomboids and latissimus dorsi, which primarily function to stabilize the shoulder joint. If an athlete's regular sport training involves repetitive external rotation or pushing motions, muscular imbalances between the anterior and posterior upper body may be exacerbated. While some power exercises use shoulder muscles that are involved in internal and external rotation, very few power exercises work the rear deltoids, rhomboids, and latissimus dorsi. When programming upper body power exercises, equalize the volume for muscle groups that push and pull, or address the volume inequalities in the athlete's traditional resistance training routine to prevent muscular imbalances that can lead to rotator cuff injuries (28).

Rotational Exercises

Research suggests that isometric core strength is related to injury prevention and athletic performance (17, 29, 34, 35). This, along with concerns that dynamic abdominal exercise exacerbates low back pain, has led to programming solely isometric core exercises, such as a plank, to improve abdominal strength (34). However, research addressing the role of the trunk muscles in sport performance suggests that dynamic training of the lateral core musculature (e.g., obliques) allows for effective transfer of forces from the lower body and increases power development of the upper body (18, 43). While performance research indicates that athletes should train using the movements they will perform in their sport, practitioners should also individually assess the history of lower back injury and the athlete's training status and then choose exercises accordingly. In addition, it may be prudent to consider the sport-specific pattern of momentum transfer. For instance, lower limb strength deficits have been reported to disrupt the kinetic chain and contribute to impingement syndrome in the shoulder (25, 28). For additional information on rotational training and trunk strengthening, see chapter 7.

UPPER BODY POWER EXERCISES

Choosing exercises to include in a program to train upper body power depends on many factors. Considerations include loading, the athlete's training experience, and the type of movement. To better facilitate these choices, exercises described in this chapter are categorized as ballistic, plyometric, or variable resisted exercises. Ballistic exercises aim to produce peak or near-peak power outputs (usually with moderate loads over a prolonged movement time, such as >250 milliseconds) and are traditionally defined as those in which the resistive force leaves the athlete's hands (such as a bench press throw) or the athlete leaves the ground, negating the need for deceleration during the concentric muscle action. Plyometric exercises can share commonality with ballistic exercises, but the movement times are usually <250 milliseconds. For instance, exercises such as bounding or depth jumps are ballistic (the athlete leaves the ground, and the concentric portion of the exercise is not decelerated), but in plyometric exercises, either a more complex movement pattern is used or the intensity of the exercise is increased because of an enhanced eccentric portion. Variable resistance exercises specifically use elastic bands to affect the absolute load throughout the movement.

Exercise Finder

Exercise	Exercise category	Page number
Ballistic inverted row	Ballistic	127
Band bench press	Variable resistance	132
Band push-up	Variable resistance	132
Band standing row	Variable resistance	134
Bench press throw on Smith machine	Ballistic	122

Exercise	Exercise category	Page number
Chest pass	Plyometric	129
Depth-drop push-up	Plyometric	128
Drop-catch landmine row	Ballistic	126
Jump push-up	Ballistic	121
Overhead throw	Plyometric	130
Scoop toss	Ballistic	124
Sled row	Ballistic	125
Stability ball shoulder roll	Ballistic	123

Ballistic Exercises

JUMP PUSH-UP

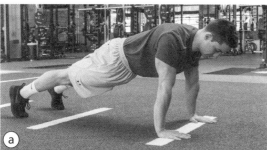

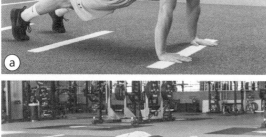

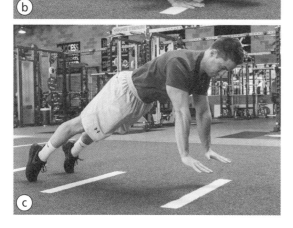

Aim

To improve upper body ballistic power.

Action

1. Start at the top of a push-up with the head in a neutral position and the arms extended (photo *a*).
2. Perform a standard push-up with a full ROM (photo *b*), while explosively extending the arms so the hands leave the ground and land in the same place (photo c).
3. Begin the next repetition immediately after landing.

Variations

See band and depth-drop push-ups. As a ballistic exercise, jump push-ups may also be done with a weight vest, if the athlete has sufficient strength and control.

BENCH PRESS THROW ON SMITH MACHINE

Aim

To allow for maximal power generation throughout the range of motion with minimal braking or deceleration at the end of the concentric motion.

Action

1. Most Smith machines come equipped with a safety lock, racks, or both that can be set to just above chest level, meaning the bar will not touch the chest. Set the safety locks at a height that prevents the bar from landing on the athlete if he or she and the spotter both fail to catch the bar.

2. Use a spotter for this exercise.

3. The start position is the same as for a standard flat barbell bench press. Carefully unrack the weight and hold it with the arms extended. The spotter helps the athlete unrack the bar. If the athlete rotated his or her hands during the unrack, the hands should be repositioned to the appropriate placement after turning the bar to unlock it from the rack (i.e., regrip). The spotter should help stabilize the bar during this process.

4. Begin by flexing the elbows and lowering bar toward the chest.

5. At the bottom of the movement, rapidly extend the elbows and release the bar when the elbows reach full extension.

6. Catch the bar in its downward path, quickly lower it to a self-selected depth, and then begin the next repetition. The spotter should help catch the bar to make sure the athlete has control, and the safety locks should be positioned so that the bar cannot touch the athlete's chest.

7. The spotter should remain diligent during the entire motion to help the athlete catch the bar.

Variations

Devices are available that attach to the bar and automatically catch the bar when it starts to descend after the throw; however, these also negate the optimized eccentric loading of the exercise.

STABILITY BALL SHOULDER ROLL

Aim

To improve ballistic upper body power generation in athletes who may not be capable of performing jump push-ups or banded push-ups.

Action

1. Lie prone with the arms and legs extended over a stability ball. The ball should be large enough that the feet touch the ground in the starting position (photo *a*).
2. Carefully flex the knees, then extend the legs rapidly while the trunk rolls over the ball.
3. Once the hands reach the floor, flex the elbows for the countermovement (photo *b*).
4. Rapidly extend the elbows and roll back to the starting position.

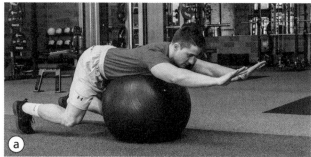

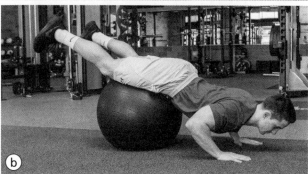

SCOOP TOSS

Aim

To improve external rotational ballistic power.

Action

1. Stand with the feet shoulder-width apart.
2. Hold a medicine ball at hip level, with the arms fully extended (photo *a*).
3. Perform the countermovement by flexing the hips and knees to approximately a half-squat position (photo *b*).
4. The athlete concentrically extends the knees and hips while externally rotating at the shoulders to throw the ball up and backward over the head in a rapid and controlled manner (photo *c*).

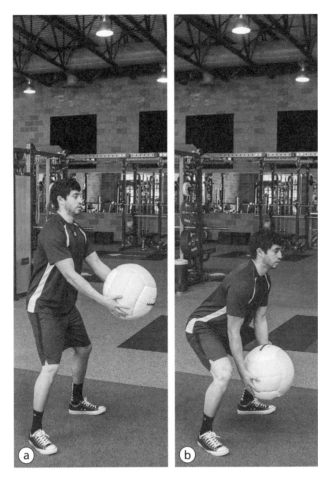
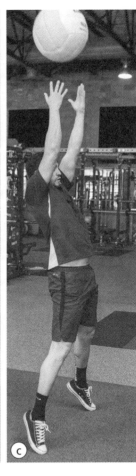

SLED ROW

Aim

To develop upper body power using a ballistic pulling movement.

Action

1. Begin by standing in an upright athletic stance, holding the attached ropes at a fully extended length (photo *a*).

2. Perform a standard row by flexing at the elbows through a full ROM, keeping the hands at midtorso level, and rapidly pull the sled toward the body while maintaining an athletic stance with the lower body (photo *b*).

3. Walk or run backward until the rope is at length again and repeat the row. Care should be taken that the rope is long enough or the sled load is heavy enough that the sled cannot be pulled the complete distance and cause a collision.

Variations

Intensity can be varied by increasing or decreasing the load on the sled. In addition, this exercise can be done with one arm.

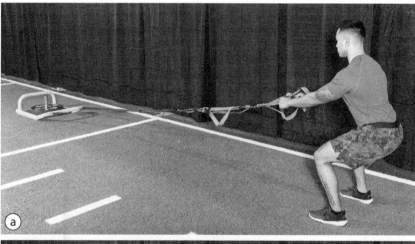

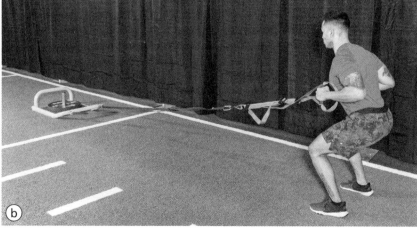

DROP-CATCH LANDMINE ROW

Aim

To develop upper body power using a ballistic pulling movement.

Action

1. Begin by standing in the standard bent-row position (slight knee flexion and hip flexion), holding the bar just underneath the collar (photo *a*).

2. Perform a standard row by rapidly flexing at the elbow through a full ROM and releasing the bar at the top (photo *b*).

3. Catch the bar while still maintaining position and prepare for the next repetition (photo *c*).

Variations

Intensity can be varied by increasing or decreasing the load on the bar, but ensure that any added plates will not come in contact with the athlete during the exercise.

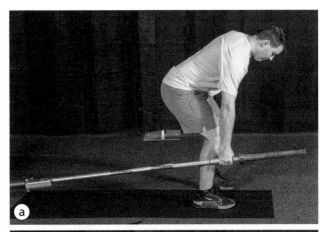

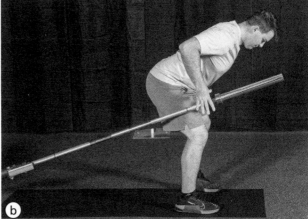

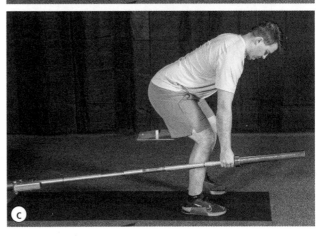

BALLISTIC INVERTED ROW

Aim

To develop upper body power using a ballistic pulling movement.

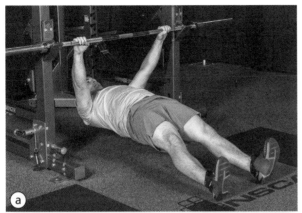

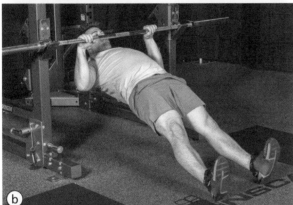

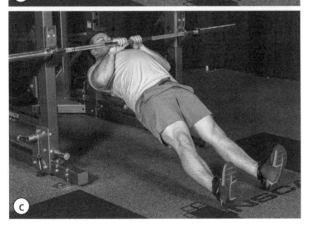

Action

1. Position a bar 2 to 3 feet (0.6-0.9 m) off the ground in a rack. Begin in a prone position, gripping the bar slightly wider than shoulder-width apart. The back should not be in contact with the ground (photo *a*).

2. Perform an inverted row by rapidly flexing at the elbows through a full ROM. The bar should be about midsternum at the end of the ROM (photo *b*). Toward the end of the ROM, release the bar and switch to a very close grip (hands should almost be touching) (photo *c*). This switch should occur before the beginning of the next concentric action.

3. Repeat the concentric action, alternating the grip-switch.

Variations

Intensity can be decreased by flexing the knees and placing the feet closer to the center of gravity. Intensity can be increased by wearing a weighted vest.

Plyometric Exercises

DEPTH-DROP PUSH-UP

Aim

To develop upper body power through enhanced eccentric loading and a short contact time with the ground. The athlete's relative strength may be a factor in keeping a short amortization phase and maintaining the plyometric nature of the exercise. For many individuals, this may be classified as a ballistic rather than plyometric exercise, due to the ground contact time being >250 milliseconds.

Action

1. Begin at the bottom of the push-up position, with the hands on raised platforms (of equal height) placed on either side of the shoulders. Generally, the height of the blocks, platforms, or sometimes bumper plates used is between 2 and 6 inches (5.1-15.2 cm) (photo *a*).
2. Begin the movement by extending the elbows, then move the hands off the platform and onto the floor (photo *b*).
3. Explosively extend the arms so that the hands leave the ground (photo *c*) and land back on the platform.

The platform height will vary depending on the intensity desired, the athlete's experience level, and the length of the athlete's arms. Higher platforms will result in greater eccentric loading and are more appropriate for experienced athletes.

Variations

- Begin at the bottom position of the push-up, with the hands on top of a medicine ball (in line with the upper chest) and the arms extended, then move the hands from the ball to the floor (approximately shoulder-width apart) and perform a push-up to the level of the ball.
- Explosively extend the elbows so that the hands leave the ground and land back on the ball.
- The height of the medicine ball will vary depending on the intensity desired, the athlete's experience level, and the length of the athlete's arms.

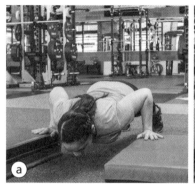
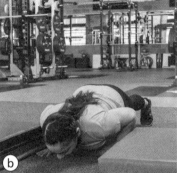
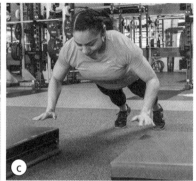

CHEST PASS

Aim

To translate increased power in sport-specific passes through a practiced shortened amortization phase time and enhanced eccentric loading.

Action

1. Stand with the feet shoulder-width apart and hold a medicine ball at the center of the chest (photo *a*).
2. Perform a countermovement by flexing the elbows before the throw, then slightly flex the knees and hips to produce a lower body countermovement (photo *b*).
3. During knee and hip extension, extend the elbows and release the ball at full extension (photo *c*).

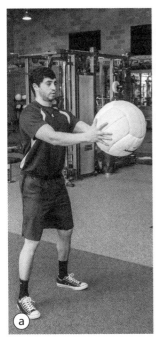 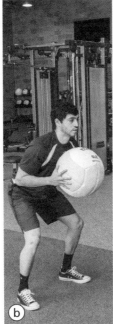 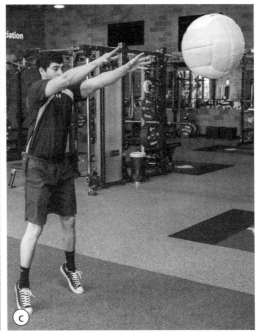

Variations

- Perform chest passes as quickly as possible with a partner to allow for enhanced eccentric loading and optimization of the SSC.
- For a deltoid exercise, throw the medicine ball straight up into the air from the center of the chest. Ensure no one else is in the immediate area in case the throw goes awry. The athlete must be prepared to catch the ball on the descent.
- To perform the exercise without a partner, throw a larger soft toss (nonbounce) medicine ball against a wall. (These balls diminish the rebound effect.) Start in the original stance on both feet. As the ball releases, explosively jump forward

off one leg and land on the opposite foot, as in a forward pass in basketball. This is an intermediate-level exercise (photo *d*).

- Perform the exercise using a rebounder, such as a vertically mounted trampoline (intermediate level).

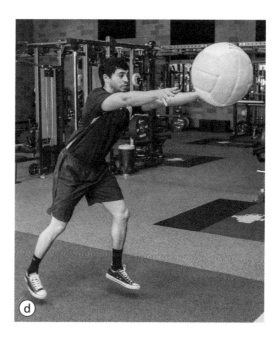

OVERHEAD THROW

Aim

To improve overhead throwing power.

Action

1. Stand with the feet shoulder-width apart, holding a medicine ball in front of the body with the arms extended (photo *a*).
2. Flex the shoulders to lift the ball over and slightly behind the head (photo *b*).
3. Keeping the elbows extended, extend the shoulders to throw the ball toward a wall, being sure to release the ball while it is still over the head (photo *c*).
4. Aim the ball at a spot on the wall so that when it rebounds, it returns to the hands, which are still positioned over the head.

Variations

- Throw for distance instead of using a wall for the rebound (novice level).
- Instead of releasing the ball over the head, maintain contact with the ball and slam it toward the ground while simultaneously flexing the knees and hips to about a quarter-squat position. This is a novice-level variation, commonly called a *medicine ball slam*; use a soft toss ball for minimal rebound.
- For an advanced variation, use a split stance and an explosive forward jump during the overhead throw, maintaining awareness of the rebound *(photo d)*.
- For an intermediate variation, use a rebounder.

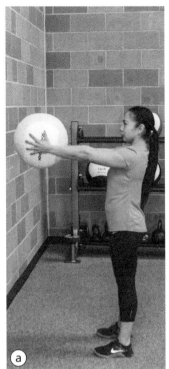
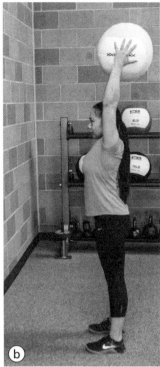
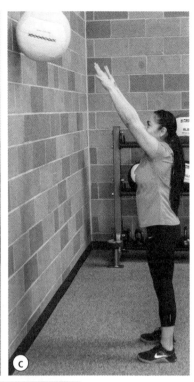

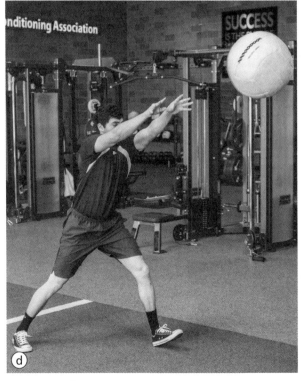

Variable Resistance Exercises

A flat band or tubing offers both resistance during the concentric muscle action and an enhanced eccentric action (as opposed to a weight or dumbbell placed on the athlete's back, which does not offer enhanced loading). As a variable resistance aid, bands allow for increased velocity at the start of the concentric phase. The enhanced eccentric loading may increase potential energy storage and concentric power.

BAND PUSH-UP

Aim

To improve eccentric loading and facilitate force generation throughout the concentric range of motion.

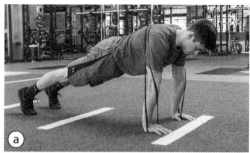
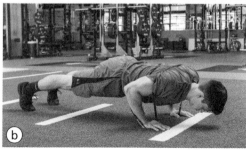

Action

1. In a push-up position, hold one end of a flat resistance band or tubing in each hand, with the band or tubing running across the upper back and rear deltoids (photo *a*).

2. Perform a standard push-up (photo *b*).

Variations

Increase intensity by leaving the ground, similar to a jump push-up.

BAND BENCH PRESS

Aim

To improve eccentric loading and facilitate force generation throughout the concentric range of motion.

Action

1. Perform this exercise using the same form as a standard flat barbell bench press.

2. Loop one end of a flat resistance band (resistance tubing is not strong enough for this exercise) on each side of the bar on the inside of the sleeve close to the weights.

3. Attach the other end of each band to a rack (newer models come with hooks on the edge of the platform near the floor) or to a heavy dumbbell placed on the floor. If dumbbells are used, they should be heavy enough that they will not be lifted during the movement. Typically, the total dumbbell weight should exceed the bar's weight.

4. Spotter duties are similar to those for the barbell bench press. However, the added resistance of the bands will increase the tension when the spotter hands off the bar and may also lead to more instability during the handoff. The spotter should release the bar smoothly into the athlete's hands. In addition, the spotter is at added risk because of the potential for the bands to snap or the dumbbells to roll.

5. The bands should be as vertical as possible when the bar is unracked and in the standard start position (photo *a*).

6. The resistance band will offer an enhanced eccentric load and more resistance at the end of the concentric action to help slow the movement velocity. This tension can lead to wavering of the bar if the athlete does not have complete control of the bar and can also lead to a rebound effect at the end of the movement when the band snaps the bar back down.

7. Focus on moving the bar explosively through a full ROM but without bouncing the bar off the chest (photo *b*).

Variations

Intensity can be adjusted by varying the weight on the bar and the length and thickness of the resistance band, as long as the athlete can move with great velocity.

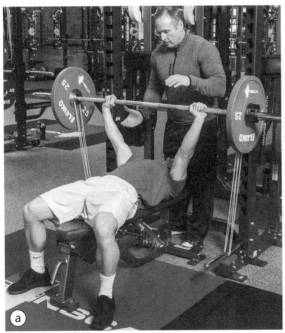
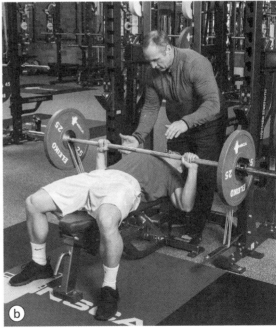

BAND STANDING ROW

Aim

To increase force generation throughout a concentric range of motion.

Action

1. Attach a resistance band to a stable rack at approximately chest level.
2. Stand with the feet shoulder-width apart and grasp the ends of the band.
3. Start the movement with the elbows fully extended and the band held taut but not stretched (photo *a*).
4. Fully flex the elbows to perform a rowing movement through a full ROM (photo *b*), then quickly return to the starting position and begin the next repetition.

Variations

- The intensity depends on the thickness and length of the band used and the distance the athlete stands from the band attachment site.
- This exercise can be varied in the same manner as a barbell or dumbbell row exercise.

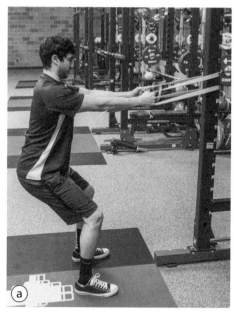 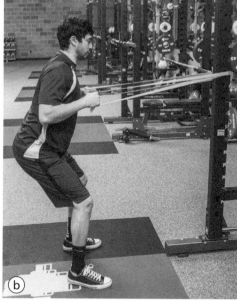

CONCLUSION

Developing upper body power is complex. Strength and conditioning professionals consider an athlete's level (i.e., novice, intermediate, or advanced) when choosing exercises and designing a program. In addition, several training aids, such as elastic bands and plyometric exercises, may enhance the intrinsic properties of power development. However, the literature neither presents a clear picture of the long-term effects of using these aids nor offers concrete evidence on establishing training intensity. Applied recommendations include training at 30% to 60% of the 1RM for optimal power development and using both ballistic and plyometric exercises in training. In addition, establishing a strength base in both the upper and lower body may lead to reduced injury and greater improvement in the transfer of momentum for sport-specific activities such as ball passing, pitching, and stick shooting.

CHAPTER 6

Lower Body Power Exercises

Bobby Smith
Brandon Burdge

Lower body power is critical for enhancing athletic performance for many sports (13). Power needs to be expressed in a variety of ways for each sport and its positional requirements. The most common movements used to develop lower body power are vertical jumping tasks. The vertical jump is one of the most versatile exercises due to the ability to add variety to the movement. Because of this versatility, vertical jumping tasks can be subdivided into ballistic (i.e., slow stretch-shortening cycle [SSC]; ground contact time [GCT], >250 milliseconds) and plyometric (i.e., fast SSC; GCT, ≤250 milliseconds). When considering tools to use, it is important to consider the process of progression to ensure athletes are perfecting the basics while adding complexity to their training regimen to include multiple qualities (i.e., force production, rate of force development, and elasticity) and patterns (vertical, linear, lateral, etc.).

When training for power, two underlying factors need to be considered: force and velocity, or work done divided by time (see chapters 1 and 2). This chapter will discuss a variety of plyometric and ballistic movements; both modalities fall on multiple areas of the force–velocity curve while involving the SSC, which is imperative for power development. Both also rely on the neurophysiological aspect (i.e., the *myotatic stretch reflex*) and elastic components associated with the SSC. In SSC-based movements, the eccentric force, reflex stimuli, and elastic contributions are greater than normal due to the rapid descent, which increases the eccentric (stretch) load. For instance, a depth jump within a training session magnifies the eccentric portion of the movement due to the height from which the athlete is dropping, increasing velocity and therefore momentum

(momentum = mass × velocity) on ground contact. The increased momentum requires a greater braking (i.e., eccentric) impulse, equivalent to the individual's momentum, to decelerate. Although a depth jump belongs more in the ballistic category due to the larger angular displacement of the joints and longer GCT, it also emphasizes the use of the myotatic stretch reflex of the SSC. On the other hand, a drop jump with reduced angular displacement and a shorter GCT will emphasize the use of the elastic components of the SSC, making it a plyometric exercise. The main difference between these exercises is that the peak knee and hip angle in the drop jump will be less than in the depth jump to allow for a quicker, more springy action from eccentric to concentric, with the drop jump being more ankle dominant and exhibiting a short GCT (e.g., <250 milliseconds).

Effective lower body power training should not only improve the way one can produce force quickly but also be able to dissipate impact force and redistribute force throughout the body when performing tasks within the respective sport. Many movements within field sports are ground based and require moving in multiple planes of motion. The body positioning and direction in which movement is occurring will determine the ability of the muscles and tendons to produce force and absorb forces, respectively. For instance, jumping sports with a run-up start (e.g., basketball, volleyball, and high jump) should consider movements that require athletes to reorganize their body position to be able to redirect and produce force quickly when moving dynamically. Coaches and strength and conditioning professionals who work with athletes in high-contact sports (e.g., football, rugby) should consider using movements or methods that expose their athletes to high forces and high rates of force development to prepare them for heavy-duty contact from another athletes. Training programs for locomotion sports (e.g., hockey, ice skating, and cycling) should include movements and methods that enhance the athletes' ability to accelerate and maneuver.

The most important consideration when applying lower body power training is the safety of the athlete. Injuries happen not only when the body is accelerating (e.g., baseball or softball players straining their hamstrings when rounding a base) but also when it is decelerating (e.g., a basketball guard cutting the rim and rupturing an anterior cruciate ligament). Deceleration mechanics, sometimes incorrectly referred to as force absorption (muscles must produce force to decelerate the athlete, based on the impulse–momentum relationship), should be a fundamental movement quality in training programs to train the deceleration (i.e., eccentric) portion of the SSC. This is very important for change-of-direction and agility movements (e.g., a running back in American football), jumping and landing (e.g., a basketball forward coming down from a rebound), and speed (e.g., a soccer midfielder maneuvering through defenders) (8). Coaches and athletes should consider unique tools for training deceleration mechanics that are relative to the sport and positional requirements (8).

Outlined in this chapter are key exercises and methods that lead to superior lower body strength, power, and elasticity. The exercises are organized into four categories: deceleration (i.e., force absorption), force production, plyometric, and ballistic. The deceleration category ties into the eccentric actions of movements, whereas the force production category ties into the eccentric and concentric actions of movements. Plyometrics and ballistics tie into the coupling of eccentric and concentric movements. The ballistic category includes two subcategories (preballistic and ballistic exercises) and provides greater detail on major considerations, methodology, modalities, and so on. Each category lists key exercises with sample progressions and regressions and is divided into four planes of motion (vertical, linear, lateral, and rotational).

DECELERATION EXERCISES

Learning to attenuate force through landing, decelerating the center of mass, and stabilizing is part of an effective training program. For sports that rely on rapid changes of direction, developing proper mechanics and power in attenuating force is critical to injury prevention and performance. Prioritizing skills in this order ensures that athletes are technically and physically prepared to tolerate the high demands of landing and cutting motions, including appropriate landing mechanics (8). In all contexts, athletes should aim to develop effective biomotor abilities, placing particular emphasis on control, motion, and strength from the earliest age possible to ensure that proper structural strength, stability, range, and movement are developed for deceleration tasks.

The biggest benefit of appropriate deceleration exercises is the ability to control body position and redistribute force throughout the body. If the body has a misalignment within the bones or joint structure, it will directly affect the muscles' function to produce force or stabilize certain joint structures throughout the *kinetic chain*—the interrelated groups of body segments, connecting joints, and muscles working together to perform movements and the portion of the spine to which they connect (14). For example, if an athlete is performing a double-leg hurdle jump and lands with excessive knee valgus (knees rotated inward toward the midline), this affects not only the ability to decelerate or dissipate force from the ground but also to produce force when jumping out of that position. There are myriad reasons why this happens (i.e., lack of body awareness, restrictions within certain joint structures, or weakness in certain muscle groups), but it is important for the strength and conditioning professional to step in and educate when the issue is relevant to the task at hand. The use of augmented feedback (e.g., video analysis) is an effective way to intervene and reassure athletes that they are executing a skill correctly (11). The skill of deceleration with appropriate mechanics (i.e., body posture) requires regular attention and practice to ensure quality of movement. The volume may vary based on the complexity of the movement and the goals of the training program. The force generated in some exercises can be very high (e.g., a snap down or a depth drop), so it is important to keep in mind that the exercise selection should match the complexity, volume, and intensity of the movement as well as the athlete's readiness and training maturity.

Exercise Finder

Exercise	Exercise category	Page number
90-degree single-leg vertical hop	Force production: rotational plane	158
90-degree vertical jump	Force production: rotational plane	157
Band- or chain-resisted hex bar deadlift	Jerk-related	173
Barbell back squat	Ballistic-related: preballistic	170
Barbell front squat	Ballistic-related: preballistic	169
Chain- or band-resisted back squat	Ballistic-related: ballistic	173
Chain- or band-resisted front squat	Ballistic-related: ballistic	172
Depth drop	Deceleration	144
Double-leg forward or backward pogo hop	Plyometric: linear plane	162
Double-leg pogo hop	Plyometric: vertical plane	160
Double-leg snap down	Deceleration	141
Dumbbell jump	Ballistic-related: ballistic	174
Hex barbell deadlift	Ballistic-related: preballistic	172
Hurdle jump	Force production: linear plane	150
Landmine rotational press	Ballistic-related: ballistic	175
Lateral or medial hop	Force production: lateral plane	155
Lateral pogo hop	Plyometric: frontal plane	163
Lateral vertical jump	Force production: lateral plane	153
Push and recover	Force production: lateral plane	156
Resisted lateral push and recover	Ballistic-related: ballistic	174
Resisted sprint	Force production: linear plane/ ballistic-related: ballistic	152
Rotational pogo hop	Plyometric: rotational plane	165

Exercise	Exercise category	Page number
Single-leg forward hurdle hop	Force production: linear plane	151
Single-leg forward or backward pogo hop	Plyometric: linear plane	163
Single-leg lateral or medial pogo hop	Plyometric: frontal plane	164
Single-leg pogo hop	Plyometric: vertical plane	161
Single-leg rotational pogo hop	Plyometric: rotational plane	165
Single-leg snap down	Deceleration	143
Single-leg vertical jump	Force production: vertical plane	148
Split jump	Force production: vertical plane	147
Split-stance snap down	Deceleration	142
Standing long jump (also referred to as the broad or horizontal jump)	Force production: linear plane	149
Vertical jump (countermovement jump)	Force production: vertical plane	145

Deceleration Exercises

DOUBLE-LEG SNAP DOWN

Aim

To train the body to effectively decelerate in a bilateral stance while maintaining control, avoiding knee valgus and excessive forward lean of the trunk when descending from a jump or plyometric exercise.

Action

1. Start with the arms above the head, standing tall on the toes (photo a).
2. Rapidly bring the arms down and behind the body, while rapidly flexing the knees, hips, and ankles to end in a quarter- or half-squatted position (photo b).

Sample Progressions

- Jump to stick
- Weighted snap down (i.e., using a weighted vest)

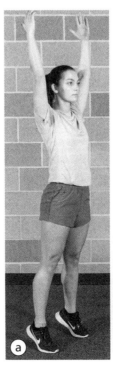
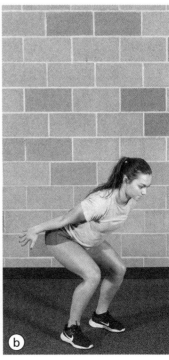

- Split-stance snap down
- Single-leg snap down

Sample Regressions

- Double-leg snap down without swinging the arms
- Box jump

SPLIT-STANCE SNAP DOWN

Aim

To train the body from a bilateral split-stance position to be able to effectively decelerate and maintain control when descending from a jump or plyometric exercise.

Action

1. Start with the arms above the head and the legs split front and back (similar to the starting position at the top of a split squat) (photo *a*).
2. Rapidly bring the arms down into a sprinter stance while rapidly flexing the knees, hips, and ankles (which ever leg is back, the arm on the same side will be forward) (photo *b*).

Sample Progressions

- Start with feet parallel, then split the feet on the snap down
- Vertical jump to split-stance stick
- Single-leg snap down

Sample Regressions

- Split squat
- Double-leg snap down

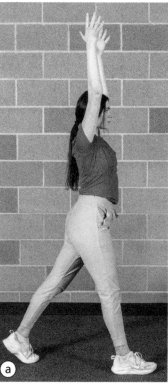
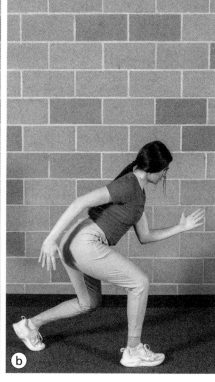

SINGLE-LEG SNAP DOWN

Aim

To train the body from a single-leg position to be able to effectively decelerate and maintain control when descending from a jump or plyometric exercise.

Action

1. Start with the arms above the head while raising one knee to 90 degrees (photo *a*). To add more complexity, the exercise can be progressed by standing on the toes of the supporting leg.

2. Rapidly bring the arms down into a sprinter stance while rapidly driving one leg back and balancing on the other leg (whichever leg is raised is the arm that is forward) (photo *b*).

Sample Progressions

- Single-leg vertical hop to double-leg stick
- Vertical jump to single-leg stick

Sample Regressions

- Single-leg squat
- Hop to box
- Split-stance snap down

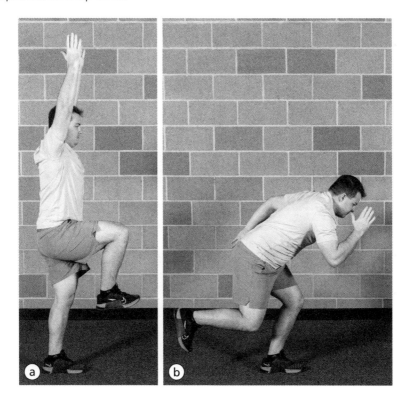

DEPTH DROP

Aim

To train the body to effectively decelerate and maintain a safe position when landing from a jump or plyometric exercise.

Action

1. The appropriate drop height is either equal to or slightly above the countermovement vertical jump height or single-leg hop height. The landing position (double leg or single leg) should fit the athlete and the goals of the training program. (Too much height can diminish the landing technique and lead to poor movement competency or potential injury.)

2. Proceed to step off the box with the arms in the air (photo *a*), then rapidly snap the arms down while landing in a quarter- or half-squatted position (photo *b*).

3. The landing should be relatively quiet, due to a compliant strategy.

Sample Progressions

- Increase the box height in small increments (such as 4 inches [10.2 cm])
- Single-leg depth drop

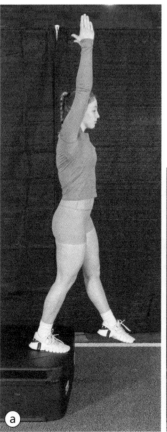

- Lateral double-leg or single-leg depth drop
- Ninety-degree rotational double-leg or single-leg depth drop

Sample Regressions

- Lower box height
- Change single leg to double leg

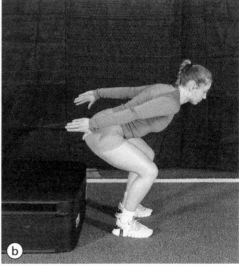

FORCE PRODUCTION EXERCISES

The angle of the joints, alignment of the bones, and plane of motion directly affect a muscle's function as it distributes force throughout the body to allow movement to occur. It is important to consider the complexity of the movement and the intensity of training, because these should determine the volume being prescribed. When progressing into force production following deceleration tasks, deceleration and propulsion should come together within an exercise, ensuring efficient use of the SSC. The emphases of force production are to achieve a medium response by the body and to introduce power training.

For ease of reference, these exercises are grouped by the plane of motion that is predominantly trained, and sample regressions and progressions are provided. The following describes the terminology used for each exercise:

- ▶ Stick: Reset after each repetition
- ▶ Jump: Push off both feet, land on both feet
- ▶ Hop: Push off one foot, land on same foot
- ▶ Bound: Push off one foot, land on opposite foot
- ▶ Mini-bounce: Small bounce between repetitions (increase volume of foot contacts with less impact on the ground and promote elastic properties of the SSC)
- ▶ Repeat: Two repetitions in a row
- ▶ Continuous: More than two repetitions in a row

Force Production Exercises: Vertical Plane

These exercises consist of jumping, bounding, or hopping in place for maximum height.

VERTICAL JUMP (COUNTERMOVEMENT JUMP)

Aim

To develop lower body bilateral power in the vertical plane.

Action

1. See "Double-Leg Snap Down" for the starting position (photo *a*).
2. Rapidly flex the hips, knees, and ankles to perform a countermovement while swinging the arms downward (photo *b*), then immediately extend the hips, knees, and ankles while swinging the arms upward to jump straight into the air (photo *c*).
3. On the descent, land back in the double-leg snap down position.

Sample Progressions

- Depth jump
- Repeat vertical jump
- Weighted vertical jump
- Weighted vest or dumbbells

Sample Regressions

- Remove the arm swing (placing the hands on the hips or holding a dowel across the shoulders)
- Squat jump (however, this eliminates the use of the SSC)

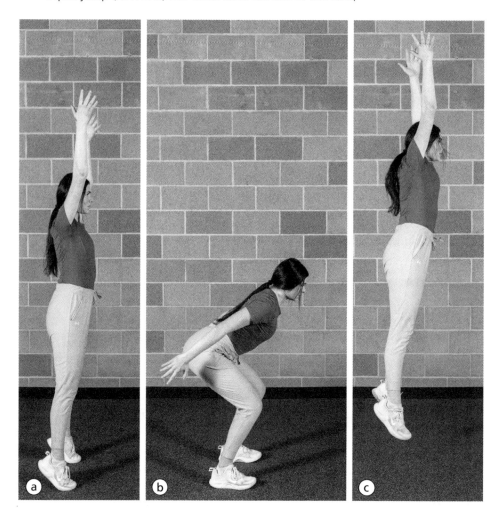

SPLIT JUMP

Aim

To develop lower body bilateral power in the vertical plane.

Action

1. See "Split-Stance Snap Down" for the starting position (photo *a*). To add more complexity, the exercise can be progressed by starting on the toes of the front foot. (The back heel should already be raised in the starting position.)
2. Rapidly perform a countermovement (i.e., a snap down into a split-stance snap down position) (photo *b*), followed by immediate and rapid extension of both legs to jump for maximal height (photo c).
3. On the descent, land back in the split-stance snap down position to attenuate the impact forces.

Sample Progressions

- Repeat split jump
- Alternating split jump (in place)
- Weighted split jump (add a weighted vest, dumbbells, medicine ball, etc.)

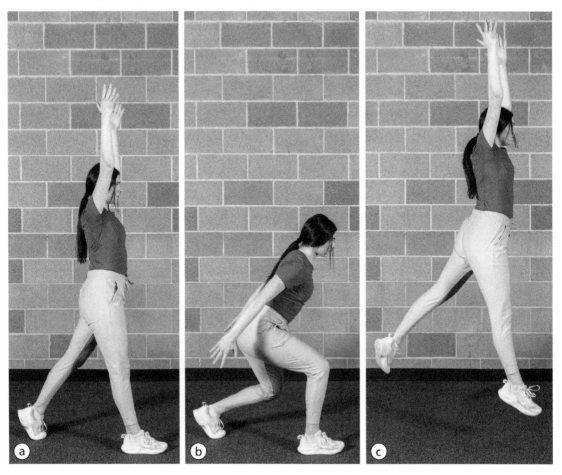

Sample Regressions

- Split jump into a double-leg landing
- Split-stance squat jump (this eliminates the use of the SSC)
- Countermovement jump

SINGLE-LEG VERTICAL JUMP

Aim

To develop lower body unilateral power in the vertical plane.

Action

1. See "Single-Leg Snap Down" for the starting position (photo *a* shows the more complex starting position of the exercise).
2. Rapidly perform a countermovement (i.e., a snap down into a single-leg snap down position) (photo *b*), followed by immediate and rapid extension of the leg to jump for maximal height (photo *c*).
3. On the descent, land in the single-leg snap down position to attenuate the impact forces. This is also a good opportunity to reinforce proper landing mechanics.

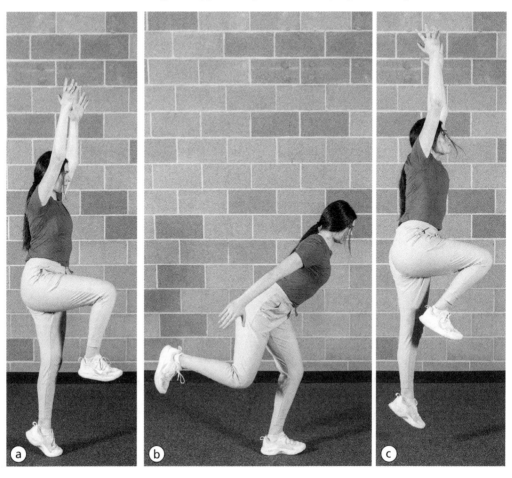

Sample Progressions
- Repeat single-leg hop
- Alternating bounds (in place)
- Single-leg depth jump

Sample Regressions
- Single-leg hop to double-leg landing (this makes the subsequent landing less demanding)
- Single-leg squat jump (however, this eliminates the use of the SSC)
- Countermovement jump

Force Production Exercises: Linear Plane

These exercises consist of jumping, bounding, or hopping for maximum height or distance in the sagittal plane.

STANDING LONG JUMP (ALSO REFERRED TO AS THE BROAD OR HORIZONTAL JUMP)

Aim
To develop lower body bilateral power in the linear plane.

Action
1. Stand with the hips and knees fully extended and the arms above the head (photo a). To add complexity and displacement (i.e., distance or height traveled) per unit of time (i.e., duration) for acceleration, the starting position can be progressed by standing on the toes.
2. Perform a rapid countermovement (photo b) and jump forward (photo c).
3. Land in the double-leg snap down position.

Sample Progressions
- Depth drop to long jump
- Repeat long jump
- Vertical jump to long jump
- Weighted long jump

Sample Regressions
- Remove the arm swing
- Long jump with no countermovement (however, this eliminates the use of the SSC)

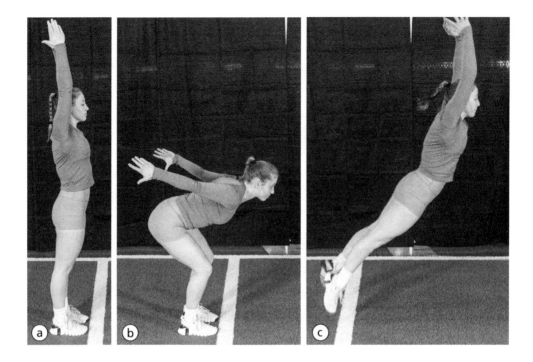

HURDLE JUMP

Aim

To develop lower body bilateral power and elasticity in the linear plane.

Action

1. Stand with the hips and knees fully extended and the arms above the head (photo *a*). To add more complexity and increase velocity during the countermovement, the starting position can be progressed by standing on the toes.

2. Perform a rapid countermovement (photo *b*) and jump over a hurdle (photo *c*). (Tucking will occur if the hurdle is higher than or relatively close to the athlete's countermovement vertical jump height, which can reduce takeoff velocity, propulsive forces, and jump height.)

3. Land in a double-leg snap down position.

Sample Progressions

- Depth drop to hurdle jump
- Repeat hurdle jump
- Hurdle jump to long jump
- Single-leg hurdle jump

Sample Regressions

- Tuck jump
- Snap down to hurdle jump

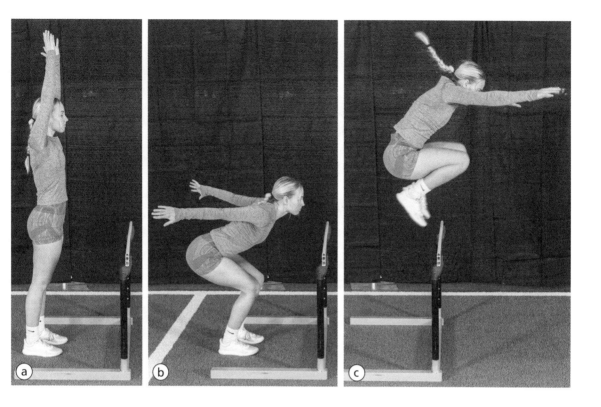

SINGLE-LEG FORWARD HURDLE HOP

Aim

To develop lower body unilateral power in the linear plane.

Action

1. Start with arms above the head and one leg raised to 90 degrees (photo *a*).
2. Rapidly perform a countermovement (photo *b*) and hop over a hurdle (photo *c*).
3. Land in single-leg snap down position.

Sample Progressions

- Repeat hurdle hop
- Alternating linear bound

Sample Regressions

- Single-leg long jump to double-leg landing
- Single snap down to hurdle hop
- Double-leg hurdle jump

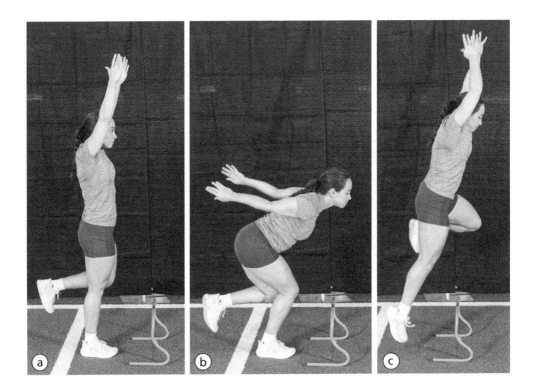

RESISTED SPRINT

Aim

To develop lower body power in the linear plane.

Action

1. Attach a sled, chain, or prowler to the body via a harness or belt and proceed to sprint as fast as possible with the applied load.

2. Choose the load and distance depending on the goal. Shorter distances (10 to 30 yards [9.1-27.4 m]) allow for high-quality effort. The load should not be heavy enough to deteriorate running mechanics. A study by Bachero-Mena and González-Badillo (1) showed the relationship between different loads accounting for 5% to 20% of the body's mass and the velocity lost within the acceleration phase. For positive effects on sprint training without diminishing or changing the sprinting mechanics, the load prescribed should not reduce the velocity by more than 10% (1). The optimal load for resisted sprinting has not been established in longitudinal studies (1). Of note, the surface friction between the sled and the ground will affect the load.

Sample Progressions

- If the distance of the sprint is being increased, consider decreasing the load to allow for high-quality effort and less strain on the body. The athlete's velocity should not be reduced by more than 10% (1).

- If the load is being increased, consider decreasing the distance to allow for high-quality effort and less strain on the body. The velocity should not be reduced by more than 10% (1).

Sample Regression

- Unresisted sprint

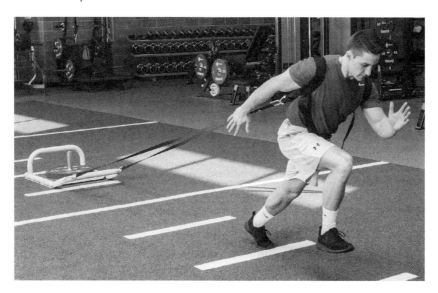

Force Production Exercises: Lateral Plane

These exercises consist of jumping, bounding, or hopping for maximum height or distance in the frontal plane.

LATERAL VERTICAL JUMP

Aim

To develop lower body bilateral power in the lateral plane.

Action

1. Stand with the hips and knees fully extended and the arms above the head (photo a). To add more complexity, the starting position can be progressed by standing on the toes.
2. Rapidly perform a countermovement (photo b) and jump up while pushing the body either left or right (photo c).
3. Land in a double-leg snap down position.

Sample Progressions

- Repeat lateral vertical jump
- Repeat lateral tuck jump
- Lateral hurdle jump
- Repeat lateral hurdle jump
- Depth drop to lateral jump
- Depth drop to lateral hurdle jump
- Depth drop to repeat lateral hurdle jump

Sample Regressions

- Lateral box jump
- Snap down to lateral jump
- Snap down to lateral box jump

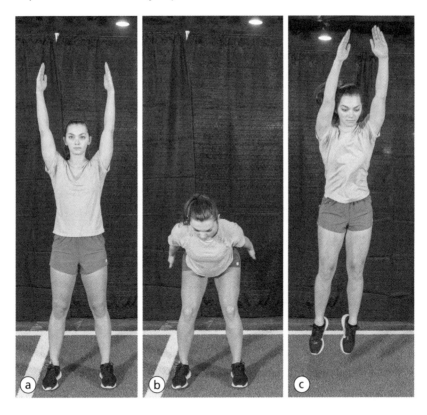

LATERAL OR MEDIAL HOP

Aim

To develop lower body unilateral power in the lateral plane.

Action

1. Start with the arms above the head and one leg raised to 90 degrees (photo *a*).
2. Rapidly perform a countermovement (photo *b*) and hop over a hurdle with either the inside or outside leg (photo *c*).
3. Land on the same leg that is hopping in a single-leg snap down position.

Sample Progressions

- Lateral or medial hurdle hop
- Repeat lateral or medial hurdle hop
- Lateral bound
- Repeat lateral bound
- 45-degree linear bound

Sample Regressions

- Lateral or medial hop to double-leg landing
- Lateral or medial hop to box
- Single-leg snap down to lateral or medial hop

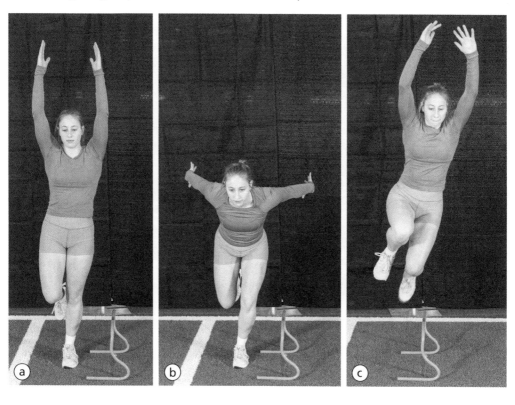

PUSH AND RECOVER

Aim

To develop total body strength and power in the lateral plane.

Action

1. Start in an athletic position (photo *a*).
2. Push hard with the outside leg while reaching with the inside leg and covering ground while staying low (photo *b*).
3. Land on the outside foot (photo *c*) and recover and reset in an athletic position for each repetition.

Sample Progressions

- Band-resisted push and recover
- Sled- or chain-resisted push and recover
- Side shuffle
- Side shuffle to sprint
- Band-resisted side shuffle
- Sled- or chain-resisted side shuffle

Sample Regression

- Step and replace

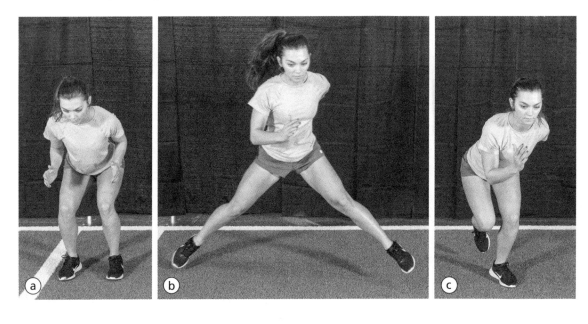

Force Production Exercises: Rotational Plane

These exercises consist of jumps, bounds, or hops for maximum height or distance in the transverse plane.

90-DEGREE VERTICAL JUMP

Aim

To develop lower body bilateral power in the transverse plane.

Action

1. Stand with the hips and knees fully extended and the arms above the head (photo a). To add more complexity, the starting position can be progressed by standing on the toes.
2. Rapidly perform a countermovement (photo b), then jump while rotating the body 90 degrees (photo c).
3. Land in the double-leg snap down position (photo d).

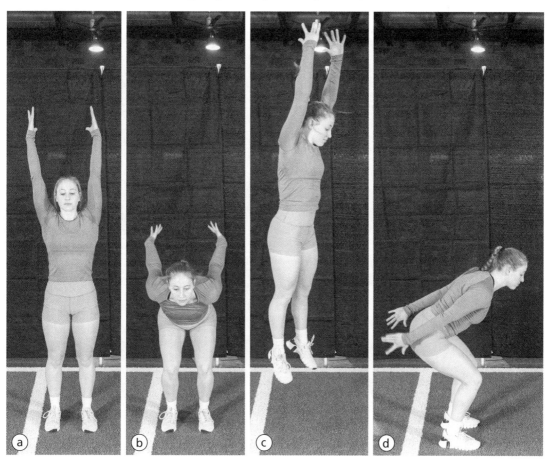

Sample Progressions
- 180-Degree vertical jump
- Repeat 90- to 180-degree vertical jump
- 90-Degree hurdle jump
- Depth drop to 90-degree vertical jump

Sample Regression
- Snap down to 90-degree vertical jump

90-DEGREE SINGLE-LEG VERTICAL HOP

Aim
To develop lower body unilateral strength and power in the transverse plane.

Action
1. Start with the arms above the head and one leg raised to 90 degrees (photo *a*).
2. Rapidly perform a countermovement (photo *b*), then hop and rotate 90 degrees while in the air (photo *c*).
3. Land in the single-leg snap down position (photo *d*).

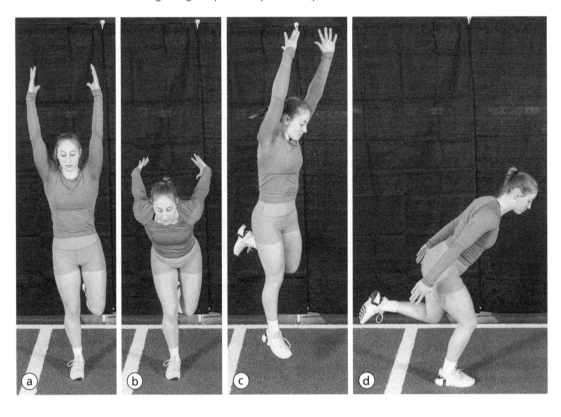

Sample Progressions

- Repeat 90-degree single-leg vertical hop
- 90-Degree single-leg vertical bound
- Repeat 90-degree single-leg vertical bound
- 180-Degree single-leg vertical hop
- Repeat 180-degree single-leg vertical hop
- 180-Degree single-leg vertical bound
- Repeat 180-degree single-leg vertical bound

Sample Regressions

- Single-leg snap down to 90-degree hop or bound
- 90-Degree single-leg vertical hop to double-leg landing
- 90-Degree vertical jump to single-leg landing

PLYOMETRIC TRAINING

The purpose of plyometric training is for speed and power athletes to recruit and develop the SSC in multiple planes of motion. It emphasizes a rapid transition from eccentric (net muscle lengthening) to concentric (net muscle shortening) movements. This type of training should be used in an athlete's training regimen to enhance the ability to jump, cut, and run efficiently.

The models associated with plyometric training are the mechanical (i.e., series elastic and parallel elastic) and neurophysiological (i.e., potentiation via stimulation of the muscle spindle) models. Within the mechanical model, the connective tissue (i.e., series elastic components [associated tendons] and parallel elastic components [fascia]) is the workhorse for plyometric exercises, with some additional contribution from the associated muscles. In this model, elastic energy in the musculotendinous components is increased with a rapid stretch and then stored. This is immediately followed up with a concentric muscle action, which increases total force production. The neurophysiological model involves neurological *potentiation*—that is, change in the force–velocity profile characteristics of the muscles' contractile components caused by the magnitude and rate of lengthening of the muscle during the eccentric phase, increasing the magnitude and rate of force production during the concentric phase. This is an involuntary response (i.e., reflex action) to an external stimulus that stretches the muscle. Muscle spindle activation occurs during plyometric exercises and is stimulated by a rapid stretch, causing reflexive muscle action and reciprocal inhibition of the antagonists. For greater detail on the mechanical and neurophysiological models, refer to *Essentials of Strength Training and Conditioning* (13).

Plyometric training should not necessarily mimic a sport movement; however, it should be used to develop the SSC relevant to the demands and positional requirements of a sport. For example, elite volleyball players may perform countermovement-style jumps, such as block jumps, jump sets, and spike jumps, 1,000 to 4,000 times per week during practices and matches. Adding sets of countermovement jumps within a training session can increase the workload for the athletes, which can be detrimental to their health and performance. The strength and conditioning professional should consider multiple possibilities that allow athletes to receive types of training they are not getting (e.g., ballistics, maximal strength training, and recovery) so that one quality is not being overemphasized. de Villarreal and colleagues (7) found that depending on the time of the year, athletes performing low (one session a week; 420 foot-contacts) and moderate (two sessions a week; 840 foot-contacts) volumes of plyometric training sessions had greater jumping and sprinting gains than those performing high volumes (four sessions a week; 1,680 foot-contacts). Of note, these volumes of plyometric tasks are high, and athletes unfamiliar with the activities should be progressively exposed to them.

Similar to the category for force production exercises, exercises in this category are grouped by the plane of motion that it is predominantly trained, and the same terminology is used. Unlike force production, the emphasis for plyometrics is a shorter GCT along with development of transitional power and elasticity.

Plyometric Exercises: Vertical Plane

These exercises consist of repeated or continuous jumps, hops, or bounds focusing on a shorter GCT and/or height in place.

DOUBLE-LEG POGO HOP

Aim
To develop and improve bilateral elasticity and tissue quality within the foot, ankle, and knee complex.

Action
1. Start with the hands either on the hips (photo *a*) or to the side of the body and the feet flat on the ground.
2. Proceed to hop straight up into the air with both feet and minimal knee flexion (photo *b*), striking the ground with the full foot. The goal is minimal GCT, and repetitions should feel springy and bouncy.
3. The body should ideally maintain a stacked position (head, neck, and spine in neutral alignment, with the ribs and pelvis stacked on top of each other).

Variations and Progressions
- Double-leg pogo hops with mini-bounce
- Continuous double-leg pogo hop to box

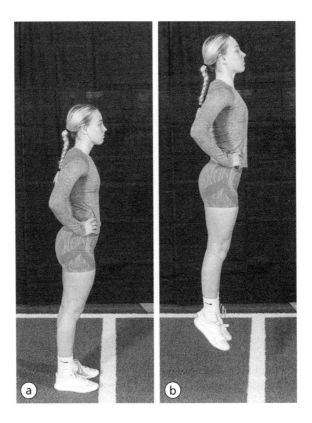

SINGLE-LEG POGO HOP

Aim

To develop and improve unilateral elasticity and tissue quality within the foot, ankle, and knee complex.

Action

1. Start with the hands either on the hips (photo *a*) or to the side of the body, with one foot raised slightly off the ground.
2. Proceed to hop straight into the air on one foot with minimal knee flexion (photo *b*), striking the ground with the full foot. The goal is minimal GCT, and repetitions should feel springy and bouncy.
3. The body should ideally maintain a stacked position (head, neck, and spine in neutral alignment, with the ribs and pelvis stacked on top of each other).

Variations and Progressions

- Single-leg pogo hops with mini-bounce
- Alternating bound in place
- Continuous single-leg pogo hop to box

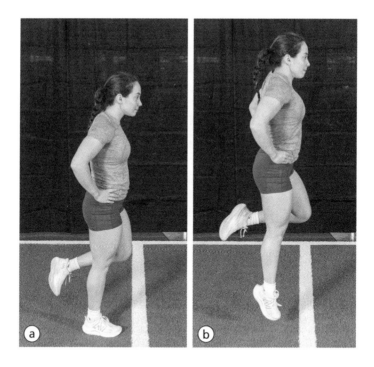

Plyometric Exercises: Linear Plane

These exercises consist of repeated or continuous jumps, hops, or bounds focusing on shorter GCT while moving forward or backward within the sagittal plane.

DOUBLE-LEG FORWARD OR BACKWARD POGO HOP

Aim

To develop and improve bilateral elasticity and tissue quality within the foot, ankle, and knee complex in the vertical plane.

Action

1. Start with the hands either on the hips or to the side of the body and the feet flat on the ground.
2. Proceed to hop straight up while moving forward or backward with both feet and minimal knee flexion, striking the ground with the full foot. The goal is minimal GCT, and repetitions should feel springy and bouncy.
3. The body should ideally maintain a stacked position (head, neck, and spine in neutral alignment, with the ribs and pelvis stacked on top of each other).

Variations and Progressions

- Double-leg forward or backward pogo hop with mini-bounce

- Continuous double-leg hurdle hop
- Continuous double-leg hurdle hop with mini-bounce
- Continuous double-leg hurdle jump
- Continuous double-leg hurdle jump with mini-bounce
- Continuous long jump (this can potentially increase the GCT due to the increasing momentum of each jump, which requires high braking and propulsive impulse)

SINGLE-LEG FORWARD OR BACKWARD POGO HOP

Aim

To develop and improve unilateral elasticity and tissue quality within the foot, ankle, and knee complex in the sagittal plane.

Action

1. Start with the hands either on the hips or to the side of the body, with one foot raised slightly off the ground.
2. Proceed to hop straight up while moving forward or backward on one foot with minimal knee flexion, striking the ground with the full foot. The goal is minimal GCT, and repetitions should feel springy and bouncy.
3. The body should ideally maintain a stacked position (head, neck, and spine in neutral alignment, with the ribs and pelvis stacked on top of each other).

Variations and Progressions

- Single-leg forward or backward pogo hop with mini-bounce
- Continuous single-leg hurdle hop
- Continuous single-leg hurdle hop with mini-bounce
- Linear bound
- 45-Degree linear bound

Plyometric Exercises: Frontal Plane

These exercises consist of repeated or continuous jumps, hops, or bounds focusing on a shorter GCT within the frontal plane.

LATERAL POGO HOP

Aim

To develop and improve bilateral elasticity and tissue quality within the foot, ankle, and knee complex in the frontal plane.

Action

1. Start with the hands either on the hips or to the side of the body and the feet flat on the ground.
2. Proceed to hop straight up while moving left or right with both feet and minimal knee flexion, striking the ground with the full foot. The goal is minimal GCT, and repetitions should feel springy and bouncy.
3. The body should ideally maintain a stacked position (head, neck, and spine in neutral alignment, with the ribs and pelvis stacked on top of each other).

Variations and Progressions

- Lateral pogo hops with mini-bounce
- Continuous lateral hurdle hop
- Continuous lateral hurdle hop with mini-bounce
- Continuous lateral hurdle jump
- Continuous lateral hurdle jump with mini-bounce

SINGLE-LEG LATERAL OR MEDIAL POGO HOP

Aim

To develop and improve unilateral elasticity and tissue quality within the foot, ankle, and knee complex in the frontal plane.

Action

1. Start with the hands either on the hips or to the side of the body and one foot raised slightly off the ground.
2. Proceed to hop straight up while moving left or right on one foot with minimal knee flexion, striking the ground with the full foot. The goal is minimal GCT, and repetitions should feel springy and bouncy.
3. The body should ideally maintain a stacked position (head, neck, and spine in neutral alignment, with the ribs and pelvis stacked on top of each other).

Variations and Progressions

- Lateral pogo hops with mini-bounce
- Continuous lateral or medial hurdle hop
- Continuous lateral or medial hurdle hop with mini-bounce
- Continuous lateral hurdle jump
- Continuous lateral hurdle jump with mini-bounce

Plyometric Exercises: Rotational Plane

These exercises consist of repeated or continuous jumps, hops, or bounds focusing on a shorter GCT within the transverse plane.

ROTATIONAL POGO HOP

Aim

To develop and improve bilateral elasticity and tissue quality within the foot, ankle, and knee complex in the transverse plane.

Action

1. Start with the hands either on the hips or to the side of the body, with the feet flat on the ground.
2. Proceed to hop straight up while rotating the hips and feet 45 degrees to the left and right with minimal knee flexion, striking the ground with the full foot. The goal is minimal GCT, and repetitions should feel springy and bouncy.
3. The body should ideally maintain a stacked position (head, neck, and spine in neutral alignment, with the ribs and pelvis stacked on top of each other).

Variations and Progressions

- Forward and backward rotational pogo hop
- Lateral rotational pogo hop
- 45-Degree forward or backward rotational pogo hop
- Repeat 90- or 180-degree rotational vertical jump
- Repeat 90- or 180-degree rotational long jump
- Repeat 90- or 180-degree hurdle jump

SINGLE-LEG ROTATIONAL POGO HOP

Aim

To develop and improve unilateral elasticity and tissue quality within the foot, ankle, and knee complex in the transverse plane.

Action

1. Start with the hands either on the hips or to the side of the body, with one foot raised slightly off the ground.
2. Proceed to hop straight up while rotating the hips and feet 45 degrees to the left or right on one foot with minimal knee flexion, striking the ground with the full foot. The goal is minimal GCT, and repetitions should feel springy and bouncy.
3. The body should ideally maintain a stacked position (head, neck, and spine in neutral alignment, with the ribs and pelvis stacked on top of each other).

Variations and Progressions

- Single-leg forward or backward rotational pogo hop
- Single-leg lateral or medial rotational pogo hop
- 45-Degree forward or backward rotational pogo hop
- 90- or 180-Degree continuous rotational vertical hop
- 90- or 180-Degree continuous rotational vertical hop with mini-bounce
- 90- or 180-Degree continuous alternating bound
- 90- or 180-Degree continuous alternating bound with mini-bounce

BALLISTIC TRAINING

The purpose of ballistic training is to increase power by applying resistance beyond body weight. While plyometric training targets fast SSC activity against a relatively low load, ballistic training targets maximal force capability with a moderate to high load. Ballistic training offers a range of loads (e.g., no external load to approximately 50% of the 1-repetition maximum [1RM]) from which to target the force–velocity spectrum to enhance the rate of force development (4, 5, 6).

There are multiple ways to program ballistic exercises. An example of a single ballistic training session per week would be performing approximately three to six exercises, with 3 to 6 sets per exercise and 3 to 6 repetitions per set. Another example for multiple ballistic training sessions throughout the week would be performing approximately one to two exercises per day, with 3 to 6 sets per exercise and 3 to 6 repetitions per set. When programming ballistic exercises, it is paramount to attend to movement quality and load. For specific programming examples, see chapters 9 and 10.

Ballistic exercises should be performed only if the athlete possesses efficient movement competency relative to the movement being prescribed. The following list gives recommendations, considerations, methods, and modalities backed by research and trends within the strength and conditioning profession.

General Recommendations and Considerations

Training Age and Experience

▶ Athletes with a low training age or lack of experience with resistance training should prioritize technique and movement quality before applying ballistic training to their training regimen.

Load Prescription

▶ Research has shown that the use of different training loads elicits different training adaptations and has further indicated load- and velocity-specific adaptations in muscular power development.

▶ It is suggested that athletes select training loads that will improve the ability to develop power against a specific resistance they often encounter in their athletic events.

▶ Multiple researchers have suggested that the loading range for ballistic training falls anywhere between 0% and 50% of the 1RM back squat (4, 5, 6), whereas in semiballistic exercises such as weightlifting, peak power output occurs anywhere between 70% and 90% for lower body exercises (3, 4).

Exercise Selection

▶ Exercise selection dictates the mechanical specificity of training. Mechanical specificity refers to the kinetic and kinematic similarity of a training exercise to the actual athletic performance. This also aligns with the principle of specific adaptations to imposed demands.

▶ Such kinetic and kinematic variables include but are not limited to force and power exerted, rate of force development, velocity of movement, movement pattern, type of muscle action, range of motion, and duration of movement.

▶ Investigators suggest that athletes include multijoint ballistic exercises or weightlifting exercises and derivatives that are mechanically specific to the actual athletic movements in their training programs to develop muscular power and enhance dynamic athletic performance.

Strength Level of the Athlete

▶ Besides the nature of the exercise, the strength level or training history of the athlete could also affect the optimal load.

▶ Researchers found that stronger athletes produced the maximal power output at a higher percentage of the maximum load (40% of the 1RM) than did weaker athletes (10% of the 1RM) in the squat jump and suggested that an upward shift in the optimal load may be present as the maximum strength levels of athletes increase (4, 5, 6, 16).

▶ Other research has demonstrated the contrary results, suggesting that stronger athletes used lower percentages of the 1RM than did weaker athletes to attain the maximum mechanical power output during the bench press throw and jump squat (4, 5, 6, 16).

▶ Based on these research results about the relationship between the optimal load and the athlete's strength level or training history, training could be expected to shift the percentage of maximum strength at which the highest power is produced (i.e., the optimal load) either upward or downward.

Program Design

▸ Periodization of training programs is important for optimum muscular power development (see chapter 3).

▸ Several investigators have demonstrated and insisted on the superiority of sequential periodized training programs, in which the training emphasis is initially on general strength with a later emphasis on more specific power development, compared with nonperiodized training programs with no or little variation (9, 10).

▸ Baker suggested that the optimal load shifts toward a higher percentage of the 1RM during phases that emphasize strength-oriented training (i.e., training with high resistance and low velocity) and toward a lower percentage during phases that emphasize speed-oriented training (i.e., training with low resistance and high velocity) (2).

Common Methods and Modalities

Dynamic Effort

▸ A widely used modality within Louie Simmons' conjugate training system (15) emphasizes using training loads between approximately 30% and 80% of the 1RM, with the intention of increasing power over a period of time (for example, back squats: 8 × 2 at 60% of the 1RM).

Accommodating Resistance

▸ Resistance bands or chains can be used to accommodate specific loads at certain parts of a movement.

▸ Loads should be reduced by 20% to 50% from what is typically assigned based on the usual repetition scheme (for example, hex bar deadlifts with 10% to 15% band resistance: 5 × 3 at 50% of the 1RM).

Contrast Training

▸ Contrast training involves pairing a high-force strength movement with a high-velocity movement (for example, performing a heavy single back squat at 90%, then immediately performing the repeat hurdle jump).

French Contrast Training

▸ French contrast training involves pairing a high-force strength movement with a high-force plyometric movement, high-force power movement, and high-velocity movement (for example, performing a heavy single front squat at 90% of the 1RM, then immediately performing a repeat hurdle jump along with a dumbbell jump and a band-assisted continuous vertical jump).

See chapters 3 and 8 for more details on programming some of the methods listed above.

Ballistic-Related Exercises: Preballistic

This section of exercises aims to improve and develop lower body movement competency and strength. It will include exercises performed without the use of elastic bands or chains. Sets can range from approximately 3 to 6 and repetitions from 5 to 10 or more (refer to the previous discussion on ballistic training or to chapters 9 and 10 for more information on programming). When choosing exercises, it is important to consider the goal of the program and the environment in which athletes are training (group-based or private). The judgement on progressing athletes from preballistic to ballistic exercises may be subjective if the athlete is working in a team environment or one-on-one with a strength and conditioning professional. The use of testing modalities may be an efficient way to know when an athlete is ready to progress to ballistic exercises.

BARBELL FRONT SQUAT

Aim
To develop lower body strength in the vertical plane.

Action
1. Begin with the bar placed across the front of the shoulders (using either a parallel or a crossed-arm position). The chest is up and out, and the head is tilted slightly upward. The feet are shoulder-width apart with the toes pointed either forward or slightly outward (photo a).
2. Descend by flexing the hips and knees while maintaining a neutral back position until the desired position is reached (photo b). (Depth will vary from athlete to athlete based on their technique and range of motion.)
3. Return to the starting position by extending the hips and knees while maintaining a neutral back position.

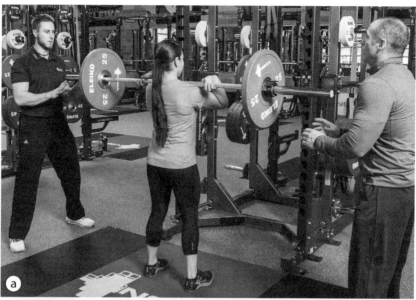

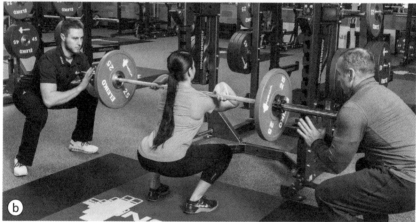

BARBELL BACK SQUAT

Aim

To develop lower body strength in the vertical plane.

Action

1. Begin by gripping the bar with a shoulder-width pronated grip and placing the bar on the upper back and shoulders (a high-bar or low-bar position can be used). The chest is up and out, and the head is tilted slightly upward. The feet are shoulder-width apart with the toes pointed either forward or slightly outward (photo a).

2. Descend by flexing the hips and knees while maintaining a neutral back position until the desired position is reached (photo b). (Depth will vary from athlete to athlete based on their technique and range of motion.)

3. Return to the starting position by extending the hips and knees while maintaining a neutral back position.

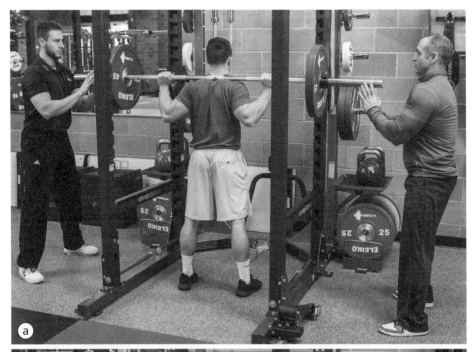

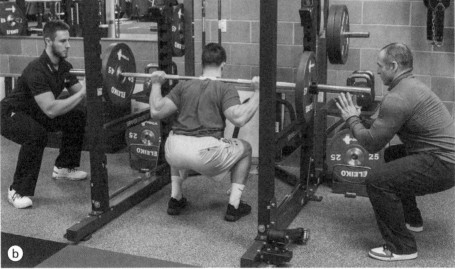

HEX BARBELL DEADLIFT

Aim

To develop lower body strength in the vertical plane.

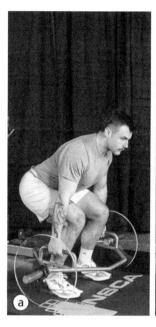

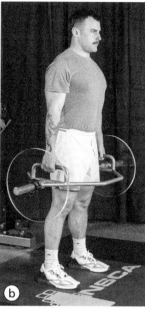

Action

1. Begin by standing in the middle of the hex bar with the handles directly to the side (high or low handles can be used). Grip the handles with a neutral and closed grip, and flex the hips and knees to get into the starting position (similar to the bottom of a squat) (photo a).

2. Stand up with the bar by extending the hips and knees while maintaining a neutral back position until the hips and knees are fully extended (photo b).

3. Return to the starting position by flexing the hips and knees while maintaining a neutral back position.

Ballistic-Related Exercises: Ballistic

CHAIN- OR BAND-RESISTED FRONT SQUAT

Aim

To develop lower body strength and power in the vertical plane.

Action

1. See the "Preballistic" section.

2. Apply rubber elastic bands or chains to the bar that equal the desired load to be trained. For example, if the prescribed load is 75% of the 1RM, including bands or chains contributing 15% toward the load, then 60% of the load should come from the weight loaded. This should allow greater acceleration from the bottom of the lift to promote higher rates of force moving toward the total vertical displacement of the movement (12).

3. The movement should feel lighter at the bottom and heavier at the top to drive more intent throughout the entire movement as the load increases when the bands stretch.

Variation

- Box front squat (add a slight pause on the box to limit SSC function)

CHAIN- OR BAND-RESISTED BACK SQUAT

Aim

To develop lower body strength and power in the vertical plane.

Action

1. See the "Preballistic" section.
2. Apply rubber elastic bands or chains to the bar that equal the desired load to be trained. For example, if the prescribed load is 75% of the 1RM, including bands or chains contributing 15% toward the load, then 60% of the load should come from the weight loaded. This should allow greater acceleration from the bottom of the lift to promote higher rates of force moving toward the total vertical displacement of the movement (17). A similar approach, but with higher loads, can be used if the primary focus is on strength development.
3. The movement should feel lighter at the bottom and heavier at the top to drive more acceleration throughout the entire movement.

Variations

- Box back squat (add a slight pause on the box to inhibit SSC involvement)
- Barbell jump squat (to develop lower body bilateral power while involving the SSC and to tolerate external loads)
- Barbell squat jump (to develop lower body bilateral power without involving the SSC and to tolerate external loads)

BAND- OR CHAIN-RESISTED HEX BAR DEADLIFT

Aim

To develop lower body strength and power in the vertical plane.

Action

1. See the "Preballistic" section.
2. Apply rubber elastic bands or chains to the bar that equal the desired load to be trained. For example, if the prescribed load is 55% of the 1RM, including bands or chains contributing 15% toward the load, then 40% of the load should come from the weight loaded. This should allow greater acceleration from the bottom of the lift to promote higher rates of force moving toward the total vertical displacement of the movement (17). A similar approach, but with higher loads, can be used if the primary focus is on strength development.
3. The movement should feel lighter at the bottom and heavier at the top to drive more acceleration throughout the entire movement.

Variations

- Hex bar jump squat (to develop lower body bilateral power while involving the SSC and to tolerate external loads)
- Hex bar squat jump (to develop lower body bilateral power without involving the SSC and to tolerate external loads)

DUMBBELL JUMP

Aim

To develop lower body power in the vertical plane.

Action

1. See "Vertical Jump" within "Force Production Exercises."

Variations

- Accentuated eccentric loaded vertical jump
- Accentuated eccentric loaded split jump
- Accentuated eccentric loaded box jump
- Accentuated eccentric loaded long jump

RESISTED SPRINT

Aim

To develop lower body power and speed in the linear plane.

Action

1. See "Resisted Sprint" within "Force Production Exercises."

Variations

- Band- or chain-resisted sprint
- Sled drag
- Sled push

Loading for a sled drag or sled push will vary based on the distance, the training age of the athlete, and the phase of the sprint that is the focus.

RESISTED LATERAL PUSH AND RECOVER

Aim

To develop lower body power and speed in the lateral plane.

Action

1. See "Push and Recover" within "Force Production Exercises."

Variations

- Band-resisted push and recover
- Sled- or chain-resisted push and recover
- Side shuffle
- Side shuffle to sprint
- Band-resisted side shuffle
- Sled- or chain-resisted side shuffle

LANDMINE ROTATIONAL PRESS

Aim

To develop lower and upper body power and speed in the rotational plane.

Action

1. Begin by placing a barbell in a landmine attachment. Face parallel to the bar (shoulders across the collar of the bar) with the outside hand supinated on the end of the barbell (the bar can start at either the hip or the shoulders) (photo a).
2. Rapidly dip the hips and knees (photo b) and accelerate the bar upward, rotating 90 degrees (photo c).
3. Return the bar back to the starting position in a controlled manner.

Variation

- Landmine rotational split jerk

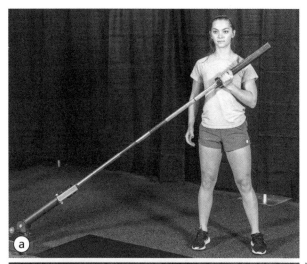

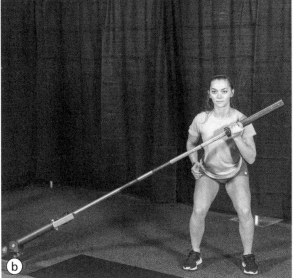

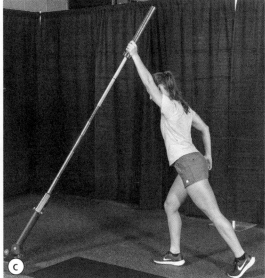

CONCLUSION

There are myriad effective exercises and methods to develop lower body power. When selecting exercises or methods, the context of the sport, the tasks associated with the sport, and the athlete's positional requirements are important considerations. Within the context of each, it is important to consider areas that need more attention and to educate athletes on the need for understanding their strengths and weaknesses.

CHAPTER 7

Anatomical Core Power Exercises

Douglas M. Tvrdy

The *anatomical core* is a general term used to describe the trunk or torso region and the muscle groups that create movement, resist movement, and protect and control the axial skeleton (rib cage, vertebral column, pelvic girdle, and shoulder girdle) and associated passive tissues (cartilage, ligaments, and joint capsules). The abdominals, internal and external obliques, erector spinae, quadratus lumborum, and multifidi are the main muscle groups involved in the anatomical core, but other groups also contribute. The anatomical core is an integral part of nearly all athletic movements and must be trained to help prevent injury and improve performance via improved lumbopelvic control.

Some researchers have shown that pre-existing anatomical core stability is not a predictor of superior sport performance (12, 13, 20). However, other researchers have shown significant improvements in sport activities (throw velocity, jump height, and running speed) after training the anatomical core over an appropriate period of time (longer than six to eight weeks), compared to standard training alone (4, 9, 14, 16, 18, 19). The results of this research justify the incorporation of anatomical core training in strength and conditioning programs to improve performance.

FUNCTIONS OF THE ANATOMICAL CORE

The functions of the anatomical core are spinal stiffness or stability, trunk movement and control, and kinetic chain linkage. *Spinal stiffness* or *stability* is the ability to resist forces acting on the spine. Trunk movement is the muscularly controlled movement of the axial skeleton. Kinetic chain linkage is the ability to maintain energy-efficient links between the upper and lower body. Improved anatomical core strength will further enhance power for sport performance (4, 9, 11, 14, 16, 18, 19) and protect against injury (11).

Spinal Stiffness

The muscles of the anatomical core, first and foremost, work in conjunction to create spinal stiffness. This is achieved by isometric muscle actions or controlled concentric and eccentric muscle actions by opposing muscle groups. Increasing spinal stiffness and stability can decrease microtrauma and macrotrauma to the sensitive structures housed within the anatomical core region (7). Also, by creating spinal stiffness and stability, the anatomical core provides the foundation upon which the limbs can move to generate force and finely detailed motor actions, which become the essence of sport movements. Without a solid foundational base, limb movements will be uncoordinated and may lead to increased injury risk of the distal segments.

Trunk Movement

The anatomical core musculature directly controls trunk movement, which occurs in all planes of movement and routinely within a combination of planes. An example of these movements occurring in multiple planes simultaneously is the swing of a bat or club. Rotation occurs in the transverse plane, with extension occurring in the sagittal plane and side-bending occurring in the frontal plane during the swing. The muscle actions creating these movements are a complex combination of concentric, isometric, and eccentric action moving in a finely tuned concert of acceleration–deceleration and isometric stability. This multifaceted responsibility of the anatomical core presents a very important yet difficult opportunity in sport performance training.

Kinetic Chain Linkage

The anatomical core is a crucial link between the lower extremities and upper body in the kinetic chains that make up functional whole-body sport movements. Commonly used in rotational movements in sports, the anatomical core is the link in transferring the kinetic energy created in the lower extremities to the upper body. A weak anatomical core allows the force or energy created by the lower extremities to dissipate before the movement is completed, resulting in suboptimal and inefficient motion. This can also be seen in lateral movements in which poor trunk control may cause malalignment of the lower extremity, leading to decreased power output. The loss of this energy will result in decreased sport performance and possible injury.

CHALLENGES AND BENEFITS OF TRAINING THE ANATOMICAL CORE

Training the anatomical core presents a unique challenge given the axial skeleton's expansive available range of motion in a variety of planes and a multitude of joints requiring simultaneous control in all aspects. The anatomical core musculature is responsible for stabilizing and moving many spinal segments that combine to create coordinated movement throughout all planes of motion. The anatomical core's interaction with and role as a link between the upper and lower extremities during movement increase the stress placed on it. Adding to the complexity of the movement, this system of muscles must continuously provide stability and stiffness to create the base of support for the limbs during dynamic sport activities. Creating controlled and coordinated movement of the anatomical core in all planes should help to prevent injury and provide forceful movements (8). The strength and conditioning professional must give equal and careful consideration to each component during the training program.

Upper Extremity Benefits of Training the Anatomical Core

During upper extremity activities, the anatomical core is essential to providing a solid link within the kinetic chain to conserve energy and force when they are transferred from the lower extremities through the trunk and into the upper extremities. During rotational movements, the anatomical core may also augment that force. Stability in the rib cage and spine allows for powerful and precise movements of the upper extremities. Researchers have demonstrated this principle, finding that participants improved handball throwing speed following an anatomical core training program (9, 16).

Lower Extremity Benefits of Training the Anatomical Core

Core stability development has also been shown to benefit lower body sport activities. Spinal stiffness provides a solid foundation proximally to allow for powerful movements in the distal segments. This is of great importance, because many lower extremity muscles have attachment points on the axial skeleton and need a solid anchor point to produce powerful contractions. These movements can be part of either an open-chain activity, such as kicking a ball, or a closed-chain activity, such as running and jumping. In an activity with a closed kinetic chain, the anatomical core enables the hip musculature to produce forces transmitted into the ground to create propulsion. Prieske (14) showed improvements in performance during both open (kick velocity) and closed (sprint speed) kinetic chain activities from an anatomical core strengthening program.

Specificity of Training

Dynamic anatomical core stabilization with limb movements that incorporate the muscle groups specific to the desired sport tend to show greater improvements than standard training, which consists of practice of the individual sport along with running, conditioning, and resistance training (22). Thus, the specificity of training is paramount to the maximization of results. Reed and colleagues (15) suggested that training muscle groups used for a specific sport or movement resulted in larger sport-specific improvements, such as golf scores. Sato and Mokha (18) demonstrated that an anatomical core stabilization program targeting the trunk and hip extensor muscle groups produced a 30-second improvement in 3.1 mile (5.0 km) running times compared with a control group. Other researchers have shown increased jump heights and sprint speed with anatomical core stabilization compared to standard training alone (4, 19). Exercise selection should be based on the model of specificity of training movements and muscle action to maximize training and produce the greatest results.

TYPES OF EXERCISES

Anatomical core exercises are placed into three categories: stabilization and postural control, dynamic control, and ballistic exercises. *Stabilization and postural control* emphasizes multimuscle contraction for spinal stiffness in proper posture and position. *Dynamic control* requires coordinated trunk and limb movement against outside forces that minimize aberrant trunk motions. *Ballistic exercises* for the anatomical core are high-velocity, multijoint trunk movements that involve the stretch-shortening cycle (10).

Stabilization and Postural Control Exercises

Stabilization and postural control exercises are the foundational exercises of the first phase of anatomical core musculature training. Stabilization exercises promote a *neutral spine* position consisting of 5 to 10 degrees of lumbar lordosis, 10 to 15 degrees of thoracic kyphosis, and 5 to 10 degrees of cervical lordosis. This posture is seen during plank exercises. Given the sensitive nature of the passive structures contained within the framework of the anatomical core (intervertebral discs, nerves, etc.), great care should be taken to avoid prolonged exposure to extreme ranges of motion to avoid possible injury. During this phase of anatomical core training, the body will begin to create neuromuscular pathways as the athlete learns these fundamental movements, and over time, the body will become more efficient in the neural economy of movement control.

Dynamic Control Exercises

Controlled trunk movements are introduced in the dynamic control category of exercise. Dynamic control exercises, such as the rollout, the Pallof press, and stir the pot, will further challenge the neuromuscular system by incorporating unstable environments or resisted limb movement (11). Control of the spine will limit microtrauma and other injuries while improving kinetic chain energy transfer. Moderate resistance in this phase of the exercise program may begin to provide the stimulus for muscle hypertrophy.

Ballistic Exercises

Ballistic exercises create high-velocity force production and incorporate movements that are similar to sport activities. Medicine ball toss exercises feature a stretch-shortening cycle and explosive actions, which are often the basis for power sports. These movements will provide the necessary resistance to further enhance muscle hypertrophy, which will increase power production.

EXERCISE PROGRESSION

Hibbs and colleagues (3) proposed a training model with a low threshold of exercise (typically <60% of the maximal voluntary contraction [MVC]) for those lower on the training scale and a higher threshold of exercise (typically >60% of the MVC) that incorporates a high dosage of dynamic and ballistic exercises to receive the maximum benefit. Thus, matching the exercise load to an athlete's current anatomical core fitness level will help optimize training and stimulate appropriate physiological changes. Far too often, the training level is either too low or too high to stimulate a physiological change. An appropriate dosage of exercise is one in which the athlete is challenged to near fatigue but still able to maintain proper form to prevent injury. If the athlete is unable to maintain proper form, the exercise should be ended. This fitness level–matched training will lead to greater power and sport performance.

Training Progression

Long-term training (more than eight weeks) that progresses to dynamic and ballistic training is most beneficial for sport-specific improvements (22). The need for long-term training is most likely due to the muscle hypertrophy and physiological muscular changes seen in endurance training that occurs over more than 16 workouts (2). This infers that a higher level of muscular force is needed to create substantial gains that result in improved sport performance. Short-term benefits of neuromuscular training have often been seen in studies, but not at the level of significant competitive gains (1, 5, 6, 17). Anatomical core stabilization is best done in sequential phases, which will progress and challenge athletes as they advance in strength and power production.

First Phase: Stabilization

The first two to three weeks focus on isometric contraction of the anatomical core musculature for stabilization, with an emphasis on form and technique training. The proper form of these exercises is characterized by maintaining a neutral spinal position, with minimal deviation into flexion and extension or a lateral side-bend of the lumbar spine, during exercises including planks and bird dogs. Technique training is the primary goal of the first phase. During this phase, the athlete will hold the exercise position for 10-second intervals, progressing repetitions and hold times as endurance and control improve.

Second Phase: Intermediate and Dynamic Control

Weeks three through seven focus on maintaining controlled anatomical core movement and stabilization with dynamic forces acting upon the trunk and limbs. An example of this would be controlling the anatomical core during lateral presses and bridges with hamstring curls. This phase transitions the athlete from isometric contractions to regulated concentric and eccentric muscle actions that prepare him or her for the final phase.

Third Phase: Explosive or Ballistic Movements

The last few weeks and beyond are focused on creating more speed and force production in a controlled fashion to replicate sport movements (chops and ball tosses). Control of the anatomical core musculature at high speeds is essential to maximize energy transfers for the different kinetic chains in the body. As part of an ongoing program, some elements from all phases should be incorporated to maintain fundamental training of correct posture and technique to enhance progressive ballistic training and injury prevention.

COMMON EQUIPMENT USED IN ANATOMICAL CORE TRAINING

Several pieces of equipment are commonly used in anatomical core training. Different types of balls, suspension straps, and bands can provide resistance to increase strength through progressive overload and provide dynamic challenges to increased neuromuscular control. Mats and padding may provide comfort and protect bony prominences.

Balls

A variety of different balls may be used in training the anatomical core. Weighted balls can provide progressive overload during ballistic movements. balls provide unstable surfaces to increase neuromuscular control. The use of balls allows for a high degree of unconstrained movement.

Medicine Balls

Medicine balls are often used in plyometric training, because they easily allow for high-speed force production in a variety of planes and positions. Different medicine balls have different levels of stiffness and the ability to rebound. Softer balls will rebound at slower speeds and may be more appropriate for beginners.

The appropriate style and size of the ball should be based on the goals and training level of the athlete.

Stability Balls

Stability balls, also called *Swiss balls*, used in anatomical core training increase anatomical core musculature activation (21). These balls provide an unstable surface that further enhances the difficulty of exercises and challenges the neuromuscular system in a controlled fashion. Using unstable surfaces incorporates reactionary movements necessary to adjust to a fluid situation that mimics the ever-changing environment of sport competition.

Suspension Straps

Suspension straps allow for a highly customizable resistance level and degree of difficulty according to the angle of the body while still allowing for a high degree of freedom of movement. These straps create an unstable environment that further enhances neuromuscular control of the anatomical core and accommodates internal and external forces rapidly.

Elastic Bands

Elastic bands provide resistance to the limbs, enhancing the spinal stiffness that provides the base for limb movements during dynamic activity. Elastic bands have a variable amount of force based on the amount of stretch that is placed on them, allowing for quick accommodation to the athlete's current abilities. This variable resistance also challenges the anatomical core throughout the range of motion to produce stability and create powerful sport-related actions.

Mats and Padding

Mats and padding provide cushioning to protect bony prominences when performing exercises. Some larger pads or cushions can also produce an unstable surface that will create a more challenging environment.

Exercise Finder

Exercise	Exercise category	Page number
Abdominal crunch toss	Ballistic	198
Bird dog	Stabilization	187
Bridge with hamstring curls	Dynamic control	188
Chest press with lateral pull (pallof press)	Dynamic control	192
Front plank	Stabilization	184
Lateral toss	Ballistic	199
Medicine ball alternating toss on wall	Ballistic	197

(continued)

Exercise Finder *(continued)*

Exercise	Exercise category	Page number
Medicine ball chop	Dynamic control	194
Medicine ball side-chop on wall	Ballistic	196
Modified prone-over-ball spine extension: "modified superman over ball"	Stabilization	186
Plank with circular upper-body stabilization on a stability ball: "stir the pot"	Dynamic control	190
Rollouts	Dynamic control	189
Side plank	Stabilization	185
Unilateral carry	Dynamic control	193
Wood chop	Ballistic	195

Stabilization Exercises

FRONT PLANK

Aim
To create abdominal strength and spinal stiffness against posteriorly directed forces.

Action
1. Begin in a prone position, with the elbows and forearms on padding or a mat as needed for comfort.
2. Raise the body up to a point where only the elbows and toes are touching the ground. The knees, hips, and shoulders should form a straight line. The spine should be held in a neutral position without allowing the hips to "sag" or "tent" in the air (see photo).
3. This position is held for a certain period of time, as discussed earlier in the chapter.
4. The body is then lowered back down to the mat to the starting position.

Variations
- Perform the plank with the feet on a stability ball. Placing half of the contact points on a ball creates an unstable environment that further challenges the anatomical core for more dynamic stabilization. Extra caution should be used when adding a ball or other dynamic implement.
- Perform the plank with the feet in suspension straps with hip abduction. Place the feet in the straps and obtain a plank position, move into slight hip abduction, and then return to the starting position. Special attention should be paid to maintaining a neutral spinal posture with the movement of the legs.
- Add leg lifts to the plank. Maintaining a plank position, alternate lifting the legs into slight hip extension.

- Add rows. In a high plank position (elbows extended rather than flexed) and holding a weight in each hand, alternate arms to perform a single-arm row from a tripod position.
- Perform planks with a weight pass back. In a high plank position, place a weight under one shoulder. Reach across the body with the other arm and move the weight across the body. Continue to pass the weight back and forth from one side of the body to the other while maintaining the plank position.

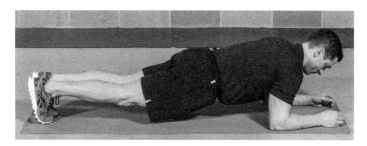

SIDE PLANK

Aim

To improve lateral musculature strength and stability, focusing on the internal and external obliques, quadratus lumborum, and hip abductors.

Action

1. Begin in a side-lying position with padding as necessary for comfort. Prop the body up on the elbow that is on the floor or mat. The elbow should be directly under the shoulder.
2. Raise the trunk and hips so that the spine is in a straight line. The only contact points with the ground are the elbow and the side of the bottom foot. The spine should be straight, with a minimal lateral side-bend (see photo).
3. Hold this position for a period of time, and perform multiple repetitions to appropriately challenge the body at its current level of fitness.
4. Lower the body back down to the mat to the starting position.

Variations

- If athletes have an issue with shoulder pain, they can perform a reverse side plank. Place the feet on a raised platform (i.e., a BOSU ball with the dome up or pads that are stacked about 8 inches [20.3 cm] high). Lie on the side of the shoulder with extra padding, as opposed to being propped up on the elbow, then perform a side plank as described before.
- While holding the side plank position, raise and lower the top leg while maintaining the neutral spine position.
- In a regular side plank position, the nonsupport arm can perform a row with a pulley or band, keeping the angle of the pull parallel to the floor while resisting the rotational pull of the pulley or band.

- With the feet in suspension straps, hold a side plank or reverse side plank position. This allows for leg movement with hip or knee flexion and extension to provide for more dynamic stabilization.

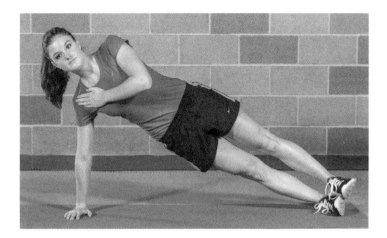

MODIFIED PRONE-OVER-BALL SPINE EXTENSION: "MODIFIED SUPERMAN OVER BALL"

Aim

To develop lumbar spine extensor strength and stabilization while working within a safe range of motion.

Action

1. Begin in a prone position with the hips on a stability ball and the feet slightly wider than shoulder-width apart, toes on the floor. Keep the head in line with the torso and the arms can either be at the sides, crossed at the chest, or extended overhead to increase difficulty.
2. For the first movement, lower the chest slightly (beyond what is shown in photo *a*); pay careful attention to avoid hyperflexing the lumbar spine.
3. Raise the chest up and hold in a slightly extended spinal position, avoiding the extreme end range of extension to limit excessive loading of the facet joints. The total arc of motion should be about 20 to 30 degrees, consisting of 10 to 15 degrees of lumbar flexion to 10 to 15 degrees of lumbar extension (photo *b*).
4. Lower to the beginning position and repeat.

Variations

- Hold weights. Assume the described position, with the feet anchored under a bar or held down by a partner.
- Add medicine ball tosses. Assume the described position, with the feet anchored under a bar or held down by a partner. Begin with the arms overhead,

and toss a medicine ball vertically into the air. Continue working with a small range of motion at the spine.

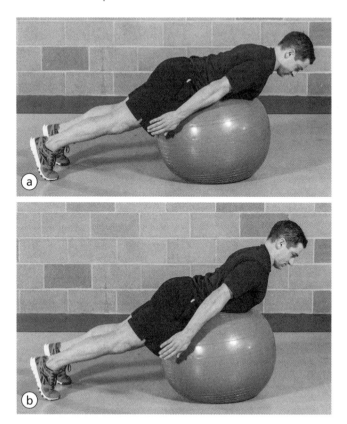

BIRD DOG

Aim

To create spinal stiffness with cocontraction of the opposing anatomical core musculature during reciprocal limb movement.

Action

1. Begin in a quadruped position with the hands and knees shoulder- or hip-width apart, using appropriate padding as needed (photo *a*).
2. The hands should be placed directly under the shoulders and the knees directly under the hips.
3. Lift the right arm and left leg up simultaneously. The contralateral limbs should be raised until they are in line with the trunk. Maintain a neutral spinal position, resisting twisting at the spine (photo *b*).
4. Lower the contralateral limbs that were raised to return to the starting position.
5. Alternate lifting the left arm and right leg, then return to the starting position. Continue alternating arm and leg lifts while maintaining a neutral spinal position for a period of time.

Variations

- Perform the bird dog as described, but add weights to the ankles and hold weights or strap weights to the wrists.
- Add dynamic movements of the raised limbs. Perform a bird dog, and while holding the contralateral limbs in the air, move the hand and foot (for example, in small circles).
- Perform a bird dog with the supporting limbs in contact with unstable surfaces. This will challenge dynamic stabilization of the anatomical core.

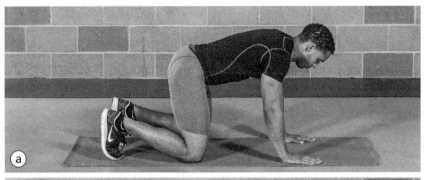

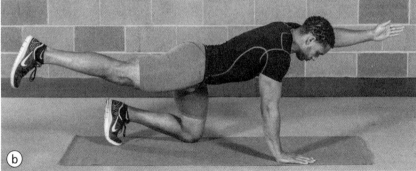

Dynamic Control Exercises

BRIDGE WITH HAMSTRING CURLS

Aim

To create increased lumbar extension and hip extension strength with dynamic control.

Action

1. Lie supine with the feet on the ball about hip-width apart and with the knees extended.
2. Press through the heels into the ball, raising the hips and lumbar spine until achieving slight hip extension with a neutral lumbar spine position. The knees should remain mostly extended (photo *a*).

3. Dig the heels into the ball, then pull the ball back toward the body, using the hamstrings to flex the knees.

4. Continue to pull the heels toward the buttocks until reaching approximately 90 degrees of knee flexion, then hold this position (photo *b*).

5. Extend the knees while rolling the ball back out. Lower the body back down to the mat, returning to the starting position.

Variation

Place the feet in the handles or stirrups of suspension straps and perform either bilateral hamstring curls or alternating unilateral hamstring curls while maintaining a bridge position.

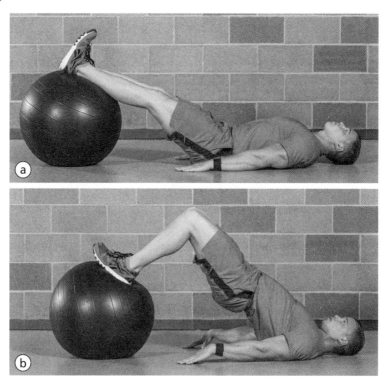

ROLLOUTS

Aim

To develop anterior abdominal and anterior hip strength and stabilization.

Action

1. Kneel on the floor in front of an ab wheel or a bar with round weights (photo *a*), using appropriate padding for the knees as needed.

2. Hold the bar or ab wheel with a pronated grip. Roll it out away from the knees, maintaining a neutral spine posture and using a slow and controlled movement.

3. Roll out as far as possible while still maintaining a neutral spine position, extending the arms overhead (photo *b*).

4. Contract the abdominal and hip flexor musculature to pull the body back to the start position, avoiding hyperflexion of the lumbar spine.

Variation

To increase difficulty, begin from a standing rather than a kneeling position and perform the rollout while keeping the knees extended.

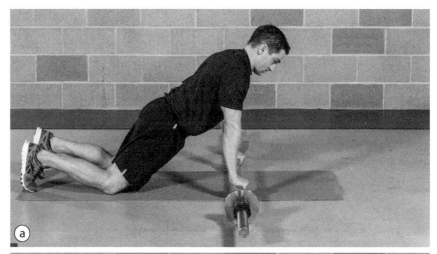

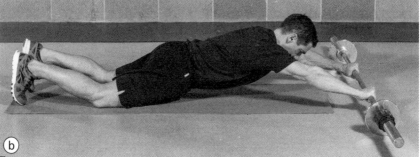

PLANK WITH CIRCULAR UPPER-BODY STABILIZATION ON A STABILITY BALL: "STIR THE POT"

Aim

To improve anterior anatomical core and abdominal activation and dynamic stabilization with upper body movements.

Action

1. Begin in a plank position, with the forearms placed on a ball about shoulder-width apart. The feet should be hip-width apart (photo *a*).

2. Circularly rotate the ball in a clockwise direction with shoulder and elbow movements. For safety, the circles should stay within the framework of the body.

3. Keep the spine in a neutral position by not allowing the hips to tent up into a flexed position or sag into lumbar extension.

4. Limit spinal rotation and side-bending by actively contracting the anatomical core musculature during the movement (photo b).

5. Repeat the movement in the counterclockwise direction.

6. Start with 10-second intervals and progress the number of repetitions as long as the ability to maintain control is maintained.

Variation

To increase difficulty, narrow the base of support by bringing the feet closer together or lifting one foot. The upper body base of support can also be narrowed by bringing the elbows closer together on the ball. Care should be taken when removing support to make sure athletes are ready for this challenge and do not injure themselves.

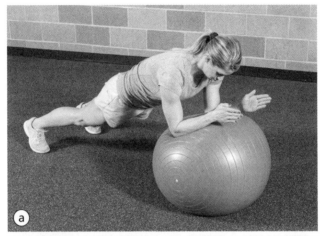

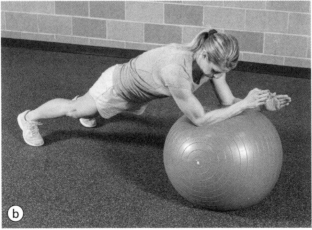

CHEST PRESS WITH LATERAL PULL (PALLOF PRESS)

Aim

To develop lateral stabilization and resistance to rotational forces with dynamic upper body movement in a standing posture.

Action

1. Begin standing in a semi-athletic posture, with the knees and hips slightly flexed and the trunk erect in a neutral spine posture.

2. Use either an elastic band or cable resistance. Hold the band or pulley handle in both hands at chest height.

3. Side-step out away from the anchor of the band or pulley stack until there is no slack in the band or cable. Maintain a semi-athletic posture with the knees slightly flexed (photo a).

4. Perform a chest-press type of motion by moving the hands away from the body (photo b), then returning to the start position. A rate of 1 repetition per 4 seconds should be used. Pay careful attention to limiting the rotation of the spine to create dynamic spinal control as the torque on the anatomical core musculature varies throughout the pressing motion.

5. Perform multiple repetitions while maintaining tension on the pulleys or band.

6. Step toward the pulley or band attachment to release the tension on the band.

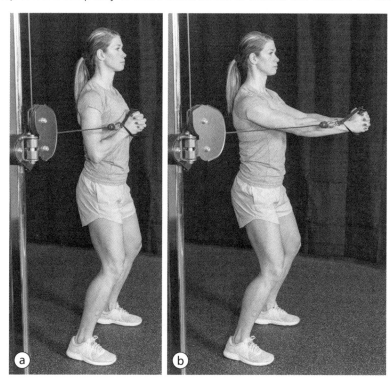

Variations

- Perform the presses in a single-leg stance position to further challenge dynamic stabilization.
- Adjust the angle of the band's pull by doing an overhead press or using a low angle to increase the difficulty.

UNILATERAL CARRY

Aim

To improve lateral anatomical core musculature strengthening and resistance of the lateral trunk bend in a standing and upright posture during a functional walking movement pattern.

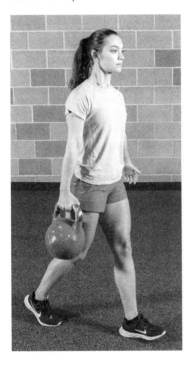

Action

1. Begin by holding a weight in one hand with a neutral grip.
2. The weight may be held in a low position, with the elbow extended and the hand next to the thigh. This allows for a heavier weight to be used while maintaining an upright posture (see photo).
3. Walk for a predetermined distance. Pay careful attention to keeping a correct posture and limiting excessive side-bending or swaying. The weight should be heavy enough that adequate activation of the contralateral anatomical core musculature can be felt.
4. Walk at a comfortable pace, approximately 2 to 3 miles (3.2-4.8 km) per hour.
5. Change the side holding the weight and walk back to the starting position.

Variations

- Hold the weight in a high position, at roughly shoulder height, which increases the lever arm so that less weight is needed to produce external torque on the anatomical core.
- Begin by holding the weight in a high position and perform overhead presses while walking, thus further challenging the dynamic ability of the anatomical core.

MEDICINE BALL CHOP

Aim

To create rotational power and dynamic control, similar to swinging a club or bat.

Action

1. Begin by standing in an athletic posture with the feet slightly wider than shoulder-width apart and the knees and hips moderately flexed. Hold a medicine ball with the arms extended in front of the body at about chest height (photo a).

2. Begin the movement by bringing the medicine ball back over the right shoulder with the left knee flexed, the right knee extended, and the trunk rotated to the right (photo b).

3. Reverse the motion by quickly rotating the trunk and hips to the left and moderately flexing both knees. Brings the medicine ball down and across the body so that it ends up outside the left knee (photo c).

4. Reverse the ball motion, bringing it back over the right shoulder.

5. Repeat the exercise using a ball path going from the left shoulder to the right knee. This should be done as quickly and forcefully as possible while maintaining control of the trunk.

Variation

Use bands for resistance, rather than a ball or weight. This requires more force at the end of the range of motion and greater eccentric control, because the resistance provided by the band increases as more stretch is placed on it.

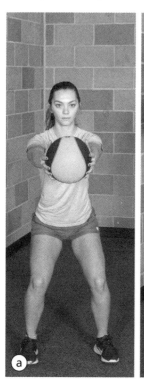
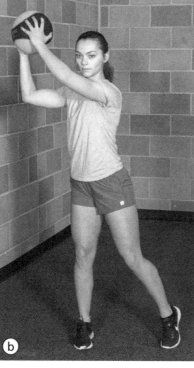
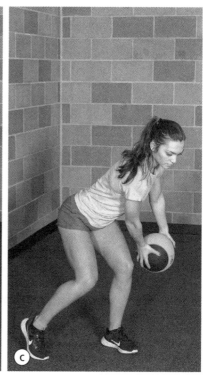

Ballistic Exercises

WOOD CHOP

Aim

To create the multiplanar, diagonal explosive force often used during throwing or other overhead sport movements.

Action

1. Begin by standing with the feet shoulder-width apart in an athletic stance, with the knees and hips moderately flexed.
2. Hold a medicine ball at chest height with the arms extended (photo *a*).
3. Rotate to one side, flexing at the waist and hips to bring the ball to knee height on that side, with the arms extended (photo *b*).
4. Quickly rotate the torso while extending the hips and knees to bring the ball overhead.
5. Without stopping, move the ball from the overhead position to now bring it down and throw it onto the ground (see photo *c*).
6. The ball should land just outside of the foot opposite to where the motion began in step 3 (photo *d*).
7. Pick up the ball and return to the start position.

Variations

- For the beginner level, start with the ball overhead and reduce the arc of motion and the countermovement.

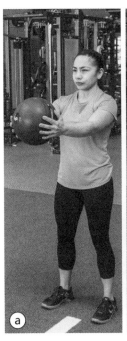
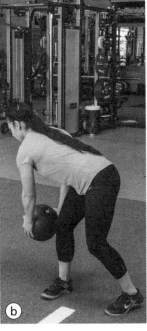
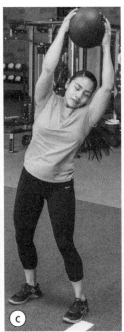
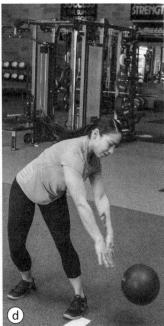

- Alternate throws to each side of the body with each repetition.
- Use a rebounder trampoline to increase the speed of the ball and add more challenge by decreasing the reaction time.
- For a more advanced version, use a large sledgehammer on a large tractor tire. The sledgehammer replaces the ball and moves in the same pattern. Special awareness of safety is needed to avoid letting go of the sledgehammer handle. The head of the sledgehammer should strike the center of the tire so that it does not bounce out of control back at the athlete or careen away.

MEDICINE BALL SIDE-CHOP ON WALL

Aim

To develop the diagonal rotational explosive force often used in swinging sport motions.

Action

1. Begin standing 1 to 2 feet (30 to 61 cm) from a wall, facing perpendicular to the line of the wall, in an athletic posture with the feet slightly wider than shoulder-width apart. Hold a medicine ball at about chest height, with the arms extended in front of the body (photo a).
2. Begin the movement by bringing the medicine ball over the left side, with the right knee flexed, the left knee extended, and the trunk rotated to the left (photo b). (Rotating to the right requires the walk to be to the left.)
3. Reverse the motion by quickly rotating at the trunk and hips and moderately flexing both knees. This accelerates the medicine ball across the body down and to the right.
4. Throw the medicine ball down to hit the base of the wall (photo c).
5. Catch the ball as it bounces or rolls off the wall.
6. Return to the starting position to reset for the next repetition.

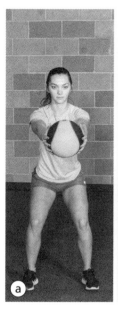
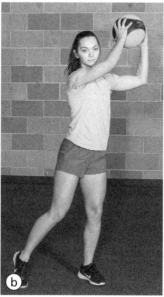
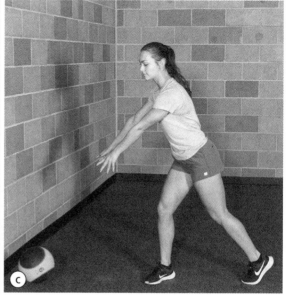

MEDICINE BALL ALTERNATING TOSS ON WALL

Aim

To create rapid contraction and relaxation of the antagonist muscle groups of the anatomical core in a dynamic environment by quickly adjusting position to track the ball and adapt to its path.

Action

1. Begin by standing 1 to 3 feet (30 to 91 cm) from a wall (depending on the softness and rebound of the medicine ball), facing perpendicular to the line of the wall. Stand in an athletic posture with the feet slightly wider than shoulder-width apart.

2. Hold a medicine ball on the outside of the hip or side of the trunk that is furthest away from the wall. The elbows are mostly extended to start this maneuver (photo a).

3. Quickly rotate the trunk by turning to face the wall. This will cause the leg closest to the wall to extend and the trailing leg to flex (photo b).

4. Using an underhand-scoop type of motion, continue moving to throw the ball toward the wall.

5. Once the ball has left the hands, switch the feet so that the hips are now facing the opposite direction (photo c).

6. Once the feet are switched, catch the ball as it bounces off the wall and bring it to just outside of the hip that is now furthest away from the wall (photo d).

7. Continue to quickly alternate throws back and forth.

Variation

Toss the ball back and forth with a partner while situated farther away from each other than if the exercise is performed using a wall.

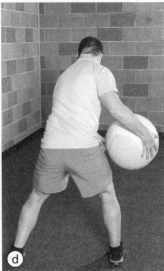

a

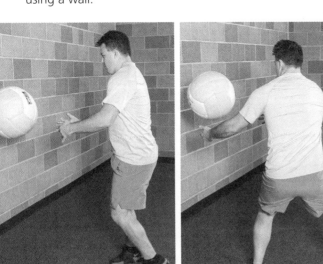

b

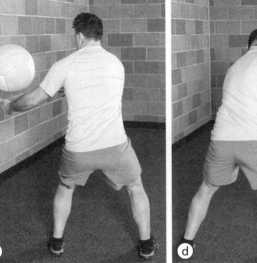

c

d

ABDOMINAL CRUNCH TOSS

Aim

To develop explosive power in the abdominal musculature.

Action

1. Begin by sitting on the floor with the knees flexed and the feet shoulder-width apart on the ground (hook-lying position).
2. The medicine ball should be held at or near the chest, with the elbows flexed (photo a).
3. A partner stands in an athletic position 1 to 3 feet (30 to 91 cm) away from the feet of the athlete performing the sit-up.
4. The athlete on the floor quickly sits up and extends through the arms to throw the medicine ball to the partner (photo b).
5. The partner catches the ball and throws it back to the athlete (photo c), who eccentrically lowers the torso back toward the ground and rests the medicine ball on the chest when contacting the ground with the back.
6. Repeat multiple repetitions quickly but in a regulated fashion.

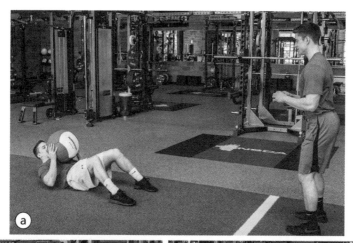

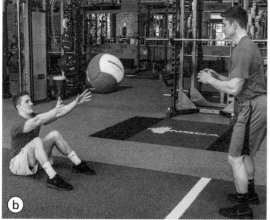

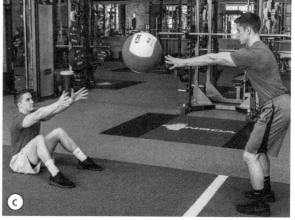

Variations

Rotational tosses: In a position similar to an abdominal crunch, begin with the medicine ball on one side of the body and have partners on either side. Perform a slight crunch with rotational throws across the body, alternating back and forth (photo *d*).

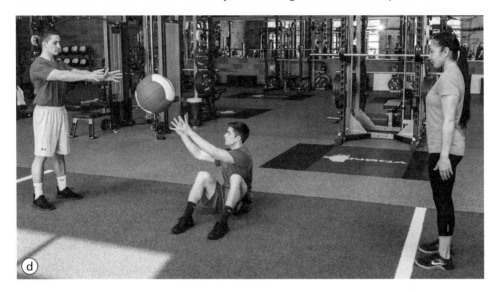

LATERAL TOSS

Aim

To develop the rotational explosive force often used in swinging motions of sports.

Action

1. Begin standing with the feet shoulder-width apart in an athletic position, facing perpendicular to the line of the wall (photo *a*). With the elbows extended, hold a medicine ball at chest height.
2. Begin the movement with a slight countermovement, rotating away from the wall and allowing for increased hip rotation and knee flexion (photo *b*).
3. Explosively extend the knees and hips to rotate the hips and torso toward the wall.
4. As the knees and hips extend and the trunk rotates, finish throwing the ball with both hands toward the wall (photo c).
5. As the ball bounces off the wall, catch it and recoil back to the position described in step 2. Repeat steps 3 and 4 for multiple repetitions.

Variations

- Vary the angle of the throws by throwing either from high or low starting positions.
- A vertical or angled trampoline may also be used to increase the speed and force of the rebound.

- Use a partner to adjust the speed and force of the ball passes.
- Vary the weight and size of the ball and the distance from the wall to change the rebound time and forces.

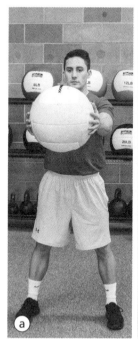
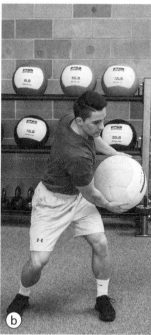
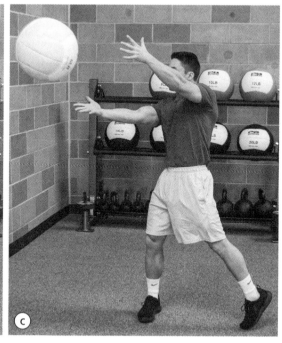

CONCLUSION

Anatomical core training has been shown to be beneficial for improving sport performance when certain training parameters are met (e.g., a progressive training period longer than eight weeks). The program should begin with stabilization exercises, then progress in intensity, and it should challenge neuromuscular control with dynamic control exercises until the athlete is able to perform high-level ballistic exercises. Selecting exercises that use muscle groups in a given sport will further enhance sport performance.

CHAPTER 8

Total Body Power Exercises

Wil Fleming
Adam Storey*

The sport of competitive weightlifting requires two multijoint, total body exercises to be performed in competition: the snatch and the clean and jerk. These exercises require athletes to exert high forces in an explosive manner to lift the barbell from the floor to an overhead position or to the shoulders in one continuous movement. During the performance of these exercises, weightlifters have achieved some of the highest absolute and relative peak power outputs reported in the literature (10-13).

Although these two competitive exercises form the basis of the training programs for competitive weightlifters, several complementary exercises that have similar movement patterns (e.g., power snatch and power snatch from a hang, power clean and power clean from a hang, snatch and clean pull, and front and back squat) are also included in training (21). The nomenclature of these exercises is used to delineate differences in starting position (e.g., *from a hang* rather than *from the floor*) or receiving position (e.g., the *power* [receiving] *position* or *catch* [receiving] *position* is performed with the knees less flexed than a full *squat clean* [receiving] *position*). These complementary exercises are routinely incorporated into the training programs of other strength and power athletes because of the kinematic similarities between the propulsive phases in both weightlifting and jumping movements (i.e., the explosive ankle, knee, and hip extension) (2, 3, 8, 9, 14-16). They are also frequently used because of the moderate to large significant relationships that exist between weightlifting ability in these exercises and power output during jumping and sprinting (1, 3, 4, 15, 24) and change-of-direction performance (15).

---

*Wil Fleming was contracted to author this chapter; Adam Storey's name was added to acknowledge his significant contribution partially retained from the previous edition.

During the snatch and the clean and jerk, weightlifters have been shown to produce peak power at loads of 70% to 80% of the 1-repetition maximum (1RM) (5-7, 17-20), which demonstrates an improved ability to generate peak power under high-load conditions. As such, other athletes who are required to generate high peak power outputs against heavy external loads (e.g., wrestlers, bobsledders, and rugby and American football players) are likely to benefit from high-load, weightlifting-style training (6).

This chapter details the purpose and teaching progressions for total body power exercises that are derived from Olympic-style weightlifting. Because of the high-speed nature and complexity of these movements, inexperienced individuals should seek the guidance of a strength and conditioning professional when attempting to learn these exercise progressions. In addition, athletes should make sure they can perform these exercises correctly before increasing the load. Derivatives of the weightlifting movements are valuable even at lower loads; thus, while learning to do the movements correctly, athletes will still derive benefits from their implementation in training. Derivatives of weightlifting movements can be used at a variety of different loads, which may have differing effects on the athletes' adaptive responses. Changes in the height of the catch position (e.g., clean versus power clean) can reduce or increase the load or barbell velocity, leading to changes in power output. A power clean catch being higher than parallel (i.e., the knees remaining lower than the hips at receiving) can lessen the load used but requires greater barbell velocity to displace the barbell to the required height. Pulling derivatives—such as the clean pull or snatch pull—or the jump shrug can be used with a wide range of loading capabilities (e.g., ≥100% of the 1RM for the clean and snatch pulls and 30%-60% of the 1RM hang power clean for the jump shrug) (6, 22, 23). Differing loads can lead to improvements in qualities such as strength or power production (6, 22, 23). Using the logical sequence of position, then speed, and then load, athletes can improve in weightlifting movements and gain the rewards of peak power generation. Such an approach also results in progressive overload, using a sequential approach.

KEY ASPECTS OF TOTAL BODY POWER EXERCISE PROGRESSIONS

The exercises outlined in this chapter are described using the following terms and positions.

Hook Grip

When gripping the barbell, the index and middle fingers wrap over the top of the thumb to apply pressure to both the thumb and the barbell (figure 8.1). The hook grip minimizes the chance that an athlete's grip will fail during the explosive pulling phase of the weightlifting exercises and their derivatives.

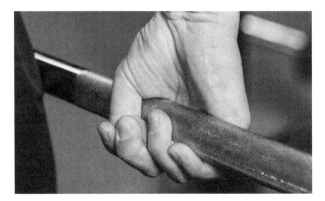

Figure 8.1 Hook grip.

Grip Placement for Snatch-Related Exercises

During snatch-related exercises, a wide overhand (also known as *pronated*) or a snatch grip should be used. The width of the grip depends on several factors, including the athlete's arm length, shoulder flexibility, and injury status. A simple method for choosing the right grip width is to stand tall with the barbell in the hands at the front of the thighs (figure 8.2a). The correct grip width is one in which the bar can rest in the crease of the hips and the hips can be flexed to 90 degrees in a standing position while the arms remain straight (figure 8.2b). This will place the bar in an optimal position in relation to the center of mass. For taller athletes, this width may be difficult to achieve, and in those cases, the grip width will be as wide as a standard barbell can accommodate.

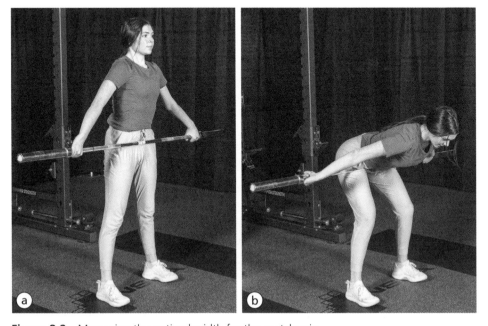

Figure 8.2 Measuring the optimal width for the snatch grip.

Straight-Arm Overhead Receiving Position

In the straight-arm overhead receiving position, the barbell is positioned over and behind the athlete's ears. When viewed from the side, the athlete's ears should not be blocked from view by the arms (figure 8.3). The bar should be in the palms of the hands with the wrists slightly extended.

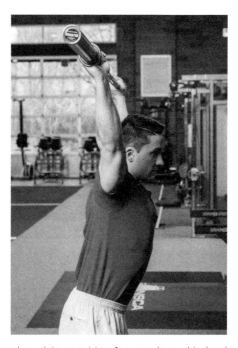

Figure 8.3 The overhead receiving position for snatch- and jerk-related progressions.

Power Variations

The power snatch and power clean are classified as exercises that are performed above the parallel thigh position. If the athlete descends below this parallel thigh position, the exercise is deemed to be a full squat snatch or a full squat clean, respectively. Although the full squat variations enable proficient athletes to lift approximately 20% more load, which is therefore the reason they are performed in weightlifting competitions, they require a greater degree of technical mastery, mobility, and strength when compared to the power variations.

Hang Variations

The hang position refers to a starting position above the knee. If an exercise is not described as using a hang position, assume that the movement is initiated from the floor. Other hang variations can be used, including high thigh (the power position), mid-thigh, and just above or just below the knee. Each position has benefits related to the length of the stretch-shortening cycle and can be implemented by coaches in specific situations in which it might be warranted.

Pull Variations

The pull variation of the snatch and clean exercises emphasizes the triple extension of the lower body, which is immediately followed by an explosive shoulder shrug. Except for the fast snatch and fast pull versions, the arms should remain relaxed and not actively engaged in an attempt to pull the bar upward; the elbows only flex after the athlete completes the lower body triple extension and upper body shrug. When the bar reaches its maximal height, it is not caught; instead, the athlete flexes the knees and hips and lowers the bar back to the starting position. This is done by letting the bar come back to the contact point in the hips and then lowering it to the ground in a controlled manner. As the bar descends to the knee level, the athlete will use a hip hinge motion; from the knee level to the starting position, the athlete will use more knee flexion in a motion similar to a squat. This controlled descent will keep the athlete in a neutral spine position. By not catching the bar, higher loads (>100% of the 1RM) can be used, thereby emphasizing the quality of strength speed (6, 22, 23). Pull variations can also be initiated from the same positions as hang variations (i.e., power position, mid-thigh, above the knee, and below the knee).

Exercise Finder

Exercise	Exercise progression	Page number
Barbell power jerk	Jerk-related	224
Barbell push press	Jerk-related	223
Barbell split jerk	Jerk-related	226
Dumbbell power clean to push press	Jerk-related	227
Dumbbell power jerk	Jerk-related	230
Dumbbell push press	Jerk-related	228
Dumbbell split jerk	Jerk-related	231
Fast clean pull from blocks	Power clean–related	222
Fast clean pull from the floor	Power clean–related	221
Fast snatch pull from blocks	Snatch-related	213
Fast snatch pull from the floor	Snatch-related	212
Heavy clean pull from blocks	Power clean–related	220
Heavy clean pull from the floor	Power clean–related	219
Heavy snatch pull from blocks	Snatch-related	211
Heavy snatch pull from the floor	Snatch-related	210
Landmine deadlift to rotational press	Jerk-related	232
Power clean from blocks	Power clean–related	217
Power clean from a hang	Power clean–related	215
Power clean from the floor	Power clean–related	218
Power snatch from blocks	Snatch-related	207

(continued)

Snatch-Related Progressions

POWER SNATCH FROM A HANG

Aim

To develop explosive power in the vertical plane. This exercise is less technically demanding than the power snatch from the floor.

Action

1. Using a wide overhand or hook grip, begin by taking hold of a loaded barbell from a lifting rack (or set of blocks) set at mid-thigh height.

2. Position the feet between hip- and shoulder-width apart and facing forward.

3. Flex the knees slightly, and with a neutral spine, flex at the hips and lean the torso forward to allow the barbell to move down the thighs to a starting position just above the knees (i.e., hang position) (photo *a*). At this position, the shoulders should be over the barbell with the elbows pointed out to the sides and the head facing forward.

4. Begin the movement by rapidly extending the hips, knees, and ankles while maintaining the shoulder position over the barbell.

5. Allow the barbell to slide up the thighs to ensure that it remains as close to the body as possible.

6. As the lower body joints reach full extension, rapidly shrug the shoulders.

7. When the shoulders reach their highest point, allow the elbows to flex to begin pulling the body under the barbell (photo *b*). The explosive nature of this phase may cause the feet to lose contact with the floor.

8. Simultaneously flex the hips and knees into a quarter squat and continue to pull the body under the barbell.

9. Once the body is under the bar, catch the bar in the straight-arm overhead receiving position described earlier.

10. Recover to a standing position while maintaining the barbell in the straight-arm overhead receiving position (photo *c*).

11. In a controlled fashion, lower the barbell by flexing at the elbows and reducing the muscular tension in the shoulders. Simultaneously flex the hips and knees as the barbell is lowered to the thighs.

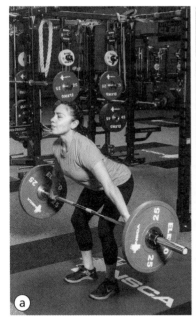 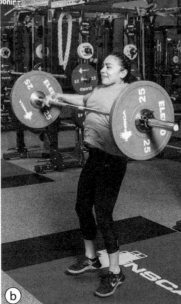 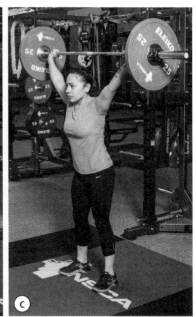

POWER SNATCH FROM BLOCKS

Aim

To develop explosive power in the vertical plane using loads that are typically heavier than those used for the power snatch from a hang. Conversely, one can use lighter loads from blocks to focus on the technical aspects of the exercise.

Action

1. Using a wide overhand or hook grip, begin with a loaded barbell on a set of lifting blocks. The height of the lifting blocks should position the barbell just above the knees.

2. At the starting position, the shoulders should be over the barbell with the elbows pointing out and the head facing forward.

3. To complete the power snatch from blocks variation (photos a-c), refer to steps 4 through 11 of the power snatch from a hang.

4. In a controlled fashion, lower the barbell by flexing at the elbows and reducing the muscular tension in the shoulders. Simultaneously flex the hips and knees as the barbell is lowered to the blocks.

Note: Use blocks of different heights to focus on different phases of the movement or to make the exercise more specific. For example, low blocks will allow a loaded barbell to be set from a starting position just below knee level, which will enable the athlete to focus on the transition phase from the first pull (i.e., from the floor to below the knee) to the second pull (i.e., from above the knee to maximal hip and knee extension). Conversely, higher blocks will allow a loaded barbell to be set from a mid-thigh starting position, which will enable an individual to emphasize a rapid hip and knee extension.

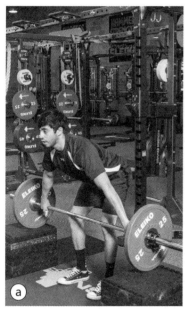 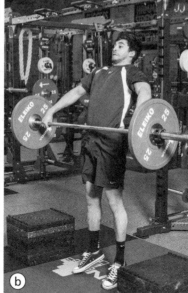 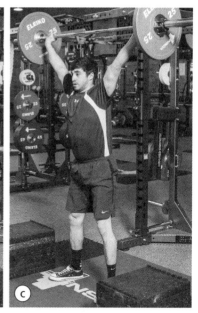

POWER SNATCH FROM THE FLOOR

Aim

To develop explosive power from the ground in the vertical plane.

Action

1. Begin with a loaded barbell on the ground.

2. From standing, position the barbell approximately a fist's width from the shins and use a wide overhand or hook grip.

3. Position the heels between hip- and shoulder-width apart, with the feet slightly turned out.

4. To achieve an ideal starting position, lower the hips, elevate the chest, point the elbows out, direct the eyes slightly upward, and align the head with the spine. The shoulders must remain over the barbell in this set position while maintaining a neutral back (photo a).

5. Begin the movement by extending the hips and knees to lift the barbell off the floor while maintaining the barbell close to the shins. This initial phase of the exercise is the first pull. During this phase, maintain a neutral spine position, with the shoulders over the barbell. Do not let the hips rise before the shoulders rise; the torso-to-floor angle must be kept constant during this phase.

6. As the barbell rises above the knees, begin the second pull by moving the knees under the barbell so it slides up the thighs.

7. Rapidly extend the hips, knees, and ankles (triple extension) while the shoulders remain in line with the barbell, and point the elbows out to the sides. The explosive nature of this phase may cause the feet to lose contact with the floor.

8. As the lower body joints reach full extension, rapidly shrug the shoulders (photo b).

9. When the shoulders reach their highest point, allow the elbows to flex to begin pulling the body under the barbell.
10. Simultaneously flex the hips and knees into a quarter-squat position while continuing to forcefully pull the body below the barbell.
11. Once the body is under the bar, catch the bar in the straight-arm overhead receiving position described earlier (photo c).
12. Recover to a standing position while maintaining the barbell in the straight-arm overhead receiving position (photo d).
13. In a controlled fashion, lower the barbell by flexing at the elbows and reducing the muscular tension in the shoulders. Simultaneously flex the hips and knees as the barbell is lowered to the floor.

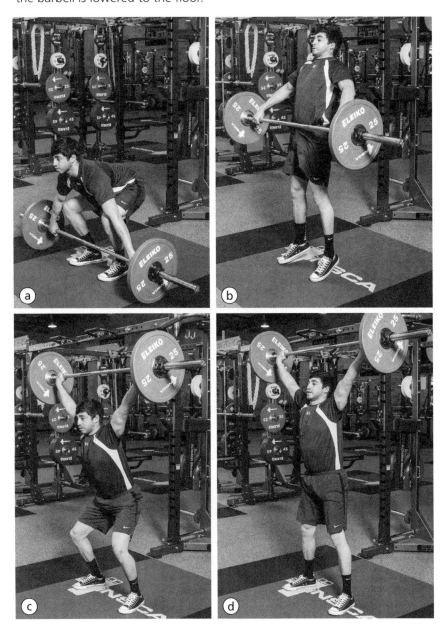

HEAVY SNATCH PULL FROM THE FLOOR

Aim

To develop strength off the floor and explosive strength during the second pull phase of the snatch.

Action

1. In a standing position, begin with a loaded barbell on the floor approximately a fist's width from the shins.

2. Position the heels approximately shoulder-width apart, with the feet and knees slightly turned out.

3. Take a wide overhand or hook grip on the bar. To achieve the ideal starting position, lower the hips, elevate the chest, point the elbows out, direct the eyes slightly upward (more than what is seen in photo *a*), and align the head with the spine. The shoulders must remain over the barbell in this set position.

4. To begin the movement, lift the barbell off the floor by extending the hips and knees while maintaining the barbell close to the shins. The spine remains in a neutral position, with the shoulders over the barbell. Do not let the hips rise before the shoulders rise; the torso-to-floor angle must be kept constant during this phase.

5. As the barbell rises above the knees, begin the second pull by moving the knees under the barbell to allow it to slide up the thighs.

6. Rapidly extend the hips, knees, and ankles (triple extension) while the shoulders remain in line with the barbell and the elbows point out to the sides (photo *b*).

7. Allow the barbell to slide up the thighs to ensure it remains as close to the body as possible.

8. As the joints of the lower body reach full extension, rapidly shrug the shoulders (photo *c*).

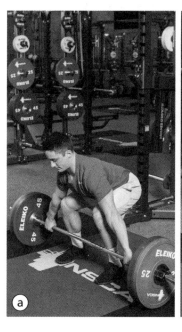
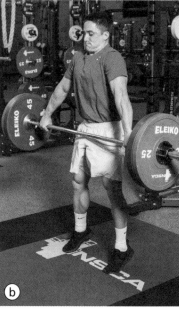
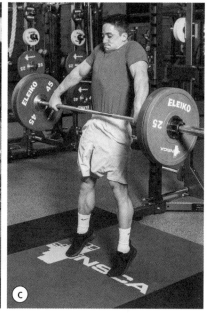

9. Allow the elbows to naturally flex in a relaxed fashion so the barbell remains close to the body as it rises in the vertical plane.

10. After the bar reaches its maximal height, flex at the knees and the hips to lower the barbell to the starting position on the floor. During this phase, the spine remains in a neutral position, with the shoulders over the barbell.

Note: During this exercise, the arms should remain relaxed and not actively engaged in an attempt to pull the bar up during the top extension phase. Emphasize the triple extension of the lower body, which is immediately followed by the explosive shoulder shrug.

HEAVY SNATCH PULL FROM BLOCKS

Aim

To develop explosive strength during the second pull phase of the snatch.

Action

1. Using a wide overhand or hook grip, begin with a loaded barbell on a set of lifting blocks. The lifting blocks should be set so that the barbell is positioned just above the knees.

2. At the starting position, the shoulders should be over the barbell, with the elbows pointing out and the head facing forward (photo *a*).

3. Rapidly extend the hips, knees, and ankles (triple extension) while the shoulders remain in line with the barbell and the elbows point out to the sides (photo *b*).

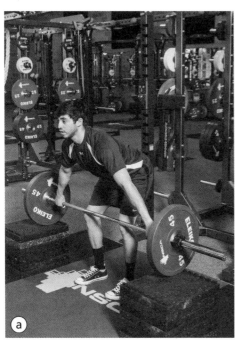
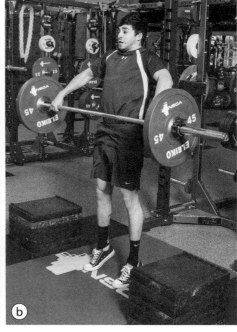

4. Allow the barbell to slide up the thighs to ensure it remains as close to the body as possible.
5. As the lower body joints reach full extension, rapidly shrug the shoulders.
6. Allow the elbows to naturally flex in a relaxed fashion so that the barbell remains close to the body as it rises in the vertical plane.
7. After the bar reaches its maximal height, flex at the knees and the hips to lower the barbell to the starting position on the blocks. During this phase, the spine remains in a neutral position, with the shoulders over the barbell.

Note: Use blocks of different heights to focus on different phases of the exercise or to make it more specific (e.g., to match the starting position joint angles of a sport-specific movement). In addition, the arms should remain relaxed during this exercise and not actively engaged in an attempt to pull the bar up during the top extension phase.

FAST SNATCH PULL FROM THE FLOOR

Aim
To develop explosive power from the floor in the vertical plane. This exercise also enables athletes to effectively train the timing and the mechanics of the transition from the explosive second pull to the "pulling under the bar" phase that occurs before moving into the overhead receiving position. The proper load can be determined by the height of the pull rather than a percentage of the 1RM, as that can vary from day to day. The correct load used for a fast pull will allow the athlete to elevate the bar to sternum height. Because of the high speed and complex nature of this exercise, it should not be performed when the athlete is fatigued. The correct form must be maintained throughout the execution.

Action
1. To complete the fast snatch pull from the floor, refer to points 1 to 8 of the heavy snatch pull from the floor.
2. As the shoulders reach their highest elevation, flex the elbows to forcefully pull the body under the rising barbell as the feet rapidly move into the receiving position. During this phase, the trunk should remain relatively upright; the chest should not lean over the barbell (photos a, b).
3. Keep the barbell as close to the body as possible during this movement and emphasize attaining a high barbell velocity. Thus, the velocity of the movement greatly dictates the load that should be used.
4. Upon completion of the rapid-pulling-under phase, flex at the knees and the hips to lower the barbell to the starting position on the floor. During this phase, the spine remains in a neutral position with the shoulders over the barbell.

Note: This exercise is ideal for athletes who are unable to achieve the straight-arm overhead receiving position of the snatch because of injury or mobility issues. However, it is not recommended for those who fail to fully extend during the second pull of the snatch-related exercises, because it can reinforce a poor technique habit (e.g., pulling the chest into the barbell). In addition, emphasize the triple extension of the lower body and immediately follow it with an explosive shoulder shrug. Avoid excessive use of the arms during this exercise and flex the elbows only after completing the lower body triple extension and upper body shrug.

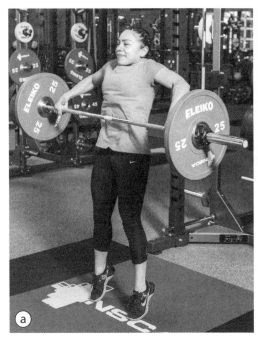 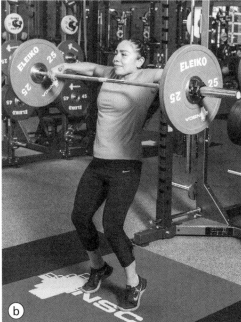

FAST SNATCH PULL FROM BLOCKS

Aim

To develop explosive power in the vertical plane.

Action

1. Using a wide overhand or hook grip, begin with a loaded barbell on a set of lifting blocks. Set the height of the lifting blocks so the barbell is positioned just above the level of the knees.

2. At the starting position, the shoulders should be over the barbell, the elbows pointing out, and the head facing forward.

3. Rapidly extend the hips, knees, and ankles (triple extension) while the shoulders remain in line with the barbell and the elbows point out to the sides.

4. To complete the fast snatch pull from blocks, refer to steps 2 and 3 of the fast snatch pull from the floor.

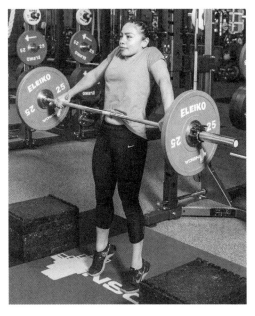

5. Upon completion of the rapid-pulling-under phase, flex at the knees and the hips to lower the barbell to the starting position on the blocks. During this phase, the spine remains in a neutral position with the shoulders over the barbell.

Note: Because of the high speed and the complex nature of this exercise, this movement should not be performed when the athlete is fatigued. The correct form must be maintained throughout the execution.

SINGLE-ARM DUMBBELL SNATCH

Aim

To develop explosive power in the vertical plane. This exercise is less technically demanding than the barbell power snatch variations.

Action

1. With the feet positioned approximately shoulder-width apart, straddle a dumbbell. The feet and knees are slightly turned out.

2. Squat at the hips and grasp the dumbbell with a closed, pronated grip. In the starting position, the shoulders should be over the dumbbell, with the arm fully extended and the head facing forward (photo a). The athlete can also initiate this exercise from a hang position, whereby the dumbbell is lifted to knee level instead of starting from the floor.

3. Begin the upward movement by rapidly extending the hips, knees, and ankles while maintaining the shoulder position over the dumbbell.

4. Allow the dumbbell to rise in the vertical plane while keeping it as close to the thighs as possible.

5. As the lower body joints reach full extension, rapidly shrug the shoulder of the arm that is holding the dumbbell. Place the other hand on the opposite hip or hold the other arm out to the side.

6. When the shoulder reaches its highest elevation, flex the elbow to begin pulling the body under the dumbbell (photo b). The explosive nature of this phase may cause the feet to lose contact with the floor.

7. Simultaneously flex the hips and knees into a quarter-squat position while forcefully continuing to pull the body under the dumbbell.

8. Once the body is under the dumbbell, catch the weight in the straight-arm overhead receiving position. In this position, the dumbbell is positioned over and slightly behind the athlete's ears (photo c). When viewed from the side, the athlete's ears should not be blocked from view by the arm. Place the other hand on the opposite hip or hold the other arm out to the side for extra balance.

9. Recover to a standing position while maintaining the dumbbell in the straight-arm overhead receiving position.

10. In a controlled fashion, lower the dumbbell to the shoulder, then to the thigh, and finally to the floor. In the hang variation of the dumbbell snatch, the dumbbell does not start on the floor or return to the floor between repetitions.

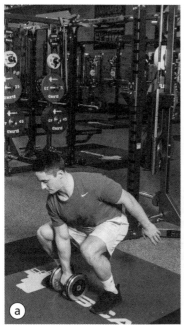 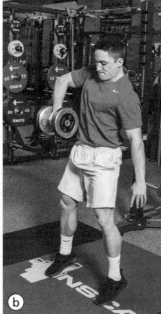 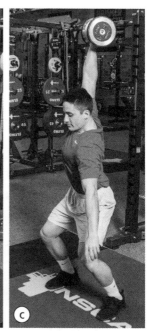

Power Clean–Related Progressions

POWER CLEAN FROM A HANG

Aim

To develop explosive power in the vertical plane. This exercise is less technically demanding than the power clean from the floor.

Action

1. Using a slightly wider than shoulder-width pronated or hook grip, begin by taking hold of a loaded barbell in a lifting rack (or set of blocks) that is set at midthigh height.
2. Position the heels approximately shoulder-width apart, with the feet facing slightly outward.
3. Flex the knees and hips to lean the torso forward, allowing the barbell to move down the thighs to a starting position that is just above the knees. At this position, the shoulders should be over the barbell, the elbows pointing out, and the head facing forward (more than what is seen in photo *a*) and in line with the spine.
4. Begin the upward movement by rapidly extending the hips, knees, and ankles while maintaining the shoulder position over the barbell.
5. Allow the barbell to slide up the thighs to ensure it remains as close to the body as possible.
6. As the joints of the lower body reach full extension, rapidly shrug the shoulders.
7. When the shoulders reach their highest elevation, flex the elbows to enable the barbell to remain close to the body as it rises in the vertical plane (photo *b*). The explosive nature of this phase may cause the feet to lose contact with the floor.

8. Rapidly move the feet and legs into a quarter-squat position while forcefully pulling the body under the barbell.

9. As the body moves under the barbell, rapidly thrust the elbows forward to catch the barbell on the front of the shoulders (photo c).

10. In the catch position, the torso is nearly erect, the shoulders are slightly in front of the hips, and the head remains in a neutral position.

11. Recover to a standing position with the barbell on the front of the shoulders (photo d).

12. In a controlled fashion, lower the elbows to unrack the barbell from the shoulders, then slowly lower the barbell to the thighs.

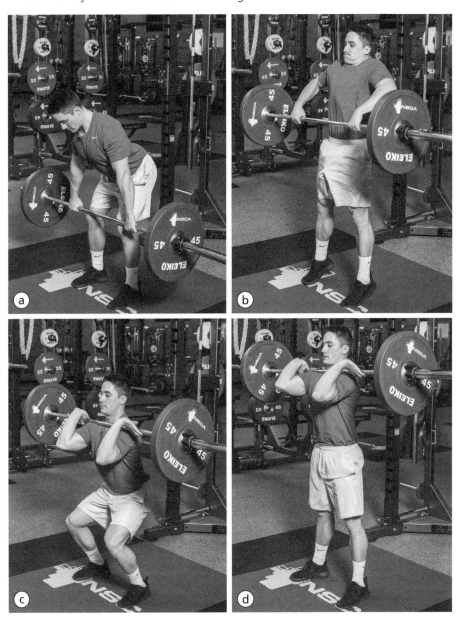

POWER CLEAN FROM BLOCKS

Aim

To develop explosive power in the vertical plane by using loads that are typically heavier than those used for the power clean from a hang. Conversely, using lighter loads from blocks allows the athlete to focus on the technical aspects of the exercise.

Action

1. Using a slightly wider than shoulder-width pronated or hook grip, begin with a loaded barbell on a set of lifting blocks. Set the height of the lifting blocks so the barbell is positioned just above the knees.
2. At the starting position, the shoulders are over the barbell, with the elbows pointing out and the head facing forward (more than what is seen in photo a).
3. To complete the power clean from blocks (photos b, c), refer to points 4 to 11 of the power clean from a hang.
4. Upon completion of the recovery phase, lower the elbows to unrack the barbell from the shoulders in a controlled fashion and slowly lower the barbell to the blocks.

Note: Use blocks of different heights so the athlete can focus on different phases of the exercise.

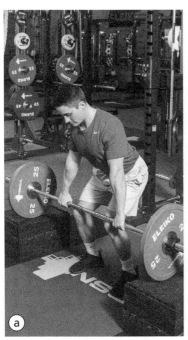
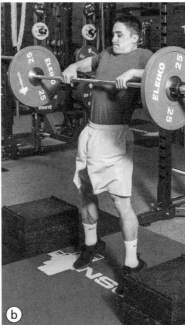
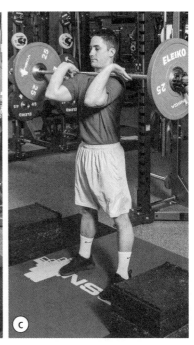

POWER CLEAN FROM THE FLOOR

Aim

To develop explosive power from the floor in the vertical plane.

Action

1. Begin with a loaded barbell on the floor.

2. Stand with the heels approximately shoulder-width apart and with the feet facing forward or slightly outward. Set the barbell approximately a fist's width in front of the shins and over the balls of the feet.

3. To achieve an ideal starting position, take a slightly wider than shoulder-width pronated or hook grip, lower the hips, elevate the chest, point the elbows out, and direct the eyes slightly upward. The shoulders must remain over the barbell in this set position while maintaining a neutral back (photo a).

4. Begin the first pull by extending the knees and hips while maintaining the shoulders over the barbell. Do not let the hips rise before the shoulders rise; the torso-to-floor angle must be kept constant during this phase.

5. As the barbell rises above the knees, begin the second pull by moving the knees under the barbell to allow it to slide up the thighs.

6. Rapidly extend the hips, knees, and ankles while the shoulders remain in line with the barbell and the elbows point out to the sides.

7. As the lower body joints reach full extension, rapidly shrug the shoulders.

8. When the shoulders reach their highest elevation, flex the elbows to enable the barbell to remain close to the body as it rises in the vertical plane. The explosive nature of this phase may cause the feet to lose contact with the floor (photo b).

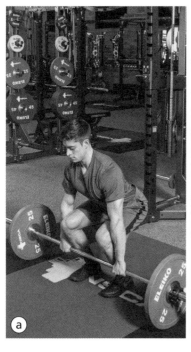 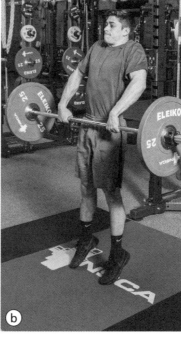 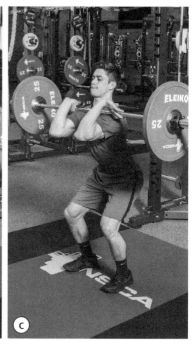

9. Rapidly move the feet and legs into a quarter-squat position while forcefully pulling the body under the barbell.

10. As the body moves under the barbell, rapidly thrust the elbows forward to catch the barbell on the front of the shoulders (photo c).

11. In the catch position, the torso is nearly erect, the shoulders are slightly in front of the hips, and the head is in a neutral position. (The grip on the bar should be more closed than what is seen in photo c.)

12. Recover to a standing position, with the barbell on the front of the shoulders.

13. In a controlled fashion, lower the elbows to unrack the barbell from the shoulders, then slowly lower the barbell to the floor.

For sample intensities, sets, and repetitions for the snatch and clean, including power variations, see table 8.1.

Table 8.1 Sample Loads (Intensity), Repetitions, Sets, and Volumes for Snatch and Clean Variations

Intensity (% 1RM)	Reps	Sets	Reps per session (i.e., volume)
70%-80%	4	4-5	16-20
80%-85%	4	3-4	12-16
90%-92%	3	3-4	9-12
≥95%	1-2	3-4	3-8

Note: If performing snatch variations, the load should be based off a 1-repetition maximum (1RM) snatch, whereas if performing power snatch variations, the load should be based off a 1RM power snatch. The same approach to determining appropriate loads should be adopted for clean variations.

HEAVY CLEAN PULL FROM THE FLOOR

Aim
To develop strength off the floor and explosive strength during the second pull phase of the clean.

Action

1. Begin with a loaded barbell on the floor.

2. Stand with the heels approximately shoulder-width apart, the feet facing forward or slightly outward, and the barbell set approximately a fist's width in front of the shins and over the balls of the feet.

3. To achieve an ideal starting position, take a slightly wider than shoulder-width pronated or hook grip, lower the hips, elevate the chest, point the elbows out, and direct the eyes slightly upward. The shoulders must remain over the barbell in this set position while maintaining a neutral back.

4. Begin the first pull by extending the knees and hips while maintaining the shoulders over the barbell (photo a). Do not let the hips rise before the shoulders; the torso-to-floor angle must be kept constant during this phase.

5. As the barbell rises above the knees, begin the second pull by moving the knees under the barbell to allow it to slide up the thighs.

6. Rapidly extend the hips, knees, and ankles while the shoulders remain in line with the barbell and the elbows point out to the sides.

7. As the lower body joints reach full extension, rapidly shrug the shoulders (photo b).

8. When the shoulders reach their highest elevation, allow the elbows to flex naturally in a relaxed fashion. This enables the barbell to remain close to the body while rising in the vertical plane.

9. After the bar reaches its maximal height, flex at the knees and the hips to lower the barbell to the starting position on the floor. During this phase, the spine remains in a neutral position, with the shoulders over the barbell.

Note: During this exercise, keep the arms relaxed and not actively engaged in an attempt to pull the bar up during the top extension phase.

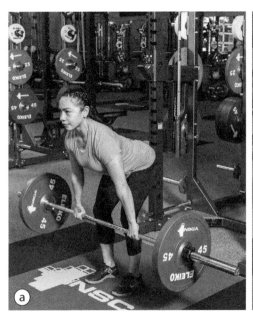 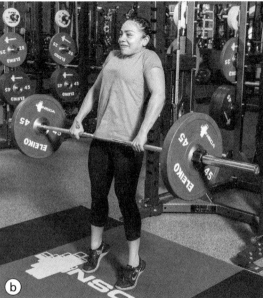

HEAVY CLEAN PULL FROM BLOCKS

Aim

To develop explosive strength during the second pull phase of the clean.

Action

1. Using a slightly wider than shoulder-width pronated or hook grip, begin with a loaded barbell on a set of lifting blocks. Set the height of the lifting blocks so that the barbell is positioned just above the knees.

2. At the starting position, the shoulders are over the barbell, with the elbows pointing out and the head facing forward.

3. Rapidly extend the hips, knees, and ankles while the shoulders remain in line with the barbell and the elbows point out to the sides.

4. Allow the barbell to slide up the thighs to ensure that it remains as close to the body as possible.

5. As the lower body joints reach full extension, rapidly shrug the shoulders.

6. Allow the elbows to flex naturally in a relaxed fashion to enable the barbell to remain close to the body as the barbell rises in the vertical plane.

7. After the bar reaches its maximal height, flex at the knees and the hips to lower the barbell to the starting position on the blocks. During this phase, the spine remains in a neutral position, with the shoulders over the barbell.

FAST CLEAN PULL FROM THE FLOOR

Aim

To develop explosive power from the floor in the vertical plane. This exercise also enables athletes to train the timing and the mechanics of the transition from the explosive second pull to the pulling-under phase that occurs before moving into the barbell-catch position effectively. Commonly performed with loads 60% to 80% of the 1RM for a clean.

Action

1. To complete the fast clean pull from the floor, refer to points 1 to 7 of the heavy clean pull from the floor.

2. As the shoulders reach their highest elevation, flex the elbows to forcefully pull the body down as it moves under the barbell and the feet move rapidly into the receiving position. During this phase, the trunk should remain relatively upright; the chest should not lean over the barbell.

3. Keep the barbell as close to the body as possible during this movement and emphasize an explosive second pull phase.

4. Upon completion of the rapid-pulling-under phase, flex at the knees and the hips to lower the barbell to the starting position from the floor. During this phase, the spine remains in a neutral position with the shoulders over the barbell.

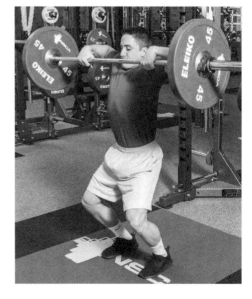

Note: This exercise is ideal for athletes who are unable to achieve the power clean catch position because of injury or mobility issues. However, it is not recommended for athletes who fail to fully extend during the second pull of the clean-related exercises, because it can reinforce a poor technique habit. Although emphasis should be on attaining a high barbell velocity during this exercise, athletes should avoid using the arms excessively. The resulting velocity of the movement greatly dictates the loads that can be used. This exercise should not be performed when fatigued, because correct technique must be adhered to at all times.

FAST CLEAN PULL FROM BLOCKS

Aim

To develop explosive power in the vertical plane.

Action

1. Using a slightly wider than shoulder-width overhand or hook grip, begin with a loaded barbell on a set of lifting blocks. Set the height of the lifting blocks so the barbell is just above knee level.

2. At the starting position, the shoulders are over the barbell, with the elbows pointing out and the head facing forward (photo a).

3. Rapidly extend the hips, knees, and ankles (triple extension) while the shoulders remain in line with the barbell and the elbows point out to the sides.

4. To complete the fast clean pull from blocks (photos b, c), refer to points 2 to 3 of the fast clean pull from the floor.

5. Upon completion of the rapid-pulling-under phase, flex at the knees and the hips to lower the barbell to the starting position from the blocks. During this phase, the spine remains in a neutral position, with the shoulders over the barbell.

Note: Because of the high speed and complex nature of this exercise, do not perform this movement while fatigued. Correct form must be maintained throughout the execution.

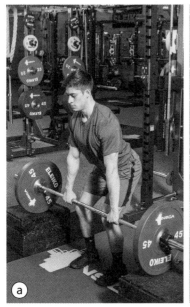
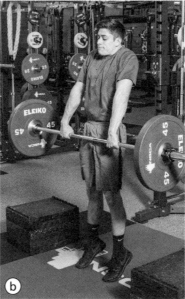
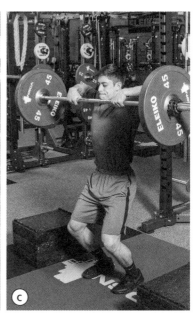

Refer to table 8.2 for sample intensities, sets, and repetitions for pulling variations.

Table 8.2 Sample Loads (Intensity), Repetitions, Sets, and Volumes for Pulls

Intensity (% 1RM)	Reps	Sets	Reps per session (i.e., volume)
PULLS FROM THE FLOOR			
80%-90%	5	3-4	15-20
90%-95%	4	3-4	12-16
95%-100%	3	3-4	9-12
100%-120%	1-2	4	4-8
PULLS FROM HIGH-THIGH OR THE KNEE (CAN BE PERFORMED WITH HIGHER LOADS DUE TO THE REDUCED BARBELL DISPLACEMENT, ALSO PERMITTING GREATER VOLUMES DUE TO THE REDUCED WORK)			
100%-140%	3-6	3-4	9-24

Adapted from Comfort and colleagues (6).

Jerk-Related Progressions

BARBELL PUSH PRESS

Aim

To develop overhead strength and explosive power.

Action

1. Using a slightly wider than shoulder-width grip, begin with a loaded barbell set across the shoulders in a fashion similar to the receiving position of a power clean (photo a).
2. Position the heels hip- to shoulder-width apart, with the feet slightly turned out.
3. While keeping the torso vertical, tuck the chin and initiate the downward movement by flexing the hips and knees. The dip should be relatively shallow, not to exceed a quarter squat (photo b).
4. At the lowest point of the dip, forcefully drive through the heels by extending the hips, knees, and ankles to raise the barbell in the vertical plane. The timing of the dip into the drive phase should be similar to that of a countermovement jump.
5. Using the momentum created by the leg drive, continue the movement by forcefully pressing the barbell overhead into a fully extended arm position. As the barbell passes the face, move the head from a chin-tucked position to a slightly forward position (photo c).
6. In the straight-arm overhead position, the barbell is slightly over or behind the ears.
7. Lower the barbell by gradually reducing the muscular tension of the arms to allow a controlled descent of the barbell to the shoulders while simultaneously flexing at the hips and knees to cushion the impact.

Note: The body remains in an extended position during the overhead pressing-to-receiving movement. This differs from the barbell power jerk, which is described next.

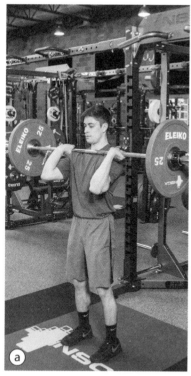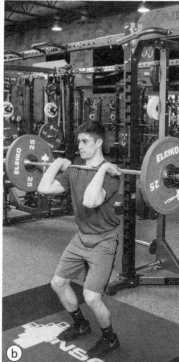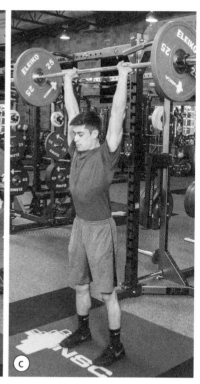

BARBELL POWER JERK

Aim

To develop overhead strength and explosive power.

Action

1. Using a slightly wider than shoulder-width grip, begin with a loaded barbell set across the shoulders in a fashion similar to the receiving position of a power clean.

2. Position the heels hip- to shoulder-width apart, with the feet slightly turned out (photo *a*).

3. While keeping the torso vertical, tuck the chin and initiate the downward movement by flexing the hips and the knees. The dip should be relatively shallow and should not exceed that of a quarter squat.

4. At the lowest point of the dip, forcefully drive through the heels by extending the hips, knees, and ankles to raise the barbell in the vertical plane. The barbell should remain in a straight vertical path during the jerk dip to jerk drive phases. In addition, the timing of the dip into the drive phase should be similar to that of a countermovement jump (photo *b*).

5. Using the momentum created by the leg drive, continue the movement by explosively driving the barbell in the vertical plane (photo *c*) as the body is driven underneath the barbell into the straight-arm overhead receiving position. As the barbell passes the face, move the head from a chin-tucked position to a slightly forward position.

6. In the straight-arm overhead receiving position of the power jerk, the barbell is slightly behind the ears, and the knees should be flexed to approximately a quarter-squat position (photo *d*).

7. Recover to a standing position while maintaining the barbell in the straight-arm overhead receiving position.

8. Lower the barbell by gradually reducing the muscular tension of the arms to allow a controlled descent of the barbell to the shoulders while simultaneously flexing at the hips and knees to cushion the impact.

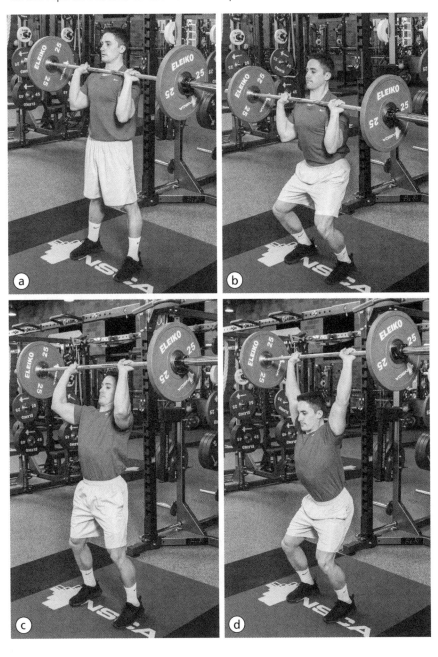

BARBELL SPLIT JERK

Aim

To develop overhead strength and explosive power.

Action

1. Using a slightly wider than shoulder-width grip, begin with a loaded barbell set across the top of the shoulders and the chest.

2. Position the heels approximately shoulder-width apart, with the feet slightly turned out (photo a).

3. While keeping the torso vertical, tuck the chin and initiate the downward movement by flexing the hips and knees (photo b). The dip should be relatively shallow and should not exceed a quarter squat.

4. At the lowest point of the dip, forcefully drive through the heels by extending the hips, knees, and ankles while driving the barbell overhead. As the barbell passes the face, move the head from a chin-tucked position to a slightly forward position. The barbell should remain in a straight vertical path during the jerk dip to jerk drive phases. In addition, the timing of the dip into the drive phase should be similar to that of a countermovement jump.

5. As the bar travels upward in the vertical plane, quickly move into the straight-arm overhead receiving position of the split jerk as the bar reaches its highest point. The feet should be positioned approximately shoulder-width apart and evenly split from the starting position to achieve a stable lockout position (photo c).

6. Determination of which foot is the lead foot is based on trial and error. Upon teaching the split position, the foot that immediately feels more comfortable should be the dominant lead foot. In many athletic applications, it is recommended that athletes alternate the lead foot on a repetition-by-repetition or set-by-set basis to avoid developing an imbalance. In the sport of weightlifting, it is suggested that athletes practice nearly exclusively with the dominant foot forward.

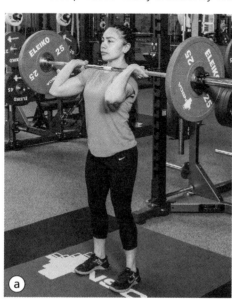
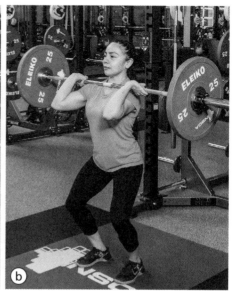

7. In the receiving or overhead lockout position, the barbell is behind the ears. In addition, the heel of the back foot is raised from the floor, and the weight is evenly distributed through both feet.

8. Recover from the split position by returning the front foot to the starting position, followed by the back foot (photo *d*).

9. Lower the barbell gradually by reducing the muscular tension of the arms to allow a controlled descent of the barbell to the shoulders while simultaneously flexing at the hips and knees to cushion the impact.

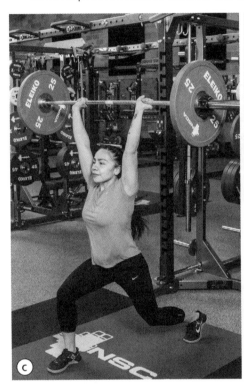
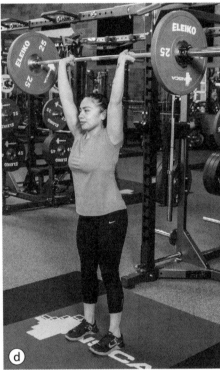

DUMBBELL POWER CLEAN TO PUSH PRESS

Aim

To develop explosive power during a full-body extension and overhead movement.

Action

1. Begin by using a neutral grip to hold a pair of dumbbells. The feet are flat on the floor between hip- and shoulder-width apart, with the toes pointed slightly outward (photo *a*).

2. With a neutral spine, flex at the hips and knees slightly so both dumbbells are at midthigh height and outside of the thighs.

3. Rapidly extend through the hips, knees, and ankles.

4. As the lower body joints reach full extension, rapidly shrug the shoulders.

5. When the shoulders reach their highest point, flex the elbows and receive the dumbbells on the front of the shoulders, using a neutral grip. During the catch phase, flex the hips and knees to absorb the impact of the dumbbells (photo *b*).

6. Immediately following the dumbbell catch phase, forcefully drive up from the dipped position through the heels to raise the dumbbells in the vertical plane.

7. Using the momentum created by the leg drive, continue the movement by explosively driving the dumbbells overhead (photo *c*).

8. In the straight-arm overhead position, the dumbbells are slightly over or behind the ears with a neutral grip, and the legs are fully extended.

9. Lower the dumbbells by gradually reducing the muscular tension of the arms to allow a controlled descent of the dumbbells to the shoulders while simultaneously flexing at the hips and knees to cushion the impact.

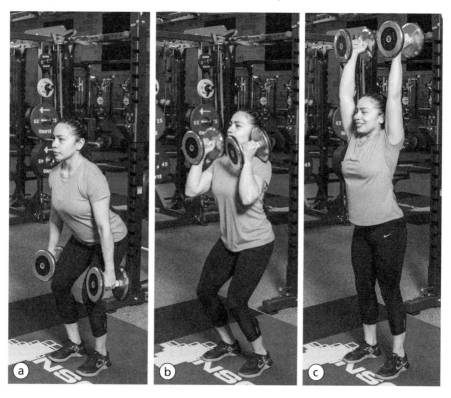

DUMBBELL PUSH PRESS

Aim

To develop full-body power with an emphasis on upper body extension.

Action

1. Begin with dumbbells at the shoulders in a neutral grip. The near head of the dumbbell can be resting on the shoulders, while the feet are flat on the ground and between hip- and shoulder-width apart. The feet can be slightly externally rotated (photo *a*).

2. With a neutral spine, flex at the hips and knees simultaneously while keeping the feet flat on the ground. It is important not to rise onto the toes during this phase of the movement.

3. The depth of the dip should be roughly 10% of total height, emphasizing dorsi-flexion and knee flexion, while maintaining an upright torso (photo b).

4. Rapidly change direction to hip and knee extension.

5. When the lower body joints reach extension, the dumbbells should be driven off the shoulders (photo c). Use this momentum and continue with the hands to drive the dumbbells, locking out overhead without re-flexing the knees or hips (photo d).

6. In the straight-arm overhead position, the dumbbells are slightly over or behind the ears with a neutral grip, and the legs are fully extended.

7. Lower the dumbbells by gradually reducing the muscular tension of the arms to allow a controlled descent of the dumbbells to the shoulders while simultaneously flexing at the hips and knees to cushion the impact.

Variation

This movement can be done with one dumbbell at a time, with the aim of improving core engagement through antilateral flexion.

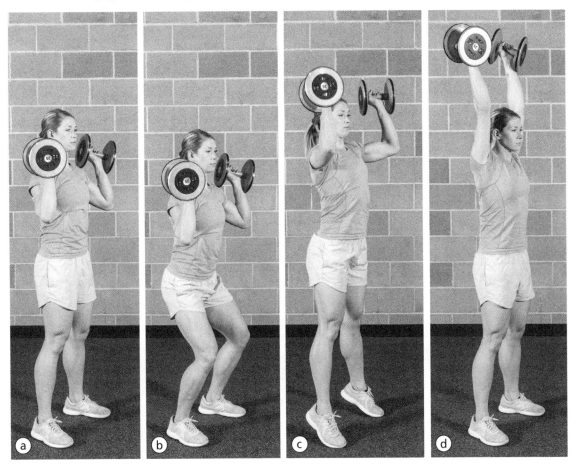

DUMBBELL POWER JERK

Aim

To develop full body power using a rapid flexion and extension cycle.

Action

1. Begin with dumbbells at the shoulders in a neutral grip. The near head of the dumbbell can be resting on the shoulders, while the feet are flat on the ground and approximately hip-width apart. The feet can be slightly externally rotated (photo a).

2. With a neutral spine, flex at the hips and knees simultaneously while keeping the feet flat on the ground (photo b). This portion of the lift should occur with the line of mass through the middle of the foot.

3. The depth of the dip should be roughly 10% of total height.

4. Rapidly change direction to hip and knee extension.

5. When the lower body joints reach extension, the dumbbells should be driven off the shoulders (photo c). Use this momentum and continue with the hands to drive the dumbbells to lockout overhead.

6. Simultaneously flex the knees and hips and resituate the feet to a slightly wider stance to receive the dumbbells overhead (photo d).

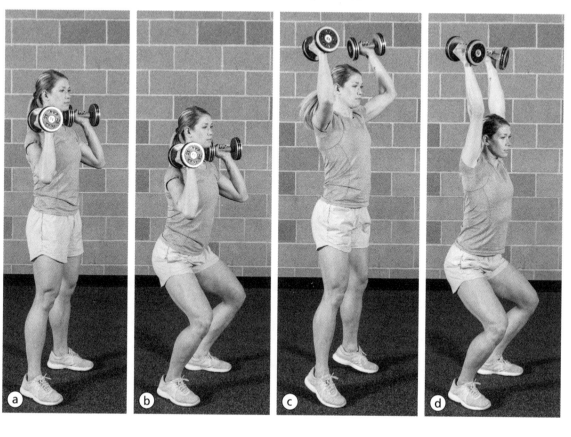

7. At receiving, meet the dumbbells firmly with the arms extended overhead, in line with or slightly behind the ears, with the feet flat on the ground.

8. Recover back to a fully standing position with the feet under the hips (not shown).

9. Lower the dumbbells by gradually reducing the muscular tension of the arms to allow a controlled descent of the dumbbells to the shoulders while simultaneously flexing at the hips and knees to cushion the impact.

Variation

This movement can be done with one dumbbell at a time, with the aim of improving core engagement through antilateral flexion.

DUMBBELL SPLIT JERK

Aim

To develop full body power using a rapid flexion and extension cycle.

Action

1. Begin with dumbbells at the shoulders in a neutral grip. The near head of the dumbbell can be resting on the shoulders, while the feet are flat on the ground and approximately hip-width apart. The feet can be slightly externally rotated (photo a).

2. With a neutral spine, flex at the hips and knees simultaneously while keeping the feet flat on the ground (photo b). This portion of the lift should occur with the line of mass through the middle of the foot.

3. The depth of the dip should be roughly 10% of total height.

4. Rapidly change direction to hip and knee extension without pausing in the bottom of the dip.

5. As the dumbbells travel upward due to the force of hip and knee extension, simultaneously push upward with the hands to extend the elbows (photo c). During this time, resituate the feet so that one foot is driven forward and the other is driven back.

6. The feet will land shoulder-width apart, with the lead shin roughly perpendicular to the ground and the foot flat on the ground. The rear leg should be flexed at the knee during receiving, with the back heel off the ground and the toes facing forward (photo d).

7. Alternate the lead foot on a repetition-by-repetition or a set-by-set basis.

8. Recover to a parallel stance, with the front foot taking a half step back prior to the rear foot taking a half step forward (not shown).

9. Lower the dumbbells by gradually reducing the muscular tension of the arms to allow a controlled descent of the dumbbells to the shoulders while simultaneously flexing at the hips and knees to cushion the impact.

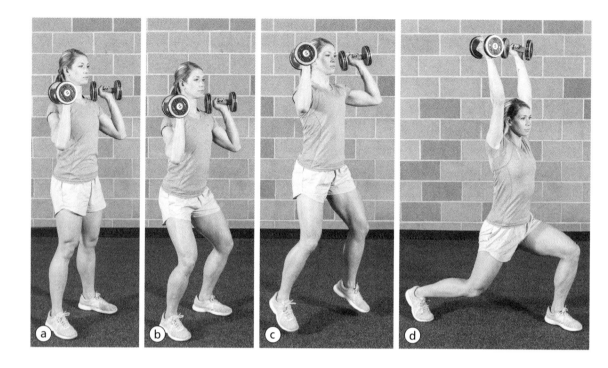

LANDMINE DEADLIFT
TO ROTATIONAL PRESS

Aim

To develop full-body power through the transverse plane.

Action

1. Secure a barbell in a freestanding or rack-based landmine attachment.

2. Assume a shoulder-width stance with the attachment point to the left or right and the sleeve of the barbell resting in front of the feet.

3. Squat down with a neutral spine and grasp the end (but not the very end) of the barbell in the hand nearest to the attachment point using an overhand (pronated) grip (photo a). The other hand should be opened and ready to receive the bar after it is lifted (i.e., step 7).

4. Lift rapidly from the ground by driving through the entire base of support in both feet. The angle of the torso should remain relatively constant as the bar moves from the ground to the mid-thigh level (photo b).

5. At the mid-thigh level, begin rotating the outside leg toward the attachment point. This rotation will continue through the remainder of the movement.

6. Extend the hips, knees, and ankles explosively.

7. As the bar reaches the level from the navel to the sternum, release the inside hand from the bar and, in its place, grasp the bar with the outside hand under the barbell to begin the push phase of the exercise (photo c).

8. Simultaneously, the lower body and now shoulders continue their rotation toward the attachment point.

9. As the bar reaches shoulder level (photo *d*), push with the arm to extension overhead.

10. While extending the arm overhead, drive the chest forward and push with the rear leg to extend the hip knee and ankle.

11. At completion, the arm will be overhead in line with or behind the ear, and a diagonal line will be created from the working arm through the rear foot (photo *e*).

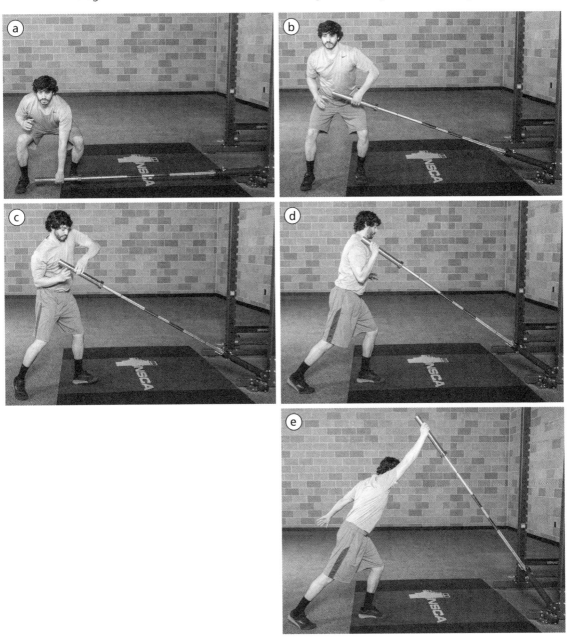

CONCLUSION

The total body power exercises described in this chapter are complex, whole-body movements that have a high degree of transference to many athletic movements, such as jumping, sprinting, and change of direction (1, 3, 4, 15, 24). Due to the complex and high-speed demands of these exercises, it is recommended to perform these movements in a nonfatigued state to ensure that correct technique is adhered to while maintaining a high-power focus during the performance of each repetition.

Similarities in set position, lifting, and receiving phases exist between the exercises described in this chapter. Therefore, acquiring an understanding of the key principles of maintaining a neutral spine, keeping the bar close to the body, and developing a strong straight-arm overhead receiving position will aid in the mastery of these movements. In addition, including lifting blocks or performing abbreviated versions of the exercises (e.g., starting from a hang position) enables individuals to focus on different phases of the movement and make the exercise more specific to their needs (e.g., to match the starting position joint angles of a sport-specific movement).

Advanced Power Techniques

Duncan N. French
Gavin C. Pratt

In the pursuit of enhanced levels of muscular power, athletes and coaches alike are adopting an ever-increasing number of novel training strategies. Some of these strategies focus on the augmentation of peak instantaneous power within a given time constant (P_{peak}), which is usually between 1 and 10 milliseconds, depending on the device sampling frequency, or on generating the maximum amount of power output that can be achieved irrespective of contraction time (P_{max}). Other individuals are exploring mean power or mean velocity within a given time constant (i.e., 1-10 milliseconds) as a proxy for power. This desire reflects the need to express mechanical power in sporting events during discrete muscle actions, where power is often considered a determinant of performance (70, 122). As discussed in previous chapters, central to many approaches to power training are exercise modalities such as plyometrics, heavy resistance training, explosive strength training, and a variety of jumps, throws, strikes, and bounds (30, 99, 121). However, as is apparent with all physical training, prolonged exposure to the same training stimuli can result in an accommodation to the imposed demands that leads to a consequent reduction in the magnitude of physiological adaption (140). Experienced athletes with a long training history who already possess high levels of muscular strength can also demonstrate a reduction in the effectiveness of training regimens that do not offer sufficient variation or overload (22, 24). In both scenarios, either when the body accommodates the training stress or when an experienced athlete does not exhibit sufficient sensitivity to a specific approach to power training, alternative or more advanced training methods must be adopted.

As discussed in previous chapters, mechanical power is derived from the force–velocity relationship. All effective power development programs are therefore underpinned by fundamental methods to increase maximal force, maximal contractile velocity, or both physical characteristics concurrently (14, 24, 72). Traditional approaches to both heavy resistance training (41) and plyometric-type high-velocity training (126) have been shown to change the characteristics of the force–velocity curve (chapter 3). These force–velocity responses are likely the result of morphological changes in the ultrastructure of muscles and tendons or specific adaptations to the neurological control of muscle activation (23). It is apparent that constituent parts of the force–velocity continuum (e.g., an increase in maximal force) can be changed through fundamental training approaches and that such changes lead to consequent alterations in the characteristics of the whole force–velocity curve. In turn, a change in the curvature of the force–velocity relationship can cause an upward shift in the mechanical power product, resulting in a training-induced shift in maximal power output (figure 9.1).

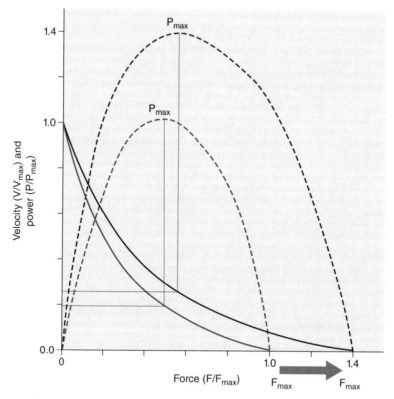

Figure 9.1 Changing the force–velocity relationship. Changing constituent parts of the force–velocity curve (e.g., increased maximum force, F_{max}) affects the associated power output.

Several studies have demonstrated the benefits of heavy resistance training on the expression of P_{max} (22, 47, 120). Other studies have indicated that high-velocity training (e.g., plyometrics) can improve maximal power output during discrete lower body jumping exercises (39, 126). However, in the applied practice of physical training, where efforts are focused on changing discrete qualities in the force–velocity relationship, there is the risk that reduced training adaptation or even staleness can occur (40, 123). Instead, to facilitate continued improvements over time that optimize athletic performance, the athlete's training strategy must be adapted to meet the specific demands of power expression within his or her sport. Therefore, it is conceivable that using only one mechanical stimulus or a single approach to resistance training may not be appropriate for advanced applications (44). In such circumstances, by using training methods that introduce more complex stimuli across the force–velocity continuum, it may be possible to target structural, local, or global factors that regulate power expression (87). As such, the introduction of advanced power training methods at the correct time and with the appropriate progression may represent the mechanism needed to achieve new gains in muscular power expression.

TRAINING PHILOSOPHY

When traditional approaches to maximal strength and rate of force development (RFD) training no longer result in the desired magnitude of physiological or performance adaptation over a specified timeframe, athletes and coaches must find alternative approaches to develop muscular power. Advanced power training methods represent the stimulus required to introduce training variety, or increased intensity, that ultimately breaks a training plateau or promotes an ongoing increase in performance enhancement through new morphological and neurological adaptation (24). Within any given training regimen, there is a multitude of opportunities to modulate the characteristics of the training stress for it to be considered advanced in its approach. However, it is critical that more complex or advanced training methods are brought into the holistic physical development program at the correct time and with the appropriate progression and that advanced methods are not simply introduced adjunct to fundamental power training methods (i.e., increasing maximal force and maximal velocity). Instead, advanced power training techniques should be considered novel strategies that complement an athlete's individual needs as or when required. When considering applying advanced methods to affect maximal power output, a highly effective approach can be to categorize the various methods using the "three Ts" paradigm: the *tools* used, the *techniques* adopted, and the *tactics* applied. Each of these categories can then be manipulated to impart an enhanced stimulus to the overall training stress (figure 9.2).

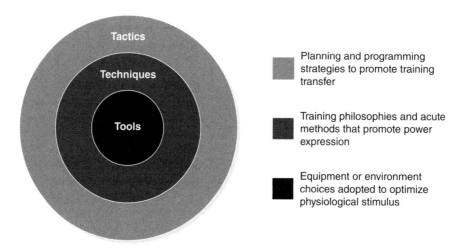

Figure 9.2 Components of advanced power training strategies: tools, techniques, and tactics.

Tools

Tools represent the equipment or environmental choices an athlete or coach can use to optimize the training stimulus beyond the methods used in traditional power training. Strength and conditioning professionals often refer to their "toolbox" as the equipment or methods they use to make exercises more challenging or complex. They also use this idea to refer to the way in which they modify equipment to better reflect the biomechanical characteristics desired and the environmental constraints placed on an athlete to challenge force–velocity characteristics. For example, within traditional power training, a decision sometimes considered by strength and conditioning professionals is to execute weightlifting variants using either a barbell or dumbbells (chapter 8). Both tools can be used to emphasize the triple extension of the hip, knee, and ankle joints synonymous with peak power outputs (17, 79). However, it is highly likely that the choice of tool and load used will affect biomechanical characteristics, motor unit recruitment, and ultimately the nature of the force–velocity relationship that is being accentuated (79).

Techniques

Power training *techniques* are philosophies and methodologies that can be applied within a given training session to promote muscular power. While all approaches to training might be considered techniques in their own right (e.g., free-weight resistance training versus plyometric training), the understanding of training science has progressed substantially over the years, such that training regimens can now be classified specifically by the techniques they adopt. For example, *eccentric strength training* is widely recognized as a training strategy in its own right, with a growing body of scientific evidence to support the morphological and performance adaptations that this technique elicits (43, 124, 133). The term *plyometrics* is also commonplace. However, within the paradigm of plyometric training, the taxonomy of exercises leads to the classification of techniques identified as *shock method training* and those simply termed *plyometrics* (132). Consequently, specific training techniques should also be considered when planning and programming advanced power training methods (see chapter 3).

Tactics

Finally, the *tactics* of advanced power training are planning and programming considerations that overarch all training methods. They are used sequentially within defined phases of training to promote the transfer and realization of power training methods into performance. The programming of advanced training is a central factor in fulfilling the likelihood that a training modality or technique will result in the desired physiological effect. In most instances, the purpose of planning and programming is to manage the fitness–fatigue relationship (i.e., overload and recovery) (67, 123). Nowhere is this more evident than when using advanced training methods, during which the optimization of the training stimulus must be apparent because of the rationale that traditional planning and programming methods were failing to impart further benefits, and thus, advanced methods were introduced.

METHODS OF ADVANCED POWER TRAINING

The manipulation of acute training variables is at the heart of any advanced training strategy. The way various tools, techniques, and tactics (i.e., the three Ts) are used by strength and conditioning professionals can profoundly affect performance outcomes. The following sections discuss the three Ts in greater detail and explore which training variables have been demonstrated to have a meaningful impact during advanced approaches to power training.

Advanced Training Tools

To understand why the use of tools or environmental constraints lends itself to advanced power training methods, force–velocity characteristics must first be examined. Resistance training methods that use external loads are generally classified as

- ▶ constant resistance, whereby the external load remains unchanged throughout the full range of motion (103);
- ▶ accommodating resistance (also termed *isokinetic resistance*), which allows muscles to contract maximally while the velocity is controlled (89); or

► variable resistance, which aligns the force-producing capabilities of the muscles with the mechanical demands throughout a given range of motion (138).

This classification becomes particularly important when exploring torque characteristics (i.e., the relationship between force and joint angle) within the human strength curve (142).

As shown in figure 9.3, the strength curve can be classified into three categories: ascending, descending, and bell shaped (89). Muscle actions with ascending strength curves express the greatest strength toward the end of the concentric phase, when joint angles tend to be at their largest (e.g., back squat). In actions with descending strength curves force is optimized in the early portion of the concentric muscle action (e.g., a prone row on a high bench). Single-joint movements such as biceps curls or leg extensions have bell-shaped strength characteristics, whereby force increases to maximum levels in the middle of the range of motion and then is reduced as the range of motion comes to completion (138). By using specific pieces of equipment that affect biomechanical features within a given movement or exercise, it may be possible to directly influence the force–velocity characteristics of respective strength curves and therefore intimately affect the stimulus placed on the muscular and nervous systems. For example, by applying variable external resistance to an exercise (e.g., with bands or chains), it may be possible for a muscle to generate consistently high levels of force throughout the movement, regardless of the nature of the mechanical strength-curve characteristics.

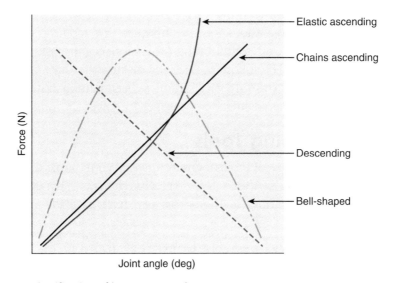

Figure 9.3 Classification of human strength curves.

Adapted by permission,from D.T. McMaster, J. Cronin, and M. McGuigan, "Forms of Variable Resistance Training," *Strength and Conditioning Journal* 31, no. 1 (2009): 50-64.

Elastic Bands

The use of elastic resistance in conjunction with body weight or free weights is a form of variable-resistance training (VRT). As shown in figure 9.3, the viscoelastic properties of an elastic band when it stretches lead to a progressive and sometimes exponential increase in tension that can be applied throughout the range of motion, regardless of joint angle (74). Elastic bands can be used to either assist or challenge human strength curves by promoting augmented neuromuscular rate coding and contractile velocity or by varying the tensile load placed on a muscle complex (27, 61, 65, 134). In modern training environments, the use of elastic resistance is becoming commonplace, and research suggests that VRT is a superior method for increasing strength, power (i.e., rate of work per unit of time), contraction time, and overall electromyography activity when compared to conventional resistance training methods (40, 134).

Training with elastic bands largely challenges ascending strength curves, and the highest resistance is experienced when the elastic is fully stretched. In human biomechanics, this typically corresponds to nearly full extension of the joint and the point of the highest force-producing capabilities (138)—for example, when the knees and hips are almost fully extended at the top of a squat. This differs from the constant resistance of free weights, where the load remains unchanged throughout the range of motion (ROM). This is an important consideration, because the mechanical properties of muscle mean there are disadvantages at various positions during a movement task due to the length–tension relationship (i.e., when a joint is in a closed position and the overlap of actin and myosin filaments does not allow for optimal crossbridge interaction) (142). With the application of elastic resistance to an ascending strength curve, the VRT properties of elastic bands allow for a lighter relative load to be applied at the point when the musculature is at its weakest (e.g., in the bottom position of the back squat) and for a greater relative load to be applied at a point in the ROM when muscle is mechanically at its strongest (e.g., in the top one-third of a back squat, where force production usually decreases and deceleration occurs). In essence, as the movement progresses toward the end of the ROM, the incremental loading associated with elastic bands complements the length–tension relationship by promoting a progressive recruitment of higher-threshold motor units (14, 33, 66). Therefore, the highest motor unit recruitment occurs at the most mechanically advantageous position within a given movement (138). Such increased muscle activation reflects the unique neuromuscular stimulus imparted by the viscoelastic properties of elastic resistance bands (3, 10).

The ability of an athlete to accelerate a load throughout a given range of motion is a critical determinant of power. When training with free weights, the force required to move a load is not the same force required to keep it moving, due to the momentum that the system mass incurs (i.e., the stimulus becomes less with increasing momentum). By using elastic bands, it is possible to affect the amount of momentum achieved within the given ROM of an exercise, such that the athlete must work to accelerate the load for a longer duration and for a larger portion of the movement. When using advanced power training strategies, this is an important consideration. The contractile element of muscle is enhanced by high contraction speeds, and the acceleration of any object is proportional to the force required to move it but inversely proportional to its mass or inertia. Owing to the way in which elastic bands vary resistance throughout the ROM (i.e., progressively increased tension), their ability to decrease or remove momentum from a system and to promote a greater demand for force would suggest they are a highly appropriate tool for developing the force–velocity capabilities required for power expression. The length–tension relationship of elastic bands varies greatly based on the band dimensions, including thickness, length, and width (134). Athletes and coaches can use variations in the length and thickness of bands to directly influence the resistance applied to the musculature within any given exercise. Table 9.1 highlights the dimensions for commonly used bands and their associated resistance.

Table 9.1 Relationship Between Dimensions of Elastic Resistance Bands and Chains and Their Respective End-Range Resistance

ELASTIC RESISTANCE BANDS, 41 IN. (104.1 CM) LONG[a]			CHAINS[b]	
Width	Thickness	Approximate resistance	Link size	Weight per foot
0.25 in. (0.6 cm)	0.2 in. (4.5 mm)	5-15 lb (2.3-6.8 kg)	0.2 in. (0.5 cm)	0.4 lb (0.2 kg)
0.5 in. (1.3 cm)	0.2 in. (4.5 mm)	20-25 lb (9.1-11.3 kg)	0.25 in. (0.6 cm)	0.7 lb (0.3 kg)
0.5 in. (1.3 cm)	0.25 in. (6.4 mm)	30-50 lb (13.6-22.7 kg)	0.3 in. (0.8 cm)	1.0 lb (0.5 kg)
1.1 in. (0.5 cm)	0.2 in. (4.5 mm)	40-80 lb (18.1-36.3 kg)	0.4 in. (1.0 cm)	1.3 lb (0.6 kg)
1.8 in. (2.8 cm)	0.2 in. (4.5 mm)	50-120 lb (22.7-54.4 kg)	0.5 in. (1.3 cm)	2.8 lb (1.3 kg)
2.5 in. (6.4 cm)	0.2 in. (4.5 mm)	60-150 lb (27.2-68.0 kg)	0.6 in. (1.6 cm)	3.8 lb (1.7 kg)
4 in. (10.2 cm)	0.25 in. (6.4 mm)	80-200 lb (36.3-90.7 kg)	0.9 in. (1.9 cm)	4.8 lb (2.2 kg)

[a]Specifications according to Sorinex Exercise Equipment's manufacturer guidelines.

[b]Adapted by permission from J. Berning, C. Coker, and K. Adams, "Using Chains for Strength and Conditioning," *Strength and Conditioning Journal* 26 (2004): 80-84.

While the use of elastic bands has primarily focused on resisting ascending strength curves, more recent exploration within applied settings has found that strength and conditioning professionals augment ascending strength curves using elastic bands to assist in overcoming gravitational forces and accelerate movement kinematics (1, 129). During such accentuated movements, harnessing the upward recoil of elastic bands improves movement velocity and has been shown to enhance jump performance when included as part of a comprehensive plyometric training program (81). While ground reaction force and takeoff impulse have been shown to decrease due to the elastic recoil of the bands, serving to "unload" an athlete (4), the increased velocity and reduced movement duration contribute to performance enhancement (69). Using elastic "assistance" to reduce bodyweight resistance by 10% to 40% has been shown to increase takeoff velocity and power output, thus leading to greater jump height both acutely and long-term with training (129). The release of elastic force at the beginning of the concentric phase of assisted jumping motions has been reported to be a critical point in avoiding impairment of acute concentric performance but also a factor that increases neural activity and produces performance enhancement adjunct to modifications in the associated movement kinetics (1, 129).

Elastic Bands: Resisted or Assisted?

When performing VRT using elastic bands, coaches and athletes have a choice of methods. The way in which they set up any exercise directly affects the potential to express maximal power output. Whether performing bodyweight exercises or in association with free weights, elastic bands can either resist or assist a given movement pattern. When using elastic resistance, rubber banding can be either positioned over the shoulders for bodyweight exercises or wrapped around the ends of a barbell and then anchored to the floor with a heavy weight or pins in the base of a power rack. The force vectors should allow vertical resistance to the floor (74). In such a setup, exercises such as the squat, shoulder press, and bench press experience the least resistance at the lowest point of bar displacement, where there is a mechanical disadvantage. This mitigates the potential effect of "sticking points" and allows the bar to be accelerated at a faster rate (i.e., resistance is lowest in the most mechanically deficient position). With ascending displacement of the bar, the elastic bands stretch, and the tension progressively increases; the mechanically strong portion of the exercise is then associated with progressive recruitment of higher-order motor units, resulting in a higher P_{peak} (59, 89). Various setups for resisted VRT are shown in figure 9.4 for lower body pushing with L-shaped bands and A-shaped bands. Simple variations in setup, including changes in bar height or anchor points, can have profound effects on the overall force–velocity characteristics of any movement pattern. (*Note*: If a rack does not have perpendicular pins, heavy dumbbells or kettlebells can be used to anchor the bands as long as they do not move during the exercise.)

In comparison to resisted VRT, assisted training methods are set up with the resistance reversed. In assisted training, the viscoelastic properties of the rubber bands augment the ascent of an athlete's body weight or a bar against gravity. By anchoring the bands at a height (figure 9.5) during descent in exercises such as assisted jumps or heavy back squats, the elastic will stretch, reducing the total load at the bottom of the squat. The bands then promote rapid movement out

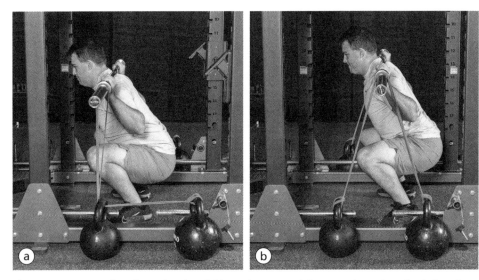

Figure 9.4 Examples of a resisted variable-resistance training exercise using elastic bands: lower body pushing with *(a)* L-shaped bands and *(b)* A-shaped bands.

of the bottom position, or in the case of "overspeed" or assisted jump training, they serve to increase momentum throughout the movement that ultimately maximizes takeoff velocity. In the case of free weights, as the athlete rises to return to standing, the magnitude of assistance is reduced throughout the ascent, and the musculature must once again take on more of the force-generating requirements within mechanically advantageous ranges. For assisted jumping movements, the momentum created by the elastic stretch in the squat position generates enhanced takeoff velocities and, ultimately, improved power characteristics. Assisted VRT methods have been shown to result in greater power and velocity output, with increased shortening rate and neuromuscular system activation reported as potential underlying mechanisms (82, 83, 117).

Programming the use of VRT techniques requires an understanding of the impact that exercise setup has on the nature of the physiological stimulus imposed. Research suggests that when used in a resistive fashion, elastic bands both complement the length–tension relationship and promote the progressive recruitment of high-order motor units. Indeed, improvements in RFD have been shown after training with resistive elastic band setups (83, 107, 134). Longer peak-velocity phases, an exploitation of the stretch-shortening cycle (SSC), and an increase in elastic stored energy were reported. In comparison, assisted VRT exercises may be more desirable during periods of heavy competition, when athlete loads may be compromised by higher levels of fatigue, or during an overspeed training phase where the speed of movement is the primary training objective (138). Assisting a movement task with the addition of elastic bands allows athletes to explode out of the bottom position of movements, such as the

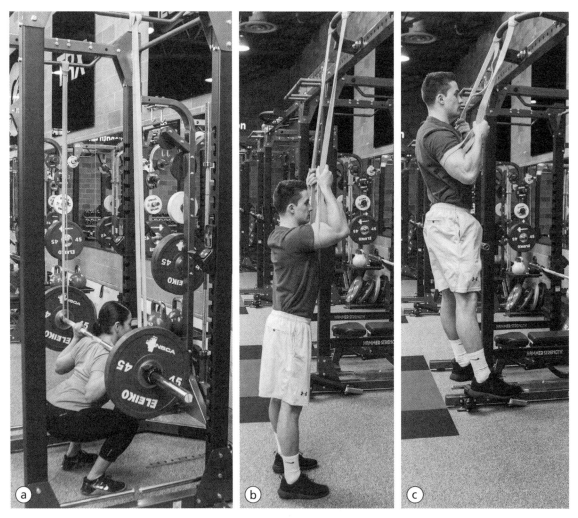

Figure 9.5 Examples of assisted variable-resistance training exercises using elastic bands: *(a)* assisted back squat and *(b-c)* assisted bodyweight vertical jumps.

squat, bench press, or vertical jump, which in turn increases task specificity, promotes high power outputs, and translates to many ballistic movements found in sport performance, such as jumping and throwing (83, 107). Examples of exercises using bands are outlined in chapters 5 and 6.

Chains

In a similar fashion to the variable-load characteristics imparted by the addition of elastic bands, heavy metal chains also represent a valuable method to influence the force–velocity characteristics of resistance training exercises. The addition of heavy metal chains to alter the force profile of popular exercises such as squats, shoulder presses, and bench presses has been popular within strength and power training for many years. The popularity of these aids has now spread to the strength and conditioning community, where they are being used for sport performance. As a result, custom-made chains are now commercially available for this specific purpose, and much like elastic bands, chains come in a variety of lengths and link thicknesses that influence the loading properties (see table 9.1). As with elastic bands, the characteristic feature of heavy chains is the ability to vary the resistance directed against a targeted muscle or muscle group over the range of an athletic movement (i.e., VRT) (118).

The use of heavy resistance to develop muscular power is vital, because strength is strongly correlated with power output (8). However, using heavy resistance often entails low velocities (100, 137). This can reduce the expression of muscular power (14, 28, 86)—although the higher load does increase the work performed, it also increases the duration (power = work divided by time). Exercises that promote higher contractile velocities throughout the ROM are therefore preferred for the development of P_{peak} within advanced power training methods. As previously discussed, strength curves approximate the torque production capabilities within a given movement. In ascending-strength-curve exercises, maximum torque production occurs near the apex of the movement (see figure 9.3); therefore, the addition of metal chains that unfurl from the floor as a barbell rises should, in theory, provide increasing resistance to match the changing torque capabilities of the neuromuscular system (73, 90). At the start of the ascending strength curve (e.g., at the bottom of a squat, shoulder press, or bench press), the additional load provided by chains is small, because the chain weight remains largely coiled on the floor. As a consequence, athletes are better able to accelerate out of the bottom portion of an exercise, imparting greater bar velocity and momentum into the system. As the ROM increases and the bar moves farther from the ground, the chains unfurl, adding additional load to the system mass but also resulting in augmented muscle stimulation, greater motor unit recruitment, and increased firing frequencies (11, 33). This combination of increased velocity and momentum imparted at the start of the strength curve of a given exercise, added to the progressive increase in muscle activation in the latter portions of the exercise due to the progressive loading, acts to induce higher P_{peak} outputs (8).

Chains: Optimizing the Stimulus

Increasing amounts of research and anecdotal evidence suggest that the setup of VRT with metal chains is critical in affecting the loading characteristics throughout the ascending strength curve (8, 11). Traditionally, a linear hanging technique has been adopted, in which chains are directly affixed to either side of a barbell and then are allowed to hang to the ground (96). This linear technique results in a significant portion of the heavy chain hanging as static weight. Only the lower portion of the chain provides variable resistance as it comes into contact with the floor. In contrast, many practitioners are now experimenting with a double-looped or positioning chains approach. Using this method, smaller chains are first affixed to the barbell. Then, heavier chains are looped through the smaller ones. Neelly and colleagues (96) report that when using the double-looped method, 80% to 90% of the chain weight load experienced at the top of a back squat is completely unloaded at the bottom of the squat. This means that during the ascent of the bar, 80% to 90% of the chain weight is progressively added to the total system load as the chain unfurls from the floor. In contrast, in the linear hanging method, only 35% to 45% of the total chain weight is added to the ascending strength curve; the rest of the chain simply hangs as static weight (96). These findings suggest nearly a twofold difference in the amount of variable resistance provided between the double-looped and the linear hung method. When considering the additional resistance offered by chains to optimize performance, Swinton and colleagues (125) indicate loads of 20% to 40% of the 1-repetition maximum (1RM) are effective, with higher loads potentially being more advantageous.

Bands or Chains?

A host of research has highlighted the differences between elastic bands and chains, with elastic bands exhibiting a curvilinear tension–deformation relationship and chains exhibiting linear mass displacement (8, 89, 90, 118, 134). The characteristics of these length–tension relationships should guide strength and conditioning professionals in their decisions regarding the choice of advanced power training tools. For example, muscle actions in which force characteristics are accumulative toward the end of a movement (e.g., a punch in boxing, a vertical jump in basketball) might be better suited to elastic band VRT, while sporting actions requiring a consistent application of force (e.g., scrummaging in rugby, a block start in sprinting) might be better suited to chain VRT. By choosing the appropriate methodology, it is likely that the intermuscular specificity will more closely resemble the force–velocity characteristics experienced during the discrete sport performance.

Although a meta-analysis by Soria-Gila and colleagues (118) has reported the comparative effects of VRT using bands or chains on maximal strength, a similar comprehensive analysis of maximal power adaptations has not been conducted. This makes comparing the benefits of each VRT method difficult. However, what is apparent is that VRT is not recommended for untrained individuals, because the increase in force characteristics that this population achieves using such methods of training are similar to the gains experienced with traditional free-weight training alone (22). This supports the use of VRT as an advanced power training method, with trained athletes experiencing improved force–velocity characteristics above those of traditional training (3, 8, 118).

ADVANCED POWER TRAINING TECHNIQUES

Advanced power training techniques are used in the day-to-day training environment and emphasize particular biomotor characteristics associated with the expression of high-power outputs. When using advanced approaches to training, considering the classification of training modalities relevant to the techniques adopted can bring clarity and focus to the holistic planning process. By focusing training on the implementation of specific training techniques, it is possible to better understand the impact that a particular training intervention has on maximal power output and how it ultimately affects performance outcomes.

Ballistic Training

In simple terms, what differentiates an exercise that develops strength from one that develops power is whether the exercise entails acceleration of a load throughout most of the ROM; this results in faster movements, and thus, higher power outputs (i.e., the same or greater work performed in a reduced time) (5, 99). Power exercises are often characterized by high-velocity movements that accelerate the athlete's body or an object throughout the ROM with a limited braking phase and little, if any, slowing of contractile velocity. A comprehension of full acceleration and movement speed is important within the paradigm of power training, because athletes are often instructed to move a load as fast as possible, often using lighter relative loads to be powerful. However, the problem with conventional resistance training techniques is that even when using lighter loads, power decreases in the final half of a repetition for the athlete to decelerate the bar or external load and for the load to achieve zero velocity by the end of the exercise motion (99). This is so an athlete can maintain his or her grip and bring the load (e.g., barbell, dumbbells, or medicine ball) to a static position under control at the end of the ROM. When resistance exercises are performed in this traditional fashion, Elliot and colleagues (35) report that the deceleration of a barbell accounts for approximately 24% of the movement with a heavy weight and 52% of the movement with a light weight. Furthermore, this deceleration phase is accompanied by a significant reduction in the electromyographic activity of the primary agonist muscles recruited in the movement (35, 99). Therefore, in any one movement, one-fourth to one-half of the full ROM is actually spent slowing down rather than trying to generate explosive contractile force (i.e., muscular power).

In *ballistic training*, an athlete attempts to accelerate a weight throughout the full ROM of an exercise, which often results in the weight being released or moving freely into space with momentum. Examples of ballistic exercises are shown in table 9.2 and are described in more detail in chapters 5 and 6.

Investigating the bench throw exercise, Newton and colleagues (99) report that ballistic movements produce significantly higher outputs for average velocity, peak velocity, average force, and most importantly, average power and peak power than traditional methods. Furthermore, during ballistic training, an external load (e.g., barbell) can be accelerated for up to 96% of the movement range, causing greater peak bar velocities and allowing the muscles to produce tension over a significantly greater portion of the total concentric phase. Even when ballistic movements are performed under heavier loading conditions (e.g., >60% of the 1RM), which may severely limit an athlete's ability to release a weight into free space, the intent to propel a load into the air is superior to traditional resistance training methods for the development of maximal power output (21). For this reason, it is essential that any coaching or cueing given to an athlete performing ballistic exercises focuses on the need to move a load "explosively" immediately after the onset of the movement and throughout the movement pattern.

Table 9.2 Resistance Training Exercises and Equivalent Ballistic Exercise (Power) Variations

Resistance training exercise	Ballistic exercise (power) variation
Squat	Jump squat
Split squat	Alternating lunge jump
Single-leg squat	Single-leg hop
Deadlift	Power clean, snatch, fast clean pull
Bench press	Bench throw
Seated row	Bench pull
Military (shoulder) press	Push jerk
Push-up	Ballistic push-up

Training to maximize power output using advanced training techniques should entail not only slow, heavy-resistance training exercises for strength development but also high-velocity ballistic exercises in which acceleration of an external load is promoted throughout the entire ROM (5, 97). Perhaps the most common ballistic exercises used in athletic performance training are the loaded countermovement jump (CMJ) for the lower body (e.g., jump squat) and the Smith machine bench throw for the upper body (5, 7, 98, 99). Further, there are many medicine ball exercises in which balls of varying loads and dimensions can be tossed, slammed, thrown, or released at the end of the ROM in a variety of different movement patterns to emphasize whole-body power (e.g., lateral shuffle rotational throw, squat throw for distance) or upper body (e.g., punch throw) and lower body (e.g., sprint start throw-and-chase, supine kickback) power in isolation (chapters 5 and 6). Plyometrics (39) and weightlifting (58) can also be considered ballistic because they too encourage full acceleration throughout a movement. In the case of weightlifting, bar velocities are affected only by gravity. For example, the low contractile velocities involved in powerlifting exercises (i.e., back squat, deadlift, and bench press) have been shown to generate approximately 12 W/kg of body weight in elite weightlifters (46). In comparison, the second pull of weightlifting movements (e.g., clean, snatch) produces, on average, 52 W/kg of body weight in the same population of athletes (46). These data are largely a consequence of the ballistic nature of weightlifting movements in which athletes try to accelerate a barbell for up to 96% of the movement (e.g., clean, snatch) in an attempt to impart momentum into the bar before dropping under it as it continues to rise in free space, thus allowing the athletes to move into the catch, or receiving, position (130) (see also chapter 8).

The mean velocities of ballistic movements are greater than those of nonballistic movements because there is no deceleration, or braking, phase. This is supported by Frost and colleagues (44), who observed that significantly higher power measures are found during ballistic exercises, largely due to their higher mean velocity. Lake and colleagues (76), however, challenged the superiority of lower body ballistic exercises for power development. Studying moderately well-trained men, they suggested that while a higher mean velocity (14% greater) is seen in ballistic exercise, there is sometimes no difference between ballistic and traditional training methods when comparing the RFD during an exercise. Data such as these continue to challenge the understanding of the kinematics related to ballistic training methods. It is apparent, however, that consideration must be given to the manner in which ballistic exercises are interpreted. If the instantaneous P_{peak} is recorded, it is likely that the impact of ballistic exercise on power characteristics may be equivocal between moderately trained and well-trained people. If, however, mean power is a more important variable to pursue, Frost and colleagues (44) suggest it may better differentiate well-trained from moderately trained people. Such comparisons once again lead to the conclusion that ballistic training methods are likely better suited to advanced athletes who already possess a high level of muscular strength and require substantial complexity and variation within their training program to augment the desired adaptation in force–velocity characteristics.

Velocity-Based Training

When developing advanced training strategies, athletes and coaches should consider the time available within discrete motor skills in which to produce peak force. While most weight room–based resistance training exercises take several seconds to complete a single repetition, rarely in sport is time sufficient within athletic movements to achieve maximal force, with instantaneous peak force instead largely occurring between 0.101 and 0.300 seconds (table 9.3). Therefore, velocity specificity should be a central consideration when training to develop muscular power, with the physiological adaptations being velocity dependent (66, 86) and the greatest adaptations occurring at or near the training velocities (102). The evaluation of movement velocity consequent to rapid force production (i.e., force–velocity profiling using dynamic or rapid isometric force expression) is therefore required to evaluate where deficiencies may lie within a movement pattern relative to given sport skills. Owing to technological advancements and improved diagnostic techniques (e.g., linear displacement transducers, force plates, and inertial measurement units), the opportunity to gain insight into the force–velocity characteristics of discrete exercises and movement patterns has increased. As a result, velocity-based training (VBT) is becoming a popular way to prescribe resistance training loads using real-time biometric feedback that reports repetition-to-repetition performance. More specifically, monitoring the velocity of each repetition helps to evaluate whether the load or resistance used during the exercise should be altered. The intent to move at high speed and maintain a desired repetition velocity, even with an altered load or resistance, can enhance the relative and absolute power output in the concentric phase of muscle actions (106). The value of velocity-based resistance training has been supported by several research studies (89, 90, 105, 106). However, the measurement error of the device should be considered when setting any velocity loss thresholds.

Table 9.3 Time Constraints of Explosive Force Production Within Discrete Sporting Movements

Sport and motion	Time to peak force (s)	Reference
Sprint running	0.101 (males) 0.108 (females)	Mero and Komi (91)
Long jump	0.105-0.125 (males)	Zatsiorsky (141)
High jump	0.15-0.23 (males) 0.14 (females)	Dapena (29)
Platform diving	1.33 (standing takeoff) 0.15 (running dive)	Miller (92)
Ski jumping	0.25-0.30	Komi and Virmavirta (71)
Shot-putting delivery	0.22-0.27 (male)	Lanka (77)

Why Velocity-Based Training?

Historically, strength and conditioning professionals have prescribed resistance training loads based on a percentage of a previously determined repetition maximum (e.g., 1RM, 3RM, or 6RM). Exercises are then performed and progressed at various submaximal intensities of these absolute loads or the calculation of a

1RM absolute load from a multiple repetition maximal load (e.g., a loaded CMJ at 40% of a 1RM back squat). Guppy and colleagues (52, 53) have demonstrated the consistency of repetition maximums as highly accurate in the evaluation of muscular strength expression, illustrating that these measures are stable across a week. However, while sound in principle and shown to have lower measurement error than does barbell velocity (52, 53), using a percentage of the 1RM can be challenging from a practical perspective. Unless regular maximums are established (e.g., 1RM, 3RM), training at a specific percentage of the RM may be flawed. Testing for absolute or training maximums can take extra time, making it logistically difficult to schedule into a program on a day-to-day or week-to-week basis. In comparison, VBT relies on instantaneous repetition-to-repetition feedback relating to the velocity of a barbell or weight. Through the simple setup and easy application of many VBT technologies, bar velocity can be very simply evaluated within any training environment. This allows for the evaluation of and instantaneous variation in training loads across a training phase, with external loads either increased or reduced to maintain a desired bar-speed threshold. This velocity-based training can then be related to the stimulus for a specific strength quality (figure 9.6). However, practitioners need to adopt caution when using any VBT technology and take the time to evaluate and validate the technical error of measurement for the device, because some tools may present measurement errors greater than prescribed velocity thresholds, and this can render them somewhat redundant for training load prescription.

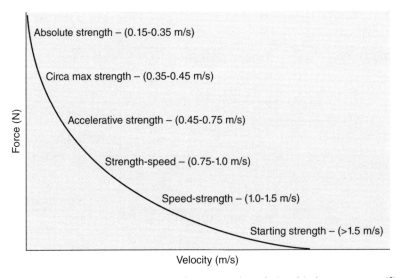

Figure 9.6 Velocity-based training curve illustrating the relationship between specific strength qualities and associated bar velocities during resistance training.

Reprinted by permission from M. Kuzdub, "Introductory Guide to Velocity Based Training," Breaking Muscle, last modified October 25, 2022, www.breakingmuscle.com/learn/introductory-guide-to-velocity-based-training.

A nearly perfect linear relationship has been reported between the percentage of the 1RM and the corresponding bar velocity (48). Therefore, monitoring the velocity of a movement can potentially be used to periodize training and promote desired neuromuscular adaptations specific to power expression. By objectively measuring bar velocity to implement neuromuscular overload rather than using the traditional percentage of the 1RM load, it is possible to use the speed of a movement as the mechanism to challenge the physiological adaptations that underpin power expression. For example, when examining figure 9.6, 40% to 60% of the 1RM is representative of both strength-speed and speed-strength qualities, with peak velocities (inclusive of both qualities) between 0.75 and 1.50 m/s (28). While both traits require the expression of high levels of muscular power, they are discrete properties and can be discerned by velocity, a major advantage of VBT. Strength-speed is defined as moving a moderately heavy weight as fast as possible (i.e., moderate loads at moderate velocities) and has been shown to exist at 0.75 to 1.0 m/s (60, 64). In comparison, speed-strength exercises include velocities ranging from 1.0 to 1.5 m/s and are best described as speed in the conditions of strength or speed prioritized over strength (60, 64), thus allowing lighter loads to be moved at a high velocity. Once again, it is important that practitioners consider experimental error when using technologies to prescribe exercise thresholds, and VBT represents such a modality; if the error of a device is larger than the thresholds of performance being prescribed, inappropriate progression or regression schemes may be deployed, potentially placing athletes at elevated risk of injury.

Overcoming Isometrics and Accentuated Eccentrics

While most power-based training strategies promote the use of ballistic-type exercises that focus on strength-speed and speed-strength qualities, eccentric resistance training, including *accentuated eccentrics* and *overcoming isometrics*, has also been shown to improve measures of muscular strength, as have jumping, sprinting, and change-of-direction performance (13, 15). Accentuated eccentric loading is a training method in which greater load is applied during the eccentric phase of a movement in comparison to the concentric phase. This technique is often performed using dumbbells (athletes hold a dumbbell in each hand during the eccentric phase of a movement and then drop the dumbbells before commencing the concentric phase of the movement), eccentric flywheels that overload negative portions of movement patterns, or eccentric hooks that hang from a barbell to create accentuated load but fall away as they come into contact with the ground, releasing from the barbell and allowing the athlete to complete the concentric portion of an exercise with a reduced external load. Elsewhere, overcoming isometrics (i.e., maximal intent) is a technique in which athletes try to move an immovable object with maximum effort (e.g., a hex bar deadlift secured in a deep squat position using rack pins), usually for 2 to 3 seconds. A similar approach could be used for upper body exercises—for example, a bench press with the bar fixed at a set height in a power rack or Smith machine. For clarity, popular coaching terminology refers to pushing isometric muscle actions as *overcoming isometrics* and to holding isometric muscle actions (i.e., submaximal efforts, usually of longer duration, such as 10-30 seconds) as *yielding isometrics* (111).

The premise behind the use of accentuated eccentrics and overcoming isometrics is that high force production during maximal isometric contractions and heavy eccentric muscle actions are associated with greater recruitment of the higher-order, fast-twitch muscle fibers (75) and a reduced neural inhibition that would lead to greater concentric force generation (135). These training modalities have also been shown to reduce coactivation of antagonist muscles (13), which may impair complete activation of the agonist, reducing specific tension and leading to decreased force production. By reducing the coactivation of the antagonist, as occurs through accentuated eccentric training and overcoming isometrics, more activation of the agonist is possible, resulting in greater force and power production without associated hypertrophy (13). Using these techniques may therefore represent an effective way to induce longitudinal neuromuscular training adaptations that are conducive to the expression of enhanced muscular power outputs. *Accentuated eccentric exercise* can be performed using a variety of modalities, including tempo eccentrics that modify the movement cadence (e.g., 5 seconds-0 seconds-2 seconds for the eccentric-isometric-concentric portions of an exercise), flywheel inertia (i.e., eccentric overload induced by the mass, radius, and angular acceleration of a flywheel device), accentuated loading schemes that overload the eccentric portion of an exercise using elastic bands or drop weights (e.g., 115% of the 1RM for the eccentric portion and 90% of the 1RM for the concentric portion), and plyometrics (124, 133). For overcoming isometrics, without an obvious outcome and finishing point to an exercise (i.e., the action is static in nature), the appropriate intent and state of arousal to execute an all-out effort can be difficult to comprehend for both novice and even highly trained and motivated athletes; therefore, a rating of perceived effort is perhaps the most appropriate way to manage exercise prescription (e.g., set 1 at 75% effort, set 2 at 90% effort, and sets 3 and 4 at 100% effort).

Cueing Power Training Techniques

Cueing is a critical component that is often undervalued but can serve to optimize the potential benefits of advanced power training techniques. Effective coaching cues should emphasize two essential factors regarding exercise technique: executing any movement pattern or exercise with the correct biomechanics and form and reinforcing the way in which athletes perform a given exercise (i.e., with intent to express high power outputs). First, it is essential to comprehend that the biomechanics (i.e., movement characteristics) of an athlete directly affect the performance outcome, or kinetics, of an exercise. Correct body position and joint alignment and the ability to brace and transfer force are contributors to outcome characteristics and directly influence power expression. When functional movement and biomechanics (i.e., exercise technique) are not cued correctly, poor movement quality can compromise the optimization of any given power training exercise. In addition to biomechanics, cueing should also address the kinematics of power training exercises, ultimately focusing on the manner or fashion in which exercises are performed. As briefly discussed in this chapter, emphasis should be placed on the intent or desire to perform movements forcefully and powerfully, maximizing both speed and strength (9). To generate high levels of muscular power, athletes should consciously strive to accelerate their body or an external resistance as hard and as fast as possible. Cueing can be used to reinforce these principles, with cues such as "be explosive," "accelerate the bar as fast as possible," and "push or pull all the way through the movement" becoming a highly motivational strategy to focus an athlete's intent. As previously discussed, VBT technologies can further reinforce the use of coaching cues, with in-the-action feedback supporting the effectiveness by which various cues improve or negate the performance of any given repetition or exercise.

ADVANCED POWER TRAINING TACTICS

The ability to stimulate specific physiological and performance adaptations optimally is in part predicted by the ability to vary training demands and induce novel stimuli at appropriate times (123). Power production is a consequence of efficient neuromuscular processes, and therefore, the effectiveness of power training is largely related to the quality with which each repetition is performed, the magnitude of fatigue-related remnants that influence contractile characteristics, or both. Baker and Newton (7) suggest both that it is important to avoid fatigue when trying to maximize power output and that performing a low number of repetitions (e.g., 1-5) with an appropriate rest interval (e.g., 2-5 minutes, depending on the demands of the exercise) optimizes power training. When developing an approach to optimize muscular power production, the ability to logically and systematically introduce appropriate training variations that complement the development of specific physiological attributes is essential (54). When implementing a periodized advanced power training program, one can introduce variation at many levels, including manipulation of the overall training load, the number of sets and repetitions, the number of exercises, the exercise order, the focus of the training block, and the rest interval between sets (see chapter 3). Therefore, strength and conditioning professionals must appropriately consider the planning and programming tactics they can implement if they are to significantly affect adaptive processes consequent to training.

Cluster-Set Training

To promote the development of maximal power output, repetitions of a given exercise should achieve ≥90% of the maximal power output and velocity for the stimulus to be considered beneficial (40). Achieving such high-intensity thresholds becomes critical, and the way exercises are prescribed becomes fundamental in determining their effectiveness. In a classic sense, training sets normally comprise a series of 3 to 20 repetitions performed continuously. When examining this traditional set configuration, however, it is apparent that bar velocity, peak power output, and bar displacement all decrease with each subsequent repetition in a set, largely as a result of accumulating fatigue (45, 55). One must therefore introduce alternative methods to maintain the performance standard for each repetition.

The ability to perform power training in a nonfatigued state, whereby a more optimal training stimulus can enhance neural adaptations, is a central philosophy behind the use of *cluster-set* training. Strength and conditioning professionals can modify the structure of a cluster set to target specific physiological and performance characteristics. Specifically, in advanced power training regimens, cluster sets provide an important tactic that optimizes the development of muscular force–velocity capabilities.

While cluster sets often focus on allowing for the development of P_{peak} within individual repetitions of a given set, a cluster-type method known as *high volume power training* (HVPT) has been used to develop the expression of repeat muscular power for sports requiring multiple high-power outputs and fatigue resistance (49, 95). Using a motor-unit firing pattern, which decreases the interference effect of antagonist cocontractions to enhance the rate of muscle contraction and relaxation (62, 88), HVPT aims to improve the average power output for repeat high-intensity efforts via high-volume repetition schemes at low to moderate loads, usually targeting 30 to 100 total repetitions per session (see table 9.4 for prescription recommendations) (94, 95).

Table 9.4 High Volume Power Training (HVPT) Prescription Guidelines

Frequency, sessions per week	Loading, % 1RM	Sets	Reps per set	Reps per session	Intraset rest (s)	Interset rest, min
2-3	30-40	3-5	10-20	30-100	5-10	2-3

Intraset rest periods, loading, and volume prescriptions can all be progressively overloaded to suit the desired adaptation. The short rest periods aim to drive the athlete's intent within a session to maintain the desired targets, with a long-term goal of maintaining these results at heavier loads. For example, a 10-second intraset rest period may be reduced to a 5-second duration under the same loading conditions across a four-week training block, with the target of maintaining average power output and peak velocity across all clusters (94). It is the intraset rest period that permits high-quality and high-velocity movements by allowing some recovery between repetitions.

While fatigue and optimal performance are said to exist at opposite ends of the fitness–fatigue relationship (108), exercise selection and loading prescriptions influence the total mechanical work performed during HVPT tactics. For example, ballistic exercises of 0% to 40% of the 1RM loads have been shown to be effective for developing power output and postactivation potentiation if repetitions are kept to ≤6. However, these positive effects may be diminished at heavier loads due to the onset of neuromuscular fatigue (24, 93, 127). Therefore, repetitions may remain identical across a training block, with the intent to gradually increase the loading prescription (i.e., percentage of the RM or total load) as the athlete adapts to the training conditions. For example, a prescription of 3 × 5-5-5 at 30% of the 1RM for two weeks may progress to 3 × 5-5-5 at 40% of the 1RM for the final two weeks of a four-week training phase. Alternatively, volume can also be an acute training variable targeted for progressive overload, whereby 3 × 5-5-5 progresses to 3 × 6-6-6 in the final two weeks of the program, using the same percentage loading conditions of 30% of the 1RM throughout. Use of monitoring tools such as VBT then becomes a critical quantitative component when prescribing HVPT to ensure that interrepetition targets are met and fatigue has not altered the desired training outcomes.

Postactivation Performance Enhancement

The performance characteristics of skeletal muscle are transient in nature and can be intimately affected by contractile history (110). French and colleagues (42) report that following heavy loading, the strength and power characteristics of subsequent muscle actions can be temporarily improved under the influence of an increased excitability of the central nervous system. This increased neural excitation is the result of an acute physiological adjustment referred to as *postactivation potentiation* (PAP) (57, 128). The PAP phenomenon is widely accepted in strength and conditioning literature. The underlying premise is that prior heavy loading can maximize subsequent explosive activity by inducing a high degree of neural stimulation that results in greater motor unit recruitment and high-frequency rate coding. The application of this premise is commonplace as an advanced training method. The underlying mechanisms associated with improved contractile properties are attributed to the phosphorylation of myosin regulatory light chains, which make the contractile proteins of actin and myosin in muscle fibers more sensitive to calcium. Calcium is a central regulator of neural activity, meaning that each nervous signal sent within a motor unit has a direct impact on a muscle's capacity to contract (57, 101). Increased recruitment of larger fast-twitch motor units has also been proposed as a potential determining factor for enhanced force production (128). If used effectively, PAP can be implemented into a power training program for the purpose of enhancing the magnitude of the training stimulus of other explosive movements (24, 87). Research suggests that the effects of PAP are observed as a positive bias for subsequent muscle actions (51), with the magnitude and decay characteristics of the performance bias intimately related to the intensity and duration of any conditioning precontractions (116).

Preconditioning activities, while enhancing PAP, also fatigue skeletal muscle (19, 128). The balance between PAP and fatigue and their effects on subsequent explosive contractions is therefore a delicate one. The optimal window for affecting performance depends on the amplitude and the rate of decay of both PAP and fatigue. Peak PAP occurs immediately following a preconditioning activity, although this is unlikely to be the time at which peak performance is evident, because it is also the time of peak fatigue. Similarly, the greater the time between conditioning activity and subsequent performance, the greater the recovery from fatigue and the greater the decrement in PAP (63).

An optimal recovery time is required to realize *postactivation performance enhancement* (PAPE) and diminish fatigue. PAPE is the manifestation of PAP after fatigue has reduced sufficiently for enhanced performance to be realized. Gullich and Schmidtbleicher (51) and Gilbert and colleagues (47) reported no change in the isometric RFD immediately following conditioning contractions; however, following sufficient recovery of 4.5 to 12.5 minutes and up to 15 minutes, increases of 10% and 24%, respectively, were observed. Similarly, Kilduff and colleagues (68) demonstrated a 7% to 8% increase in CMJ peak power 8 to 12 minutes after conditioning contractions, while Chatzopoulos and colleagues (18) showed that 30-meter sprint performance increased 2% to 3% 5 minutes afterward. These results differ from those of French and colleagues (42), who did not use a recovery period but still observed significant increases in both drop-jump height and acceleration impulse knee-extension peak torque immediately following 3 sets of 3-second isometric maximum voluntary contractions. Chiu and colleagues (20) were unable to detect significant improvement in the peak power of three CMJs or three loaded squat jumps at 40% of the 1RM, even when performed after recovery periods of 5, 6, and 7 minutes following 5 individual repetitions of back squats at 90% of the 1RM.

An important consideration for advanced power training techniques is the magnitude of individual PAPE responses and how they are influenced by characteristics of individual athletes, including muscular strength, fiber-type distribution, training history, and power–strength ratios. In elite rugby players already possessing high levels of muscular strength and a long training history, Kilduff and colleagues (68) reported a positive correlation between stronger athletes (absolute and relative) and peak power output during a CMJ test 12 minutes after they each performed potentiating 3RM back squats. Gourgoulis and colleagues (50) indicate that individual strength levels are important when trying to maximize the PAPE effect, reporting a 4% increase in CMJ in stronger participants able to squat more than 160 kilograms (over 350 lb) compared to an increase of only 0.4% in weaker athletes squatting less than 160 kilograms (under 350 lb). Such strength-based comparisons are supported by cellular-level characteristics, with people exhibiting predominantly fast-twitch muscle fibers (type II) able to elicit a greater PAPE response than people with high numbers of slow-twitch (type I) fibers (56). However, people with predominantly type II fibers also elicited the greatest fatigue response following conditioning contractions (56), highlighting the importance of administering PAP protocols. An athlete's training history is also an important consideration for the expression of PAP. When comparing athletes who were training to compete in sports at a national or international level to those who undertook recreational resistance training, Chiu and colleagues (20) found significant differences in the nature of the PAPE–fatigue relationship. Following 5 sets of 1 repetition of back squats at 90% of the 1RM and 5 to 7 minutes of subsequent recovery, the advanced training group exhibited a 1% to 3% increase in CMJ and squat jump performance, whereas the recreational trainers experienced a 1% to 4% reduction in performance.

The opportunity to use the physiological characteristics associated with PAPE is an attractive consideration for athletes and coaches seeking to enhance the mechanical power stimulus associated with explosive training modalities. However, because of the number of influencing factors, it can be challenging to effectively optimize PAP (114). Inconsistent results from research further challenge the clarity with which this training methodology should be implemented. As illustrated earlier, advanced athletes who train at higher levels and have greater muscular strength, a greater fast-twitch fiber distribution, and a lower power–strength ratio are likely to benefit from the inclusion of PAPE techniques in their training program. Coaches and athletes can take advantage of PAPE techniques both in training (see the "Complex Training" and "Contrast Training" sections later in this chapter) and immediately before a competition or sporting skill that requires high levels of muscular power expression, commonly referred to as *priming* (e.g., before a jump performance or a push start in the bobsled) (see chapters 10 and 11 for examples). With results showing the potential for a 2% to 10% increase in performance following PAP strategies, the value of these methods certainly warrants acknowledgement for advanced performers. To promote the expression of PAPE, the following recommendations are given:

▶ Effective application of PAPE requires determining the optimal application for each athlete before using it within competition environments or heavy training phases.

▶ Maximal contractions and heavy external loads appear to offer the best opportunity to elicit PAPE, and while no definitive optimal load is evident, loads should directly recruit type II muscle fibers and thus will need to be ≥85% of the 1RM.

▶ Optimal rest periods vary among athletes and depend on the interaction between potentiation and fatigue. Practitioners and athletes should determine the appropriate rate of recovery following a conditioning activity for each athlete. If this is not feasible in a team sport setting, 4 minutes is recommended.

▶ Only experienced athletes with an extensive training history should use PAPE strategies for precompetition priming or as a training stimulus.

▶ Contrasting loads that provide a strength–power potentiating complex within a training regimen may be an effective way to use PAPE when the expression of muscular power is a critical outcome of the training phase. PAPE complexes can be performed in a variety of practical applications: in a "contrast" exercise sequence, high-load and low-load (high velocity) exercises are alternated in a set-by-set fashion within the same session; in "ascending" complexes, several sets of low-load, higher-velocity exercises are completed before several sets of high-load exercises within the same session; and in "descending" complexes, several sets of high-load exercises (e.g., back squat) are completed before several sets of low-load, higher-velocity exercises (e.g., vertical jump) within the same session (25, 26, 84).

Complex Training

The neuromuscular phenomenon of PAPE can be harnessed in a training environment with the objective of intensifying a neuromuscular stimulus. *Complex training*, or the use of strength–power potentiation complexes, is an advanced programming strategy that involves alternating biomechanically similar, high-load weight training exercises with plyometric-type exercises (25, 26, 113-115), with the completion of the heavy sets first followed by lighter power and plyometric exercises. Complex training was first presented by Verkhoshansky and Tatyan (131), who postulated that resistance exercise would have a performance-enhancing (i.e., potentiating) effect on plyometric activity by increasing power output and SSC efficiency. More recently, Ebben and Watts described the effectiveness of combining resistance training and plyometric activities and presented strategies for including both of these divergent strength characteristics in the same workout session (34). For example, a complex training strategy may involve 3 × 5 heavy back squats at 87.5% of the 1RM followed by 3 × 6 jump squats at body weight.

The fashion in which complex training sets are structured reflects the mechanism by which potentiation of the neuromuscular system augments explosive muscle actions following preconditioning contractile activity. Examination of the various conditioning activities used for lower body strength–power potentiation complexes reveals that the back squat or power clean is most commonly used (112, 115). However, Seitz and colleagues (115) suggest that the power clean results in significantly greater sprint performance when compared to the back squat. Regardless of the exercise protocol adopted, the general format of the conditioning activity typically uses heavy-load or ascending protocols that go up to approximately 90% of the athlete's 1RM (table 9.5).

Table 9.5 Sample Strength–Power Potentiating Complexes

Potentiation-inducing activity	Workout assignment	Recovery time (min)	Performance activity
Heavy-load squat	3 reps at 90% 1RM	4-5	40 m (43.7 yd) sprint
Heavy-load power clean	3 reps at 90% 1RM	7	20 m (21.9 yd) sprint
Heavy-load squat	3 reps at 90% 1RM	7	20 m (21.9 yd)sprint
Heavy-load squat	3 reps at 90% 1RM	3-6	Squat jump
Ascending-load squat	5 reps at 30% 1RM 4 reps at 50% 1RM 3 reps at 70% 1RM	4-5	40 m (43.7 yd) sprint
Ascending-load squat	5 reps at 30% 1RM 3 reps at 50% 1RM 3 reps at 70% 1RM 3 reps at 90% 1RM	4-5	5 horizontal plyometric jumps
Ascending-load squat	2 reps at 20% 1RM 2 reps at 40% 1RM 2 reps at 60% 1RM 2 reps at 80% 1RM 2 reps at 90% 1RM	4-5	Vertical jump

Based on Seitz and colleagues (112, 115), Gourgoulis and colleagues (50), McBride and colleagues (86), and Yetter and Moir (139).

Several studies have demonstrated how enhanced motor performance during plyometric training can occur when combined with traditional weight training (2, 38, 78). Maio Alves and colleagues (80) demonstrated such training responses after six weeks of complex training in elite youth soccer players, with increased performances found in 5 meter (5.5 yd) (7%-9.2%) and 15 meter (16.4 yd) (3.1%-6.2%) sprint times as well as squat jump height (9.6%-12.6%). Like all programming strategies that aim to augment PAP responses, complex training program design must always consider important variables such as exercise selection, load, and rest between working sets (32).

Complex training is not a new approach to power training. Early studies of strength–power potentiating complexes reported them to be effective for both the upper body (36) and lower body (104) and to be more effective in men than women (104). Both the prerequisite strength and the intensity of the load used in the resistance training portion of the complex appear to be important regulators in eliciting the complex training effect during subsequent plyometric conditions (140). While more research is required, some studies have reported that children and female athletes show inconclusive responses to complex training when compared to fundamental resistance training programs (37, 104, 143). This lack of a significant difference between methods is likely a reflection of the fact that specific population groups that lack the prerequisite strength will probably experience limited benefit from the effects that complex training (i.e., PAP) might offer (20, 34). In contrast, in well-trained National Collegiate Athletics Association Division I football players who were engaged in a periodized resistance training program for one to five years, complex training methods were found to promote significantly more improvement in vertical jump performance than traditional training methods (16). Similar changes in jumping ability following complex training stimuli have been reported elsewhere within the literature (80, 140).

When programming strength–power potentiation complexes as part of a periodized training plan, consider where in the program these types of advanced tactics are best suited. Typically, they are used in phases that target power output or when transitioning from maximal strength development to power-orientated strategies. They are typically used in the specific preparatory phase (109, 113). However, because strength–power potentiation complexes are mixed-methods activities that target strength and power simultaneously, they may also be useful during the precompetitive and main competition phases of an annual training plan.

Contrast Training

Similar to complex training, contrast training is also a planning and programming strategy that aims to accentuate the neuromuscular characteristics associated with PAPE. Unlike complex training, contrast training uses sets of biomechanically similar movements but with very different loads to create a stark and purposeful divergence in contractile velocities. Complex training uses multiple sets, or complexes, of heavy-resistance exercises followed by several sets of plyometric exercises. Contrast training instead relies on alternating heavy and light exercises; a set of high-velocity muscle actions follows each set of heavier, high-force exercises (105). In principle, this approach alternates sets of heavy-resistance loads with sets of plyometric exercises—for example, using 1 × 5 back squats at 87% of the 1RM followed by 1 × 6 jump squats at 30% of the 1RM for 3 sets. Like complex training, contrast training adopts heavy resistance, which appears to create a greater activation and preparation for ensuing maximal effort in subsequent explosive movements (108, 128, 140). Perhaps the most recognized approach to contrast training is the *French contrast* method (25, 84). French contrast training is a subset of contrast training in which a series of similar exercises is performed in a sequence within a single session. The session begins with a heavy compound exercise (e.g., back squat, clean), which is then followed by a low-load, high-velocity plyometric exercise (e.g., repeat hurdle jumps), after which the athlete performs a light-to-moderate load compound exercise that maximizes movement speed and external power output (e.g., loaded jump squat). The sequence finishes with a plyometric exercise that is often assisted (e.g., band-assisted vertical jumps). With exercise loads often varying between approximately 85% of the 1RM, 30% of the 1RM, and band assisted loads, the French contrast method effectively potentiates the neuro-muscular system to augment P_{peak} within high-velocity movements (25, 84).

While the most effective methodology for optimizing PAPE in both complex and contrast training regimens remains to be fully elucidated, researchers and practitioners generally agree that combining high-resistance loads with lighter, high-velocity movements produces optimal gains in power output (25, 26). In comparing the respective benefits of both approaches, Rajamohan and colleagues (105) showed better effects in contrast-trained athletes in both strength and power parameters when compared to complex-trained athletes after 12 weeks of training. Changes in explosive power were interpreted as gains in both vertical and horizontal jump performances, with contrast training indicating a 3.2% and 5.9% increase over complex training methods, respectively.

While contrast training has traditionally involved very heavy loads followed by lighter loads or bodyweight exercise, Sotiropoulos and colleagues (119) inves-tigated using a contrast training protocol adopting a predetermined load that maximized mechanical power output in resisted jump squats (P_{max}), a 70% P_{max} load, and a 130% P_{max} load. These data were then compared to repeated vertical jumps at body weight. These authors reported that the load that maximizes external mechanical-power output compared with a heavier or a lighter load, using the jump squat, is not more effective for increasing jumping performance afterward. These data perhaps reinforce that the intensity of the loading strategy used for any preconditioning activity that is trying to harness the neuromuscular characteristics of PAP is critical in determining a beneficial outcome. In explor-ing data such as these, it is apparent that science has yet to fully elucidate the exact mechanisms that support PAP during contrast training methods. While research continues to investigate this complex question, applied practitioners continue to engage with the anecdotal benefits to performance observed during advanced training strategies.

IMPLEMENTING ADVANCED TRAINING METHODS

As discussed within this and previous chapters, the ability to generate maximal muscular power is multifaceted, with many contributing factors affecting power expression (23). The manner in which coaches and athletes impart a training overload on the neuromuscular system regulates the development of muscular power. While power training strategies have been shown to effectively improve muscular power in some people, they have not in others (23, 24). Therefore, it is critical that the implementation of advanced training methods is conducted in a fashion that will meet the specific needs of the individual athlete.

In the early stages of power training, it is likely that changes in the force–velocity relationship are the consequence of increased muscular strength (22, 23, 24). However, with advancing years of training history, athletes can exploit the gained adaptations in neuromuscular synchronization and increased type IIa fibers to further enhance power expression through training methods that harness these new physiological attributes. Heavy resistance training improves maximal power output in relatively untrained or weak people (2, 22, 23, 24, 136, 137) but not in stronger, more experienced athletes (98, 136). Instead, stronger athletes who possess greater levels of basic strength appear to best develop ongoing muscular power expression by increasing complexity in their training stimulus, specifically the addition of velocity-based exercises (5). While continuing to maintain high levels of maximal strength, advanced athletes should use exercises that promote the maximal shortening properties of muscle (i.e., maximal velocity) to alter the characteristics of the neuromuscular system. In turn, this will change the profile of the force–velocity curve and affect the muscular power product. The inclusion of principles of advanced power training into the training program of well-trained athletes has the capacity to promote ongoing increases in maximal power output.

CONCLUSION

This chapter presented tools, techniques, and tactics one can implement into advanced training programs to develop muscular power. By understanding human strength curves, one can introduce advanced power training methods in a way that affects muscular force production within given exercises. The strength and conditioning professional's equipment choices can significantly affect how the neuromuscular system is activated to express muscular power. Beyond that, by comprehending the importance that full acceleration throughout the ROM has for power output, ballistic exercises then offer a unique challenge to advanced athletes. During this process, it is prudent to cover a wide range of loading schemes in an effort to challenge the expression of instantaneous P_{peak} rather than focusing on an athlete's maximal power output. In doing so, the ever-changing resistance and velocity will better reflect the power expression characteristics experienced in sporting competition. Modulating training program structures through distinct changes in exercise prescription (e.g., cluster sets, complex training, and HVPT) may be an efficient means to enhance power output by managing fatigue, promoting physiological phenomena that optimize power output (i.e., PAPE), or both. At a minimum, programming strategies provide clarity in the organization of power training that will help an athlete understand how the neuromuscular system should be challenged in order to elevate optimal thresholds of muscular power development. Chapters 10 and 11 present examples of these programming strategies.

CHAPTER 10

Training Power for Team Sports

Dave Hamilton
Nicholas Ripley

This chapter discusses sample power training sessions and training programs for specific team sports. These sample sessions highlight the link between key performance assessments and training. Coaches and athletes can use the samples here to help guide the development of training programs and individual training sessions. The reader should also review the practical case studies and examples presented in chapter 2 ("Assessing Power and Individual Training Needs"), chapter 3 ("Periodization and Programming for Maximizing Power"), and chapter 4 ("Adapting Power Training to Special Populations").

These sample programs are presented in the context of training power, and for the most part, they do not include extensive details on other aspects of the training plan. When putting together an overall training program, it is critical to consider the other aspects of training that will affect the development and optimization of muscular power, as well as overall sports performance. The aspects of long-term planning discussed in chapter 3 also need to be considered when designing power assessments (see chapter 2) and training programming.

Understanding the specific needs of the sport with which an athlete is involved is necessary for designing position-specific training programs for power development. An important factor in training for team sports is the substantial differences in power needs between positions within a sport. For example, in a sport such as rugby union, clear differences exist in the demands of a winger compared to those of a front-row forward. In American football, a lineman has different physical requirements than a wide receiver. A goalkeeper in soccer

The authors would like to acknowledge the significant contribution of Mike R. McGuigan to this chapter.

requires a different training approach than a midfield player. Prescribing training programs and exercises based on the demands of a position prepares the athlete for the specific demands of his or her role in competition and facilitates optimal performance. Along with selecting appropriate tests and measures of physical capacity (chapter 2), the needs analysis should also include performance analysis of athletes during competition. This allows the coach to develop individualized training programs to meet the specific demands of the sport.

Another consideration when developing a training program for team sports is the complexity of the competitive season. Numerous competitions and long seasons can make designing a training program difficult. Additional factors must be considered: training age, game exposure, strengths and weaknesses (determined from physical performance testing), injury history, and fluctuations in the recent training load. All these factors should influence the specific, individual plan for a player from a training (e.g., content and load) and game exposure perspective.

When using the templates and examples, it is critical to include an adequate warm-up for each training session.

RUGBY UNION

Power is a critical component of high-level performance in collision-based sports such as rugby. Specifically for the collision aspect of sports such as rugby, it is likely that momentum (mass × velocity) has the greatest impact; where a player's velocity can be increased by improvements in lower body power output while maintaining body mass, the increased momentum into collision situations would lead to more successful outcomes (2, 8). One approach to maximizing strength and power is to use a program template that emphasizes strength development one day and power development another. Table 10.1 shows a six-week in-season training program for an intermediate-level rugby union player using a linear progression across the weeks. Exercises can be rotated in and out of the program using an appropriate combination of sets, repetitions, and loads (usually a percentage of a 1-repetition maximum [1RM]). For example, on day 1, the back squat could be replaced with any other squat variation that provides a sufficient load. For athletes who regularly compete once a week during the competition phase, high-force contrast training consisting of strength-speed one day and speed-strength another day can be used to manage the training intensity and volume-load through a week (i.e., a speed-strength emphasis results in a reduction in volume-load for that session) (4). Using appropriate loading for both sessions could be "heavy," but the emphasis is on alternating stimuli and volume-load within a training week to see a notable decrease in volume-load when approaching competition to minimize fatigue. This would be an effective method for improving performance over a short training phase during the competitive season (1).

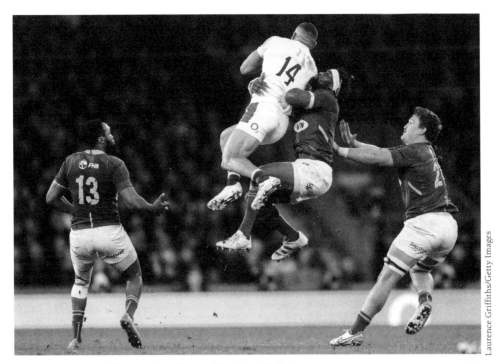

Power is a critical for rugby players like Siya Kolisi.

Table 10.1 Six-Week, Two Days per Week Training Program for an Intermediate-Level Rugby Union Player

DAY 1: STRENGTH						
Exercise	Week 1	Week 2	Week 3	Week 4	Week 5	Week 6
Bench press	3[a] × 6[b] (65%)	3 × 6 (75%)	3 × 6 (80%)	3 × 5 (85%)	3 × 3 (87.5%)	3 × 3 (90%)
Bench row	3 × 6 (65%)	3 × 6 (75%)	3 × 6 (80%)	3 × 5 (85%)	3 × 3 (87.5%)	3 × 3 (90%)
Back squat	3 × 6 (65%)	3 × 6 (75%)	3 × 6 (80%)	3 × 5 (85%)	3 × 3 (87.5%)	3 × 3 (90%)
Barbell push press	3 × 5 (65%)	3 × 5 (75%)	3 × 5 (77.5%)	3 × 5 (80%)	3 × 5 (85%)	3 × 5 (87.5%)
DAY 2: POWER						
Exercise	Week 1	Week 2	Week 3	Week 4	Week 5	Week 6
Jump squat	3 × 5 (30%)	3 × 5 (35%)	3 × 3 (40%)	3 × 5 (BW)	6 × 3 (BW)	10 × 2 (BW)
Front squat	3 × 6 (70%)	3 × 5 (75%)	3 × 5 (80%)	3 × 3 (82.5%)	3 × 3 (87.5%)	3 × 3 (90%)
Bench press throw	3 × 6 (30%)	3 × 5 (32.5%)	3 × 5 (35%)	3 × 3 (37.5%)	3 × 3 (40%)	3 × 3 (42.5%)
Push jerk	3 × 6 (65%)	3 × 5 (70%)	3 × 5 (75%)	3 × 3 (80%)	3 × 3 (82.5%)	3 × 3 (85%)

Note: % = prescribed percentage of the 1-repetition maximum; BW = body weight.
[a]Sets. [b]Repetitions.

BASKETBALL

The strength and conditioning professional is faced with notable challenges when programming for team sports. Sports such as basketball require a range of physical capacities in addition to power; however, considering the intense playing schedule and high-intensity matches, training should focus on aspects of physical performance that are not trained by the sport. Table 10.2 outlines a sample in-season power training session for basketball players of all positions. A relatively small number of exercises is prescribed, and repetitions are kept low to enable to the athlete to maximize power and velocity over the set while minimizing fatigue. The session involves low-intensity (extensive) bilateral plyometrics, because matches typically incorporate high-intensity unilateral plyometric landing tasks, and the prescribed volume can vary based on the training load. Strength and conditioning professionals could also incorporate an exercise that uses higher loads (≥85% of the 1RM) to aid in strength development, because this is another physical characteristic that would not be trained by the sport. This is a good example of a mixed-methods training approach that has been shown to be an effective strategy for improving power in athletes (4, 9, 10).

Table 10.2 Sample Power Workout for Basketball Players

Exercise	Sets × reps	Intensity
Low repeated box jump	3 × 6-8	BW
Hang pull	4 × 3	85% 1RM
Belt squat	4 × 3	85% 1RM
Tall kneeling dumbbell press	3 × 5	70% 1RM

Note: 1RM = 1-repetition maximum; BW = body weight.

Figure 10.1 shows a dynamic strength index (DSI) profile for a basketball player. Based on the results of the testing, the athlete has good strength levels (as indicated by the isometric mid-thigh pull peak force) but below-average jump height (bilaterally and unilaterally), which has resulted in a low peak propulsion force (in the bilateral countermovement jump). This profiling reveals the athlete's specific physical characteristics that require attention, including a focus on either ballistic (a DSI of <0.60) or maximal resistance (a DSI of >0.80) training or a concurrent approach (a DSI between 0.60 and 0.80) (5, 13, 14). Based on the profile, the strength and conditioning professional may also decide to implement more single-leg training to overcome any imbalance revealed during the testing.

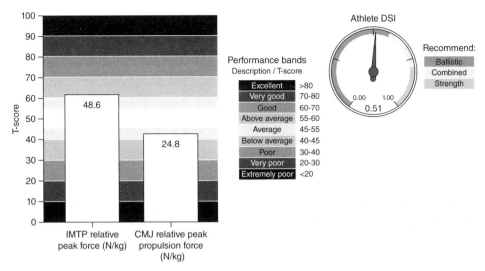

Figure 10.1 Dynamic strength index profile comparing an athlete's strengths and weaknesses using standardized T-scores.

VOLLEYBALL

In a similar fashion to basketball athletes, volleyball athletes complete a large volume of power-type movements (i.e., jumping, accelerating, and decelerating) in training and competition. Strength and conditioning professionals need to be aware of this when designing power training programs for this sport. A substantial volume of plyometric movements is not necessary in gym-based training sessions during the season, when athletes perform hundreds of these movements in technical and tactical training sessions and matches. It would be recommended to increase the volume during the off-season or early preseason to ensure that athletes are physically prepared to cope with the in-season volume of plyometric and landing tasks. Loaded triple extension–based exercises (such as squat jumps) and weightlifting-based exercises can be an effective way for athletes to improve jump performance by improving their ability to produce high forces in short epochs (periods of time).

As an example, a collegiate volleyball player weighing 70 kilogram (154 lb) underwent a six-week in-season training program to increase her jump performance by incorporating loaded squat jumps and weightlifting derivatives in addition to conventional resistance training exercises (table 10.3). This mixed-methods approach can lead to meaningful improvements in jumping performance (figure 10.2) when the change is greater than a previously determined minimal detectable change, with a progression from moderate loads in the jump squat (50%-75% of the 1RM) to relatively light loads (10%-40% of the 1RM) while using a variety of loads that can optimize power output in the weightlifting derivatives.

Table 10.3 Six-Week Lower Body Strength and Power Training Program for an Elite Volleyball Player

SESSION 1						
Exercise	**Week 1**	**Week 2**	**Week 3**	**Week 4**	**Week 5**	**Week 6**
Trap bar jump squat	4[a] × 4[b] (50%)	5 × 3 (60%)	6 × 2 (70%)	4 × 4 (30%)	5 × 3 (20%)	6 × 2 (10%)
Power clean	5 × 3 (70%)	5 × 3 (75%)	3 × 3 (75%)	5 × 2 (80%)	5 × 2 (85%)	3 × 2 (85%)
Front squat	4 × 5 (70%-75%)	4 × 5 (70%-75%)	2 × 5 (70%-75%), 1 × 3 (75%-80%)	4 × 3 (80%-85%)	4 × 3 (80%-85%)	1 × 5 (75%-80%), 2 × 3 (80%-85%)
SESSION 2						
Exercise	**Week 1**	**Week 2**	**Week 3**	**Week 4**	**Week 5**	**Week 6**
Trap bar jump squat	4 × 4 (55%)	5 × 3 (65%)	6 × 2 (75%)	4 × 4 (25%)	5 × 3 (15%)	6 × 2 (10%)
Split jerk	5 × 3 (70%)	5 × 3 (75%)	3 × 3 (75%)	5 × 2 (80%)	5 × 2 (85%)	3 × 2 (85%)
Reverse lunge	4 × 5 (70%-75%)	4 × 5 (70%-75%)	3 × 5 (70%-75%)	4 × 5 (75%-80%)	4 × 5 (75%-80%)	3 × 5 (75%-80%)

Note: % = prescribed percentage of the 1-repetition maximum. [a]Sets. [b]Repetitions.

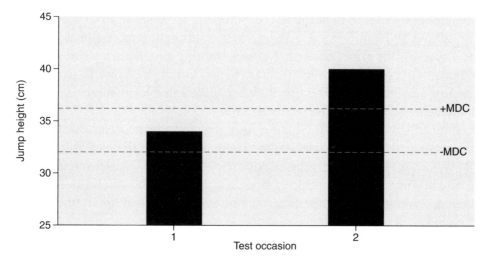

Figure 10.2 Meaningful change in jump height, with the observed change being greater than the minimal detectable change (MDC).

SOCCER

Competitive seasons for many sports are becoming increasingly longer; moreover, periods of *fixture congestion* (i.e., periods with a higher frequency of competitive matches), where it is not uncommon to have two to three fixtures in seven days, are becoming especially apparent across leagues. Another challenge posed to strength and conditioning professionals at the national level is competition scenarios (e.g., a World Cup or a continental championship), where it is not uncommon to have five fixtures in 13 days (with two-day turnarounds) (3). This presents challenges in terms of programming for power training and how to maintain it throughout the competitive season. As discussed extensively in chapters 1 and 3, it is critical to maintain strength because it is the foundation of power. Resistance training should be a regular fixture for team sports because of the strong relationships between power and sprint and jump performance (chapter 2). Table 10.4 shows an example of an in-season power training program for an elite soccer player with the goal of improving power, or at the very least, maintaining power. This program uses a wavelike approach, including a week with decreased volume to provide variety and restitution and allow for adaptations to develop (chapter 3).

Table 10.4 In-Season Power Training Program for a Soccer Player

DAY 1: POWER									
Exercise	**Week 1**	**Week 2**	**Week 3**	**Week 4**	**Exercise**	**Week 5**	**Week 6**	**Week 7**	**Week 8**
Jump squat	$3^a \times 5^b$ (25%)	3 × 5 (30%-35%)	3 × 3 (35%-40%)	4 × 3 (BW)	Jump squat	3 × 5 (25%-30%)	5 × 3 (30%-35%)	6 × 2 (35%-40%)	6 × 2 (BW)
Clean pull	4 × 4 (70%-65%)	4 × 4 (75%-80%)	4 × 4 (80%-85%)	2 × 4 (80%-85%)	Hang clean pull	3 × 3 (70%)	3 × 3 (75%)	3 × 2 (80%)	-
Back squat	3 × 6 (65%)	3 × 5 (70%)	3 × 4 (75%)	3 × 3 (80%)	Front squat	3 × 5 (70%)	3 × 5 (75%)	3 × 4 (80%)	3 × 2 (85%)
SL RDL	2 × 6	2 × 6	2 × 6	2 × 6	SL back extension	2 × 6	2 × 6	2 × 6	2 × 6
DAY 2: STRENGTH									
Exercise	**Week 1**	**Week 2**	**Week 3**	**Week 4**	**Exercise**	**Week 5**	**Week 6**	**Week 7**	**Week 8**
Trap bar deadlift	3 × 6	3 × 5 (75%-80%)	3 × 4 (80%-85%)	3 × 3 (80%-85%)	Trap bar deadlift off blocks	3 × 5 (77.5%)	3 × 4 (80%-85%)	3 × 3 (85%-90%)	3 × 2 (90%-92.5%)
Box jump (step down)*	3 × 3 (BW)	3 × 3 (BW)	3 × 3 (BW)	3 × 3 (BW)	Box jump (step down)*	3 × 3 (BW)	3 × 3 (BW)	3 × 3 (BW)	3 × 3 (BW)
Bench press	3 × 6 (70%)	3 × 6 (70%-80%)	3 × 5 (80%-85%)	3 × 3-5 (85%-90%)	Landmine press	3 × 6	3 × 6	3 × 6	3 × 6
Pallof press	3 × 5	3 × 5	3 × 5	3 × 5	Banded twist	3 × 5	3 × 5	3 × 5	3 × 5

Note: % = prescribed percentage of the 1-repetition maximum; BW = body weight; SL RDL = single-leg Romanian deadlift. *Performed as a complex with the trap bar deadlift. [a]Sets. [b]Repetitions.

AMERICAN FOOTBALL

This case study of a skill-position American football player discusses an original program and adjustments based on a power profile (figure 10.3). The athlete is a wide receiver (age, 19 years; height, 6 feet [182.9 cm]; weight, 180 pounds [81.6 kg]). His power profile toward the end of training camp in August indicates that his strength levels are adequate (isometric mid-thigh pull peak force = 3,600 N), but his force at 150 milliseconds declined from 1,750 N to 1,350 N. In addition, his modified reactive strength index during the countermovement jump (CMJ) decreased from 1.02 to 0.88. This was despite no decline in his CMJ height or his sprint ability (20 m [22 yd] time, 2.75 seconds), although these were below what was expected based off the positional average for the squad. In the four weeks before the August testing, the athlete performed three resistance training sessions per week. These sessions included a heavy strength day early in the week, a power day, and a hypertrophy day at the end of the week.

Based on the data collected as part of the fitness testing, an adjustment to the weekly training program was made. For the first session each week, the athlete performed strength–power potentiation complexes including heavy back squats with drop jumps from greater than CMJ height and heavy clean pulls with

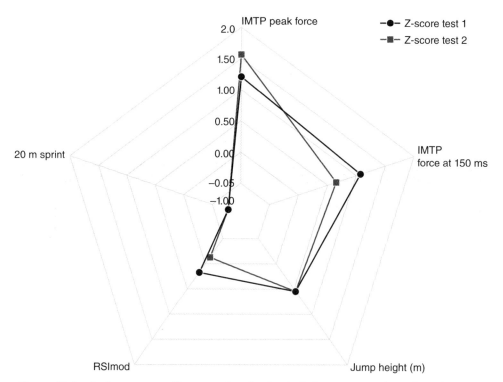

Figure 10.3 Performance profile comparing the football player's strengths and weaknesses using standardized z-scores. CMJ = countermovement jump; IMTP = isometric mid-thigh pull.

repeated broad jumps, upper body work, and accessory exercises. In the second session, the athlete completed the same power-based session, incorporating a variety of plyometric and ballistic tasks, focusing on a fast stretch-shortening cycle and high power outputs. The hypertrophy session was removed to allow for greater focus on strength and power exercises by minimizing fatigue and maximizing recovery, because the inclusion of hypertrophy training could result in residual fatigue and muscle soreness through higher volumes of training. The addition of strength–power potentiation complexes and the increase in the relative volume of jumping exercises would enable lower body power to increase in linear sprinting and jumping tasks while maintaining maximum force output (12).

BASEBALL

Baseball is another sport in which the physical demands depend on the position and the role of the player. Strength and conditioning professionals should design training programs and sessions to develop power with this in mind. Table 10.5 outlines an in-season upper body power training session for a pitcher. An alternative approach could be the use of ascending and descending power workouts, as described in chapter 3. Also, the total number of throws the pitcher performs during all training sessions and games needs to be considered when designing these programs.

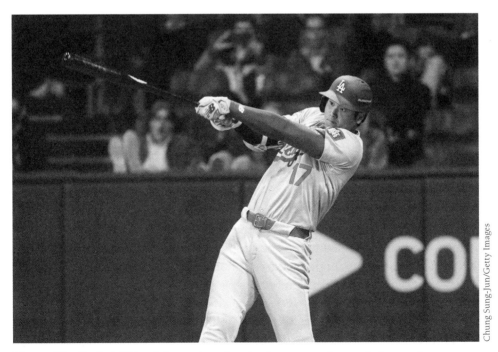

Chung Sung-Jun/Getty Images

Hitters like Shohei Ohtani depend on developing power to maximize performance.

Table 10.5 Upper Body Power Training Session for a Baseball Player

Exercise	Sets × reps	Intensity
Medicine ball drop throw	4 × 3-5	Increase loading via drop height
Band row	4 × 6	Increase loading via bands across the sets
Lateral rotational medicine ball toss (2-3 steps)	4 × 3-5	Light medicine ball with a focus on output
Single-arm dumbbell bench press	4 × 5	6/10 to 8/10 rating of perceived exertion
Single-arm dumbbell row	4 × 5	6/10 to 8/10 rating of perceived exertion

SOFTBALL

Softball has similar physical demands to baseball, highlighting that softball athletes require a range of physical characteristics that would necessitate physical development. As with baseball athletes, softball athletes need a high level of lower limb power, which is required for base sprinting (i.e., acceleration ability) and for throwing and hitting performance (including swing velocity). Therefore, training programs should be designed to develop lower limb power. Table 10.6 outlines a lower limb power training program that could be used in-season for softball athletes.

Table 10.6 Five-Week Lower Body Power Training Program for a Softball Athlete

Exercise	Week 1	Week 2	Week 3	Week 4	Week 5
Drop jump	3[a] × 3[b]	4 × 3	5 × 3	5 × 2	6 × 2
Power clean	3 × 3 (70%)	4 × 3 (75%)	5 × 3 (80%)	5 × 2 (80%)	5 × 2 (85%)
Back squat	4 × 5 (70%-75%)	4 × 5 (70%-75%)	4 × 5 (75%-80%)	3 × 3 (75%-80%)	4 × 3 (80%-85%)

Note: % = prescribed percentage of the 1-repetition maximum. [a]Sets. [b]Repetitions.

FIELD HOCKEY

Field hockey is an intermittent-effort sport requiring a myriad of high-intensity actions. Developing athletes who can tolerate repeated bouts of asymmetrical, low-to-ground actions, high speed running, rapid changes of direction, and forceful accelerations and decelerations is paramount for success. The asymmetrical movements of hockey players can be attributed to the right-handed–only sticks that players use. Holding the stick with the left hand at the top has led to several predetermined movement patterns associated with tackling, dribbling, hitting, pushing, and free running without the ball. As a result of these actions, the left and right legs can vary significantly in biomechanical qualities as well as strength and power profiles. It is critical that a training prescription looks to mitigate excessive imbalances while developing and embracing the asymmetrical nature of the sport to support optimal performance.

Despite an increase in the availability of technology, many strength and conditioning professionals have limited resources to use for performance assessment (e.g., only a jump mat and a tape measure). These constraints limit the performance assessments that can be used to determine baseline measurements. Appropriate profiling exercises could be the CMJ, squat jump (with no arm swing), and lateral hop and stick test (LHT) (left to right, then right to left). Using a ratio score of the CMJ to squat jump assessments, the eccentric utilization ratio (EUR) can be determined, and the training program can be prioritized to support either strength development (>1.1 EUR) or plyometric development (<1.0 EUR) (see chapter 2 regarding limitations of the EUR). The LHT offers insights into power production and absorption qualities in each leg and further supports training prescription to mitigate any individual leg imbalances that may have transpired due to the nature of the sport or previous injury. Table 10.7 outlines a program designed to increase power qualities for an athlete with

Table 10.7 Strength–Power Training Session for Field Hockey

Order	Exercise	Sets × reps	Intensity
	SESSION 1		
1a	Back squat	3 × 5	72%-80%
1b	SL box jump and SL landing (12-16 in. [30.5-40.6 cm] box)	3 × 5	BW
2a	BB lunge	3 × 6	70%-75%
2b	SL box drop (16-20 in. [40.6-50.8 cm] box with a 3-s eccentric landing)	3 × 5	BW
2c	BB hip extension	3 × 8	65%-75%
3a	Lateral ice skater (fast ground contact)	3 × 12	BW
3b	Bench press	4 × 8	65%-75%
3c	Pull-up (banded)	4 × 8	BW
	SESSION 2		
1a	Speed squat	3 × 15	Barbell
1b	SL CMJ	3 × 6	BW
2a	Bulgarian squat	3 × 6	70%-75%
2b	SL stability quarter squat (eyes closed)	3 × 10-20 sec	BW
2c	Nordic hamstring curl	3 × 3	BW
3a	SL DB shoulder press	3 × 6	70%
3b	SL bent-over row	3 × 6	70%

Note: % = prescribed percentage of the 1-repetition maximum; BB = barbell; BW = body weight; CMJ = countermovement jump; DB = dumbbell; SL = single leg; Order = Performing one set of each exercise (1a, 1b) in the group one after the other. After the first set is completed, go back to the first exercise in the group and do the second set of each exercise. If certain exercises call for fewer sets than others in the group, perform those sets on the back end of the grouping.

an EUR <1.02 and a complimentary lower body strength and stability program after observing high levels of landing instability during the LHT on both legs.

LACROSSE

Lacrosse is an invasion-based team sport with varying positional demands, and it requires a different training approach for each position. Therefore, when designing training programs for lacrosse athletes, the prescription should prepare the athletes for the specific demands that can facilitate optimal performance. Another consideration to make with lacrosse is that there are now three variants of the sport (field, box, and sixes), which all have unique physical, tactical, and technical demands. This case study highlights a six-week, power-orientated program for a sixes lacrosse player (age, 26 years; height, 6 foot 2 [188.0 cm]; weight, 225 pounds [102.1 kg]). The coaches were happy with the athlete's positional strength; however, they were concerned with his acceleration and speed characteristics on the field, which are integral requirements for the small-sided variant of the game (sixes).

The player's profile showed a balanced DSI of 0.64; when observing the constituent parts, the peak CMJ propulsion force was 2,677 N, and the peak isometric mid-thigh pull force was 4,188 N. The case study results highlight

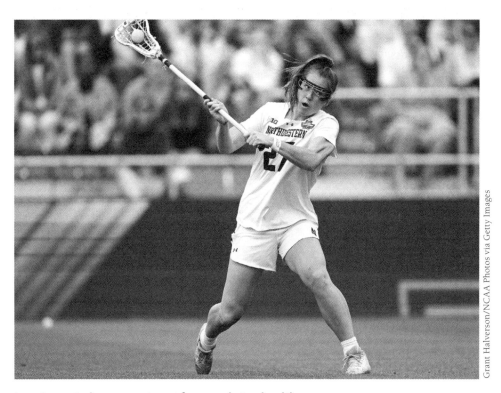

Izzy Scane trains power to perform and stay healthy.

Grant Halverson/NCAA Photos via Getty Images

that the athlete required a prescription incorporating both strength and power elements. Table 10.8 outlines a balanced in-season training program incorporating both a strength- and a power-based prescription, using a mixed-methods approach to optimize development across the force–velocity curve. As with any multidirectional sport, hamstring strain injuries are extremely prevalent in lacrosse. Therefore, both knee-dominant exercises (e.g., Nordic hamstring curl and machine leg curl) and hip-dominant exercises (e.g., Romanian deadlift and good morning) are incorporated for a balanced approach to injury risk reduction (11).

Table 10.8 Lower Body Strength and Power Training Session for a Sixes Lacrosse Player

SESSION 1						
Exercise	Week 1	Week 2	Week 3	Week 4	Week 5	Week 6
Drop jump	3a × 2b (BW)	3 × 3 (BW)	4 × 2 (BW)	4 × 3 (BW)	5 × 2 (BW)	5 × 3 (BW)
Hang power clean	5 × 3 (65%)	6 × 3 (65%)	5 × 3 (70%)	6 × 3 (70%)	5 × 3 (75%)	6 × 3 (75%)
Front squat	4 × 5 (80%)	5 × 5 (80%)	4 × 3 (85%)	5 × 3 (85%)	4 × 2 (90%)	5 × 2 (90%)
RDL	2 × 6 (65%-70%)	2 × 8 (65%-70%)	2 × 6 (70%-75%)	2 × 8 (70%-75%)	2 × 6 (75%-80%)	2 × 8 (75%-80%)
SESSION 2						
Exercise	Week 1	Week 2	Week 3	Week 4	Week 5	Week 6
Single-leg broad jump	3 × 2 (BW)	3 × 3 (BW)	4 × 2 (BW)	4 × 3 (BW)	5 × 2 (BW)	5 × 3 (BW)
Trap bar jump from below the knee	5 × 3 (10% TBDL)	6 × 3 (10% TBDL)	5 × 3 (15% TBDL)	6 × 3 (15% TBDL)	5 × 3 (20% TBDL)	6 × 3 (20% TBDL)
Bulgarian split squat	3 x 5 (70%-75%)	3 x 5 (70%-75%)	3 x 5 (70%-75%)	3 x 5 (70%-75%)	3 x 5 (70%-75%)	3 x 5 (70%-75%)
Nordic hamstring curl	3 × 3 (BW)	3 × 3 (BW)	3 × 3 (BW)	3 × 3 (BW)	3 × 3 (BW)	3 × 3 (BW)

Note: % = prescribed percentage of the 1-repetition maximum; BW = body weight; RDL = Romanian deadlift; TBDL = trap bar deadlift. aSets. bRepetitions.

PRIMING FOR TEAM SPORTS

Priming can be used the day of or the day before a match to bring about a substantial improvement in performance using a power-based prescription. Priming sessions, designed with the needs of the athlete and sport in mind, are typically performed 5 to 24 hours before a match and last just 10 to 30 minutes (6, 7). Table 10.9 shows a sample power priming session that emphasizes force and velocity for a team sport athlete 6 hours before a match and that could be performed with minimal equipment. In this session, the first two exercises are performed as a complex (sets of high-force exercises followed by sets of high-velocity plyometric exercises). The isometric exercise presented in table 10.9 could be substituted for other high-force tasks, such as heavy back squats. Other strength–power potentiating complexes and exercise pairings could also be used, as highlighted in chapter 3. However, several variables need to be considered when looking to apply priming strategies for team sport athletes, including but not limited to equipment availability, training age, recent training loads, and athlete preference. For instance, for athletes with a lower training age or lower recent training loads, prescriptions such as 2 to 3 sets of 2 to 3 repetitions for the back squat at greater than 85% of the 1RM could be detrimental for subsequent performance by inducing fatigue and muscle soreness, in contrast to athletes with a greater training age and higher acute training loads, who should be familiar with higher volumes and therefore should not experience any muscular soreness or fatigue. Moreover, athlete preference is also an important consideration, because high sporting performance requires psychological readiness, and making athletes perform exercises that are unfamiliar or toward which they have antipathetic feelings could have negative effects on sporting performance. One example of how to overcome some of the issues surrounding athlete preference is to give several options within a priming session—for instance, two to five velocity-oriented lower body exercises such as jumps, medicine ball throws, and sprints—from which athletes can choose, with similar optionality for force-oriented exercises—for instance, isometric exercises, heavy resistance training exercises (e.g., back squats), or a heavy sled push.

Table 10.9 Sample Power Priming Workout for Team Sports

Exercise	Sets × reps	Intensity
Isometric mid-thigh pull, squat, and sled push combo	3 × 3 × 3-5 second efforts	Maximum
Band-resisted jump*	3 × 3	BW
Medicine ball throw	3 × 5	Maximum speed

Note: BW = body weight.
*An isometric variation and jump could be performed as a contrast training complex with 2 minutes of rest between alternating sets of each exercise.

CONCLUSION

Strength and conditioning professionals are faced with unique challenges when designing training programs for team sports. Factors such as positional, match, and training demands, structure of the competitive season, training age, game exposure, injury history, and alterations in recent training load need to be considered. Moreover, appropriate testing methods and relevant measures can be used to determine the training needs of an athlete. It is also critical to appreciate how power training fits within the overall physical preparation of the athlete and how assessment of power can be used to inform the design of a training program.

CHAPTER 11

Training Power for Individual Sports

Dale W. Chapman
Josh L. Secomb

This chapter provides a brief overview of the key physical capacities, along with associated power training program examples, for a variety of individual sports, including independent sports, independent object sports, and combat sports (21). Specifically, the independent sports of swimming and rowing and the track and field disciplines of the throws and the heptathlon are included. The independent object sports presented with examples of power development programs include golf and tennis, the extreme sports of surfing and skateboarding, and the winter ice sliding sports of skeleton, bobsleigh, and speed skating. The chapter will explain how similar processes can be followed when working with combat sports, examining the similarities and differences when working with a purely striking athlete (boxing) compared to a grappling and throws athlete (judoka or wrestling) and providing a blended program for a mixed martial artist. As in chapter 10, these programs highlight the link between assessments of power and how the data can be used to inform training program design.

The principles discussed at the beginning of chapter 10 also apply when working with individual sports. Specifically, strength and conditioning professionals should initially perform a needs analysis and seek to improve their knowledge of the wide range of disciplines and events within each of these sports. This will allow them to be aware of the physical and physiological capacities that may limit or facilitate performance of the sport's key technical or tactical requirements and to identify an athlete's specific needs from the assessments. This knowledge and information can then be used to inform training program design—specifically, the selection of individual exercises aimed at improving power. Importantly, strength and conditioning professionals must also consider how the power training components fit within the overall training plan and determine periods of the competitive season when the focus should be to improve or maintain power.

SWIMMING

As discussed in chapter 10, a power priming session provides an acute neuromuscular and hormonal effect before competition or an important training session (14). Additionally, these sessions, commonly referred to as *microdosing* (17), provide a training stimulus that is brief and intense for less experienced athletes. When considering the structure of a typical training mesocycle and microcycle in swimming (as well as the competition meet format, which requires numerous heats and finals within approximately one week), it is apparent that the prescription of power priming sessions is of great value to strength and conditioning professionals. Physical capacities of importance for a swimmer include the concentric velocity of the countermovement jump and the pull-up, because these movements have been reported to have strong and significant relationships with block start times and freestyle paddling velocity, respectively (25). Therefore, jumping exercises and velocity-based upper body pulling exercises should be included in power priming sessions. Table 11.1 outlines a power priming session for a sprint swimmer 24 hours before a meet.

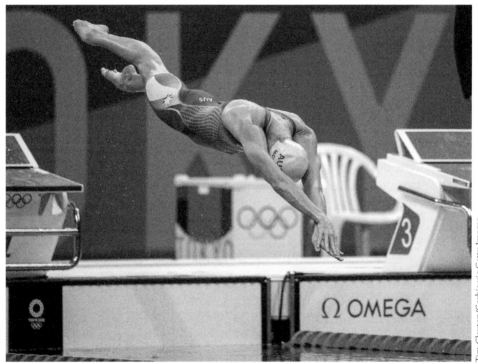

Tim Clayton/Corbis via Getty Images

Power is essential for swimmers like Emma McKeon for a strong start off the blocks.

Table 11.1 Sample Power Priming Workout for a Sprint Swimmer

Exercise	Sets × reps	Intensity
Squat jump	4 × 3	Body weight
Plyometric push-up	4 × 3	Use a 12 in. (30.5 cm) box for each hand
Depth jump	3 × 3	Use an 18 in. (45.7 cm) box
Band-assisted pull-up	3 × 4	Use a band; focus on concentric velocity
Assisted jump	3 × 3	Use a band

Developing power priming sessions requires a systematic process of trial and error early in the periodized program due to individual athlete differences in their physiological response to and psychological perception of such sessions. Specifically, it has been identified that individuals with greater relative strength are more likely to experience a meaningful increase in power output and performance following a priming session (22). Therefore, it is recommended to identify and construct different types of individualized sessions that can be tested before less important competitions and training sessions. This will increase the chances that the desired positive performance effect is optimized but also that the athlete and coach understand and value the session, enhancing buy-in and trust. To determine which power priming session is of most benefit for the athlete, the strength and conditioning professional should consider both objective data (positive change in performance) and subjective data (the athlete's perception of benefit).

ROWING

It is well established that athletes in endurance sports can benefit from resistance training (1, 2). The sport of rowing has traditionally required very well-developed aerobic endurance, muscular strength, and power qualities. With a reduction in the Olympic racing distance from 2,000 meters (2,187 yd) to 1,500 meters (1,640 yd) for the 2028 Olympic games, it has been hypothesized that the importance of the first 250 meters (273 yd) for overall performance outcomes could increase, but systematic supporting evidence is required. Traditionally, the first 250 meters is where the athlete must develop maximal repeated power to accelerate the boat to race speed before then seeking to maintain boat position and speed. For individual rowing events, the boat weighs approximately 33 pounds (15.0 kg), and this increases to approximately 250 pounds (113.4 kg) for an eight-person boat. Thus, when the weight of the boat is combined with the mass of the athlete or athletes, it is evident that overcoming substantial inertia will be required to effectively accelerate the boat in this initial 250 meters. For endurance sports such as rowing, high repetitions with low loads are of little value, will not improve power, and are extremely unlikely to improve overall performance (18). Therefore, the power training principles discussed in previous chapters apply here. Table 11.2 shows a six-week training program for an elite

Table 11.2 Six-Week, Two Days per Week Training Program for a Rower

DAY 1: STRENGTH						
Exercise	Week 1	Week 2	Week 3	Week 4	Week 5	Week 6
Bench press	3[a] × 6[b] (65%)	3 × 6 (75%)	3 × 6 (80%)	3 × 5 (85%)	3 × 3 (87.5%)	3 × 3 (90%)
Bench row	3 × 3 (90%)	3 × 3 (87.5%)	3 × 5 (85%)	3 × 6 (80%)	3 × 6 (75%)	3 × 6 (70%)
Back squat	3 × 6 (70%)	3 × 6 (75%)	3 × 6 (80%)	3 × 5 (85%)	3 × 3 (87.5%)	3 × 3 (90%)
Barbell push press	3 × 6 (65%)	3 × 5 (70%)	3 × 5 (75%)	3 × 3 (80%)	3 × 3 (82.5%)	3 × 3 (85%)
DAY 2: POWER						
Exercise	Week 1	Week 2	Week 3	Week 4	Week 5	Week 6
Squat jump	3 × 5 (30%)	3 × 5 (35%)	3 × 3 (40%)	3 × 5 (BW)	6 × 3 (BW)	8 × 2 (BW)
Bench pull	3 × 5 (65%)	3 × 5 (55%)	3 × 5 (45%)	3 × 3 (45%)	3 × 3 (40%)	3 × 2 (55%)
Front squat	3 × 6 (55%)	3 × 6 (60%)	3 × 6 (62.5%)	3 × 5 (65%)	3 × 4 (70%)	3 × 3 (75%)
Bench throw	3 × 5 (30%)	3 × 5 (32.5%)	3 × 5 (35%)	3 × 3 (37.5%)	3 × 3 (40%)	3 × 2 (42.5%)

Note: % = prescribed percentage of the 1-repetition maximum; BW = body weight. [a]Sets. [b]Repetitions.

rower who is transitioning from a general preparation strength phase to a power development phase. The program highlights the benefit of using cluster sets with higher loads for these athletes. Figure 3.22 and table 3.2 on pages 77 and 78, respectively, show examples of configurations for cluster sets.

The body positions required to perform the rowing stroke, and thus where power is developed, are similar to positions attained during the power clean, squat jump, and bench pull. As an example case study, a rower was tested using a 1-repetition maximum (1RM) bench press, bench pull, power clean, peak concentric velocity on a bench press and bench pull with 40 kilogram (88 lb), and an unloaded and loaded (40 kg [88 lb]) squat jump. The results indicated a difference between pushing and pulling strength and below-average peak concentric velocity for both the bench press and bench pull with 40 kilograms (88 lb). Furthermore, the squat jump performance highlighted a deficit in the ability to dynamically express the strength qualities when performed under load. This indicates that the emphasis of subsequent training should be to incorporate more pulling movements, such as rows and bench pulls. In addition, an increased focus on transitioning the developed strength capacities into a dynamic power expression using reduced loads moved at greater velocity or an intention to move faster should be implemented.

TRACK AND FIELD

This case study discusses a junior-level shot-putter (age, 18 years; height, 5 foot 9 [175.3 cm]; weight, 187 pounds [84.8 kg]). The technical coach and the strength and conditioning professional have identified that the athlete needs to improve explosiveness, because they believe this will help achieve a performance improvement. The athlete's power profile during November testing indicated a moderately high strength level (back squat 1RM = 130 kg [287 lb], approximately 1.5 × body weight). However, average to below average explosive capabilities during the 40 kilogram (88 lb) squat jump (relative peak power, 14 W/kg), bodyweight squat jump (relative peak power, 21 W/kg) and drop jump (reactive strength index, 1.3) were recorded and compared to historical training values (20). During each of the four weeks before the November testing, the athlete had been performing one heavy strength session that included back squats, deadlifts, and snatch pulls from blocks on Mondays, followed by a power day consisting of full snatches, front squats, and power cleans later in the week (e.g., on Thursdays), in addition to a moderately heavy strength session that included upper body exercises (table 11.3).

Based on the results of the testing, the strength and conditioning professional adjusted the athlete's lower body resistance training program. In the new program, the athlete's first session each week consisted of heavy back squats, snatch pulls, and push presses (5 sets of 3 repetitions). The second session continued the same power session as before, but with the addition of a 30-50 kilogram (66-110 lb) loaded countermovement jump (4 sets of 3 repetitions). This training program was performed for three months. The results of the follow-up testing

Table 11.3 Four-Week, Two Days per Week Training Program for a Shot-Putter

DAY 1: STRENGTH				
Exercise	Week 1	Week 2	Week 3	Week 4
Back squat	4[a] × 5[b] (83%)	4 × 6 (83%)	4 × 4 (87%)	4 × 3 (90%)
Deadlift	3 × 6 (80%)	3 × 5 (82.5%)	3 × 4 (85%)	3 × 3 (90%)
Snatch pull from blocks	4 × 4 (82.5%)	4 × 5 (82.5%)	4 × 4 (85%)	4 × 5 (85%)
Incline DB bench press	3 × 6 (80%)	3 × 5 (82.5%)	3 × 6 (82.5%)	3 × 5 (85%)
DAY 2: POWER				
Exercise	Week 1	Week 2	Week 3	Week 4
Snatch	4 × 5 (80%)	4 × 4 (83%)	4 × 3 (87%)	4 × 2 (90%)
Power clean	3 × 4 (83%)	3 × 4 (85%)	3 × 4 (87%)	3 × 3 (90%)
Front squat	3 × 6 (75%)	3 × 6 (77.5%)	3 × 6 (80%)	3 × 5 (83%)
Barbell push press	3 × 3 (50%)	3 × 4 (55%)	3 × 5 (55%)	4 × 4 (60%)

Note: % = prescribed percentage of the 1-repetition maximum; DB = dumbbell. [a]Sets. [b]Repetitions.

are outlined in figure 11.1. The athlete continued to increase their strength (1RM squat = 140 kg [309 lb], approximately 1.6 × body weight) and power capabilities during the 40 kilogram (88 lb) squat jump (18 W/kg) and maintained bodyweight squat, countermovement, and drop jump (reactive strength) performance. Most importantly, throwing distances in training improved by an average of 2% to 3%. It appeared that the training program modifications improved the athlete's strength and loaded-power capabilities while maintaining light-load velocity and power capabilities, which translated into increased sport performance. Focusing on how physical training can improve sport performance is the key for strength and conditioning professionals.

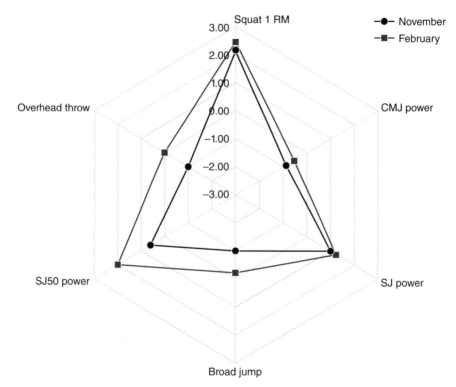

Figure 11.1 Power profile comparing the athlete's strengths and weaknesses using standardized z-scores. SJ50 power = loaded static jump (50 kg [110 lb]).

Multi-events present significant challenges to coaches, who must manage the technical skill demands of the different events when scheduling the various disciplines during training sessions. Table 11.4 outlines a power training program for a heptathlete. In this sample program, the power-focused sessions are scheduled early in the week while the athlete is relatively fresh. The second session later in the week retains a focus on power but also seeks to develop strength.

Table 11.4 Eight-Week Preseason Power Training Program for a Heptathlete

DAY 1: POWER								
Exercise	**Week 1**	**Week 2**	**Week 3**	**Week 4**	**Week 5**	**Week 6**	**Week 7**	**Week 8**
Squat jump	3[a] × 5[b] (25%)	3 × 5 (30%-35%)	3 × 3 (35%-40%)	4 × 3 (0%)	3 × 5 (25%-30%)	5 × 3 (30%-35%)	6 × 2 (35%-40%)	6 × 2 (0%)
Back squat	3 × 6 (65%)	3 × 6 (70%)	3 × 5 (75%)	3 × 3 (80%)	3 × 6 (70%)	3 × 5 (75%)	3 × 3 (80%)	3 × 2 (85%)
Fast snatch pull from blocks	4 × 5 (60%)	4 × 5 (65%)	4 × 5 (70%)	-	3 × 3 (70%)	3 × 3 (75%)	3 × 2 (80%)	-
Dumbbell power clean to jerk	3 × 5 (20 kg [44 lb])	3 × 3 (30 kg [66 lb])	3 × 3 (35 kg [77 lb])	3 × 2 (40 kg [88 lb])	3 × 5 (25 kg [55 lb])	3 × 3 (30 kg [66 lb])	3 × 3 (35 kg [77 lb])	3 × 2 (35, 40, 45 kg [77, 88, 99 lb])
Overhead throw[c]	3 × 5 (4 kg [8.8 lb])	3 × 3 (5 kg [11 lb])	3 × 3 (6 kg [13 lb])	3 × 2 (4 kg [8.8 lb])	3 × 5 (4 kg [8.8 lb])	3 × 3 (3 kg [6.6 lb])	3 × 3 (5 kg [11 lb])	3 × 2 (4 kg [8.8 lb])
DAY 2: STRENGTH AND POWER								
Exercise	**Week 1**	**Week 2**	**Week 3**	**Week 4**	**Week 5**	**Week 6**	**Week 7**	**Week 8**
Front squat	3 × 6 (70%)	3 × 6 (70%-80%)	3 × 5 (80%-85%)	3 × 3-5 (85%-90%)	3 × 6 (72.5%)	3 × 6 (70%-80%)	3 × 5 (80%-87.5%)	3 × 2-3 (90%-92.5%)
Jump squat[d]	3 × 3 (BW)	3 × 3 (BW)	3 × 3 (BW)	-	3 × 3 (BW)	3 × 3 (BW)	3 × 3 (BW)	-
Band bench press	3 × 6 (70%)	3 × 6 (70%-80%)	3 × 5 (80%-85%)	3 × 3-5 (85%-90%)	3 × 6 (72.5%)	3 × 6 (70%-80%)	3 × 5 (80%-87.5%)	3 × 2-3 (90%-92.5%)
Ball drop	3 × 5 (5 kg [11 lb])	3 × 3 (7 kg [15 lb])	3 × 2 (10 kg [22 lb])	-	3 × 5 (5 kg [11 lb])	3 × 3 (7 kg [15 lb])	3 × 2 (10 kg [22 lb])	-

Note: % = prescribed percentage of the 1-repetition maximum (0% means that no external weight is used); BW = body weight. [a]Sets. [b]Repetitions. [c]Performed as a complex with the dumbbell power clean to jerk. [d]Performed as a complex with the front squat.

GOLF AND TENNIS

Power is important in golf and tennis (23), as it is for many similar team sports that use an implement with a rotational skill application (e.g., field hockey, lacrosse, and baseball). Measures of both lower body power (countermovement jump [CMJ] variables) and rotational power (side medicine ball throw) have been found to be related to the speed of the club head in golf and to serve speed in tennis, which are characteristics of higher-level athletes in each sport (6, 25).

Specifically, a faster golf club head speed will increase driving and iron distance potential, and a greater tennis serve speed will either enhance the opportunity to win points with an ace or increase the ability to play attacking shots during a rally.

The ability to store and release elastic energy is a critical component of an effective golf swing and tennis serve. Importantly, during these rotational movements, the athlete is required to produce a stretch-shortening cycle (SSC) action, whereby the trunk muscles are stretched rapidly to increase the storage and release of this elastic energy. However, it must be noted that the golf swing is recognized as a slow SSC activity (contraction time of approximately 300 milliseconds). Therefore, golf athletes may benefit from rotational power training exercises that focus on maximizing the impulse created when using light to moderate resistances (2-8 kg; 4.4-17.6 lb) (13). Table 11.5 outlines a training session that could be used to improve a golfer's power. Other options for upper body and anatomical core exercises are given in chapters 5 and 7.

Table 11.5   Sample Training Session for a Golfer

Exercise	Sets × reps	Intensity
Loaded jump squat	4 × 3	20%, 25%, 30%, 35% 1RM
Bench press throw	4 × 5	30%, 35%, 40%, 35% 1RM
Wood chop (low to high)	3 × 5	8 kg (17.6 lb)
Push press	3 × 3	50%, 55%, 60% 1RM
MB side toss	3 × 4	3 kg (6.6 lb)

Note: % = prescribed percentage of the 1-repetition maximum; MB = medicine ball.

EXTREME SPORTS (SURFING AND SKATEBOARD)

Across the globe, extreme sports such as surfing and skateboarding have experienced an exponential increase in funding and high-performance support. This is primarily due to their inclusion in the Olympic Games beginning in Tokyo 2020. Both sports require extensive durations of aerobic-based locomotive activity (paddling for surfing and pushing and gliding for skateboarding), which are interspersed with the execution of explosive, powerful technical maneuvers. These technical maneuvers are the only components considered by the judges in the subjective scoring criteria; regardless, performance in each sport requires a broad spectrum of physical qualities, which can present challenges for the strength and conditioning professional in training prescription.

Part of the challenge is that surfing and skateboarding are typically lifestyle sports, whereby the athlete often performs the sport for recreation as frequently as for intentional technical skill practice. This contrast in performance contexts allows the strength and conditioning professional to primarily focus on improving the physical qualities that underpin the performance of the explosive technical maneuvers, because minimal prescription is required for the development and maintenance of the aerobic-based locomotive activity. However, although the aforementioned paddling efforts in surfing are not a component of the scoring criteria, a high sprint paddling velocity is necessary to successfully catch waves and enter the wave with a greater speed. Together, this promotes the performance of more highly-scored technical maneuvers and should be considered by the strength and conditioning professional. Specifically, it has been identified that a 1RM pull-up of ≥1.3 times body weight is the threshold to maximize transference between upper body pulling strength and sprint paddling velocity potential (7, 31). Once this performance threshold has been achieved, training should then target improved velocity and RFD variables of upper body pulling, similar to swimming.

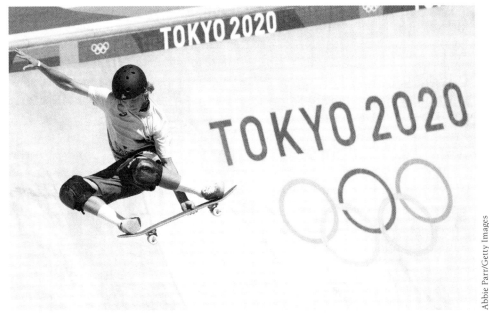

Figure 11.2 Example of the large internal-rotation range of motion of the hip required to perform skateboarding maneuvers.

In competitive surfing and the *park* discipline of skateboarding, athletes are required to perform explosive, powerful maneuvers in succession during a single wave or run, whereas in the *street* discipline of skateboarding, athletes perform a single maneuver during a run. Turning maneuvers are not typically scored as highly as aerial maneuvers in competitive surfing or skateboarding, but they are performed more frequently and with a higher completion rate in surfing

(11, 12). Greater absolute isometric and dynamic strength has been associated with scoring potential of turning maneuvers in elite-level male surfers, and thus, it should be profiled in these athletes (29). Trunk rotational power is also of great importance to the surfing and skateboarding athlete, due to the need to accelerate and decelerate the trunk and lumbopelvic complex to control the trunk throughout these maneuvers. Therefore, many of the training principles applied to sports with a rotational power application, such as golf and tennis, and to combat sports are also fundamental when working with extreme-sport athletes (see chapter 7 regarding anatomical core power).

The most highly scored technical maneuvers in surfing and skateboarding are aerial maneuvers (11, 12). These maneuvers require athletes to maximize jump height through explosive triple-extension of the lower body to provide themselves with sufficient time to manipulate their body into a variety of specific positions and postures that include extreme ranges of motion (ROMs) in the ankle and hip joints (figure 11.2). Once the apex of the aerial maneuver height has been achieved, the athlete must immediately prepare for and perform a rapid reabsorption of high-magnitude landing force through the lower body (figure 11.3). It is advantageous for the landing component to be performed quickly to allow the athlete an immediate transition to the next maneuver, increasing adherence to the scoring criteria. As such, athletes must integrate the capacity to generate a large magnitude of lower body power, with highly developed sensorimotor proficiency and the ability to effectively control their limbs through these large joint ROMs. A key consideration for a training prescription is that elite-level surfing and skateboarding athletes are typically observed as hypermobile and with hip dysplasia, similar to dancers and gymnasts, due to the similar hip ROM required for performance (32). Therefore, the key areas of focus for strength and conditioning professionals working with these athletes are to improve lower body power and eccentric force production, ensure adequate joint ROM, and enhance the ability to control the limbs through the ROM. Table 11.6 outlines example power training sessions for a competitive surfing athlete.

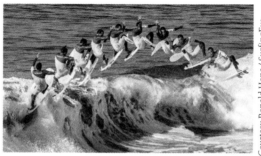

Courtesy Ronald Hons / SurfingEye Images

Figure 11.3 Example of the triple extension required to produce and then absorb power in a typical aerial surfing maneuver.

Table 11.6 Sample Power Training Sessions for a Surfing Athlete

Exercise	Sets × reps	Intensity
DAY 1		
Snatch balance	2 × 5	20-40 kg (44-88 lb)
Snatch from floor	3 × 3	75%, 80%, 85% 1RM
Front squat	4 × 3	85% 1RM
Lateral hurdle jump*	4 × 4	Body weight; use 6 in. (15.2 cm) hurdles
Side MB rotational throw	3 × 5	6, 7, 8 kg (13.2, 15.4, 17.6 lb)
Drop depth jump	3 × 3	12 in. (30.5 cm) box
DAY 2		
Hang clean	4 × 4	75%, 77.5%, 80%, 82.5% 1RM
Accentuated eccentric (DB release) box jump	4 × 3	Use DBs equal to 20% of body weight; use a 20 in. (50.8 cm) soft plyometric box
MB slam from overhead	3 × 5	10 kg (22 lb)
180-Degree rotational vertical jump	3 × 4	Body weight
Plyometric push-up	3 × 5	Body weight

Note: % = prescribed percentage of the 1-repetition maximum; DB = dumbbell; MB = medicine ball.
*Performed as a complex with the front squat (three-minute rest between exercises).

WINTER SPORTS

Power is an important physical quality for a large variety of winter sports, particularly for the sliding sports of skeleton and bobsleigh (4, 28). Of importance to either a skeleton or a bobsleigh athlete's overall performance is the sprint push start performed to initiate the timed run. These starts require maximal-effort sprints for approximately 100 feet (30.5 m) while pushing the sled downhill (slope of approximately 7 degrees) on ice. The athlete needs to generate a nearly maximal sprint velocity in this distance before immediately transitioning to either laying prone and headfirst on the sled (skeleton) or loading into and sitting in the bobsled. Athletes who can perform these sprint push starts faster have a competitive advantage over their competitors, because the ability to develop high initial velocity and downhill momentum is associated with a faster final race time (33). As such, a key focus for the strength and conditioning professional is to enhance the underpinning physical qualities related to faster sprint push start performance in these sports. However, other important considerations in the power training prescription for these athletes are the extreme hip flexion position required to perform the sprint start in the skeleton and the mass of the bobsled (360 pounds [163.3 kg]) in the bobsleigh. Specifically, skeleton athletes will require a large ROM in hip flexion and adequate lower body posterior chain strength to reduce the risk of injury during acceleration, whereas a bobsleigh athlete must be able to produce sufficient power to overcome and accelerate the external mass of the bobsled. Examples of simple low-load exercises that can assist with promoting the development of the necessary hip ROM include the following gluteal exercises: double-leg bridge, side-lying hip abduction, quadruped lower-extremity lift, side-lying gluteal clam at 60 degrees, prone single-leg hip extension, bodyweight squat, and hip abduction in quadruped ("dirty dog"), as described by Crow and colleagues (8).

Table 11.7 provides an example training session for a skeleton competitor. The strength and conditioning professional used a 3RM back squat and vertical jump to assess the athlete's strength and power. The most recent athlete testing identified that maximum strength was above average for this athlete, but the jump height was below average, indicating that power was an issue that needed to be addressed. One of the implemented sessions was a complex session to maintain strength but also increase power. Strength–power potentiation complexes can also be used in these types of sessions, with examples shown in table 3.3 on page 81.

Table 11.7 Sample Power Training Session for a Skeleton Athlete

Exercise	Sets × reps	Intensity
Back squat	4 × 3	90% 1RM
Squat jump[a]	4 × 3	Body weight
Heavy snatch pull from floor	3 × 3	85% 1RM
Broad jump[b]	3 × 3	Body weight
Barbell power jerk	3 × 5	80%-90% 1RM
Depth jump	3 × 3	Use of a 16 in. (40.6 cm), 18 in. (45.7 cm), or 20 in. (50.7 cm) box

[a]Performed as a complex with the back squat (three-minute rest between exercises).
[b]Performed as a complex with the heavy snatch pull (three-minute rest between exercises).

SPEED SKATING (SHORT TRACK)

Short-track speed skating requires athletes to complete a designated number of laps around the 111 meter (365 ft) oval track in an anticlockwise direction as fast as possible. The three events in individual speed skating are the 500-meter (546.8 yd), 1,000-meter (1,093.6 yd), and 1,500-meter (1,640.4 yd) races, all of which require the athlete to possess high sprint-skating velocity and well-developed tactical knowledge. To generate high sprint-skating velocity, the athlete must apply a large concentric impulse into the ice surface through the combination of hip extension, abduction, and external rotation along with ankle plantar flexion (9, 27). In both speed skating and ice hockey, sprint skating performance has been significantly related to a variety of lower body strength and power variables, including CMJ height and relative peak force, broad jump distance, relative 1RM squat, and isometric and dynamic knee extension and hip abduction strength (3, 10, 19, 30). As such, the strength and conditioning professional should seek to incorporate this wide variety of physical qualities into the training program for a speed skating athlete.

Analysis of elite-level 500-meter (546.8 yd) speed skating competitions has revealed that the athlete who wins the race typically enters the first turn of the race before all other competitors (16). This is due to substantial difficulty in successfully overtaking competitors during the remainder of the race while also avoiding the potential to lose balance when jostling for position and to then crash out (23). As such, the sprint start is of great importance for these athletes, because it can dictate their competitive success. Previously, researchers have suggested that both lower body plyometric exercises and off-ice sprinting can provide meaningful improvements in the sprint-start component of speed skating (15, 16, 19). Additionally, during the propulsive phase of the skating stride, force is applied through one leg while the other leg acts as a support. Therefore, high levels of strength and power in single-leg and split-leg positions are highly relevant for these athletes. The strength and conditioning professional should seek to enhance both the force and velocity components of power to optimize the concentric impulse that can be applied into the ice surface. To do so, contrast training can be of great value for short-track speed skating athletes.

An example power training program for a speed skating athlete is provided in table 11.8. The strength and conditioning professional used a 1RM Bulgarian split squat, a CMJ, and a seated single-leg vertical jump (SSLJ) on a portable force plate to assess the athlete's strength and power. It was interpreted that the athlete demonstrated sufficient lower body unilateral strength and bilateral lower body power (CMJ height, >18 in. [45.7 cm]) and dynamic strength (CMJ relative peak force, >2.5 N/BM) to maximize transference to speed skating performance. However, the athlete was benchmarked as below average for unilateral lower body power (SSLJ concentric impulse, <160 N/s for each leg) and dynamic strength (SSLJ relative mean force, <1.4 N/BM for each leg). These unilateral metrics are key foci for the strength and conditioning professional, because they may limit the speed skating athlete's ability to apply the required concentric impulse into the ice surface to maximize sprint skating performance. It is important to note that in this example, relative peak force values were applied due to the practical nuances of the sport; there can be substantial body size differences in short-track speed skating athletes, and relative values provide greater clarity between athletes, not as pseudo indicators of other possible metrics derived from jump testing.

Table 11.8 Sample Power Training Sessions for a Short-Track Speed Skating Athlete

Order	Exercise	Sets × reps or time	Intensity
		DAY 1	
1a	Front squat	4 × 5	83% 1RM
1b	Broad jump	4 × 3	Body weight
2a	Skater squat	3 × 8	Dumbbell loaded; 75% 1RM
2b	Seated vertical jump	3 × 5	Body weight
3a	Isometric Copenhagen hold	3 × 15 s	Body weight
3b	Skater bound	3 × 8	Body weight
		DAY 2	
1	50 meter (or yard) hill sprint	2 × 3	10- to 15-degree incline
2	Loaded jump squat	4 × 3	35% 1RM
3a	Reverse slide split squat	3 × 6	Safety bar loaded; 75% 1RM
3b	Single-leg box jump	3 × 3	Body weight
4a	Lateral lunge	3 × 8	Goblet loaded; 73% 1RM
4b	Split jump	3 × 4	Body weight
		DAY 3	
1a	Bulgarian split squat	4 × 4	85% 1RM
1b	Seated single-leg vertical jump	4 × 3	Body weight
2a	Trap bar squat	4 × 6	82% 1RM
2b	Tuck jump	4 × 5	Body weight
3a	Banded hip abduction	3 × 8	Moderate-tension resistance band
3b	Lateral broad jump	3 × 3	Body weight

Note: Order = Performing one set of each exercise (1a, 1b) in the group one after the other. After the first set is completed, go back to the first exercise in the group and do the second set of each exercise. If certain exercises call for fewer sets than others in the group, perform those sets on the back end of the grouping.

COMBAT SPORTS

In many sports, the ability to produce power repeatedly is important (chapters 1 and 2). This has led to the belief that circuit training with a focus on high repetitions and short rest periods (metabolic conditioning) can improve power and the ability to maintain power over the course of an event. However, research to support this is lacking, and in many cases, this type of training is not relevant to the athlete, nor is it sport specific. Two sports in which this type of training is specific and regularly applied are boxing and mixed martial arts, due to the repeated power efforts required in striking with a fist or foot and the development of nearly maximal high-force power to deliver a knockout with a fist or foot. In comparison, metabolic conditioning is also required for grappling and throwing combat sports, such as judo or wrestling. Specifically, each requires well-developed isometric strength (to hold a position) and an ability to transition rapidly to an explosive, powerful throw while maintaining the ability to perform these movements repeatedly during a bout. The training challenge is the need to combine and balance these training foci. Table 11.9 shows a power training circuit for a wrestler and another for a boxer, in which the athletes rotate through various stations while maintaining power output and session quality. Across the various combat sports, the athlete should receive more than adequate amounts of sport-specific metabolic conditioning from the sport-specific training sessions, thereby allowing the strength and conditioning professional to focus on alternative performance limiters identified in testing.

Table 11.9 Sample Power Circuit for a Wrestler and a Boxer

Exercise*	Sets × reps or distance	Intensity
WRESTLER		
Jump squat	4 × 6	Body weight
Band push-up	4 × 6	Light-tension resistance band
Single-arm dumbbell snatch	4 × 5	20-30 kg (44-66 lb)
Scoop toss	4 × 5	4 kg (8.8 lb)
Squat jump	4 × 6	Body weight
Jump push-up	4 × 5	As fast as possible
Dumbbell power clean to power jerk	4 × 5	25-35 kg (55-77 lb)
Overhead throw	4 × 5	4 kg (8.8 lb)
Torsonator rotation (both directions)	4 × 4	30-40 kg (66-88 lb)
Prowler push	4 × 20 m (or yd)	Heavy load
BOXER		
Alternating split jump	3 × 8	Body weight
Band chin-up	4 × 6	Light-tension resistance band
Single-arm dumbbell snatch	4 × 5	20-30 kg (44-66 lb)
Medicine ball slam	4 × 5	10 kg (22 lb)
Squat jump	4 × 6	Body weight
Alternating single-arm wall throw	4 × 4	4 kg (8.8 lb)
Overhead wall throw	4 × 5	4 kg (8.8 lb)
Abdominal twist	4 × 6	3 kg (6.6 lb)
Landmine press	4 × 5	20-30 kg (44-66 lb); perform explosively

*The athlete takes approximately 30 seconds of rest between stations.

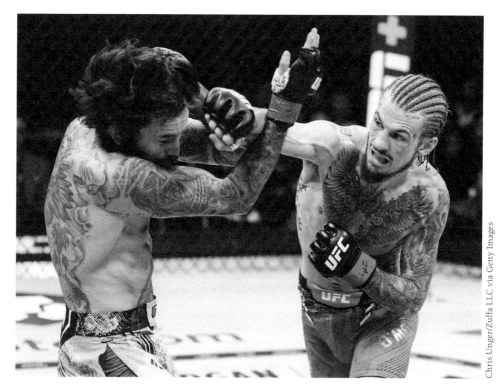

Sean O'Malley trains to develop a consistently powerful attack.

Chris Unger/Zuffa LLC via Getty Images

MONITORING POWER TRAINING

Monitoring power and other variables during training sessions with technology such as linear position transducers, force plates, and accelerometers is common practice in sport settings. As discussed in chapter 9, methods such as velocity-based training (VBT) are becoming more widely used because they provide accepted alternatives to determine optimal resistance training loads through immediate feedback. When technology that can accurately measure velocity is available, figure 9.6 provides a general guideline for establishing training zones from testing data. Also see chapter 2 regarding the assessment of power.

Strength and conditioning professionals may also use the information obtained from these technologies as an indicator of neuromuscular fatigue and the athlete's readiness to train, or more accurately, their readiness to receive their next adaptation stimuli. However, only a small body of research provides evidence-based recommendations for accurately using this type of information in practice. The following is an example of how to use this approach for a downhill skier.

Before the start of each power training session, the athlete performs a series of three squat jumps. A transducer measures mean power output for the jumps. Power testing performed early in the training cycle allows the strength and conditioning professional to determine the athlete's baseline (2,000 W) and smallest worthwhile change (140 W). Therefore, if monitoring produces a result below this threshold (1,860 W), it could indicate residual fatigue. The strength and conditioning professional considers this information in the context of other monitoring information obtained, such as results of a wellness questionnaire or simply asking the athlete how he or she feels. The strength and conditioning professional now has a decision to make: continue with the power training session as planned or modify the session. For example, the number of exercises, sets, or repetitions could be reduced to maintain the quality of the session, or the number of exercises, sets, or repetitions could be retained, and instead, the way the exercises are completed could be changed by using clusters of sets to manipulate the rest-to-recovery ratio. If available technology for monitoring the power of each repetition is used, it can provide further immediate objective information to adjust the session as it progresses through a VBT approach or simply to indicate when repetition power has dropped below the smallest worthwhile change value. The practical challenge is to apply this information without compromising the primary goal (i.e., data-informed decision making that leads to improved performance of the athlete).

CONCLUSION

Many training techniques are available to improve power in athletes who compete in individual sports. The link between testing and programming—that is, how the results of the testing influence the training program design—is crucial. Strength and conditioning professionals have a wide range of tests available to them to assess power in their athletes. However, it is essential that the selected tests relate to the key technical and tactical requirements of the sport, thereby requiring well-developed knowledge of the sport and individual events. It is also important to remember that power development is just one piece of the training puzzle, and it needs to be put in the context of the overall training prescription. Understanding how the development of this athletic quality fits with the athlete's individual needs analysis through monitoring assessments, training methods, and periodization decisions specific to the needs of the athlete and the sport will help strength and conditioning professionals optimize their training programs.

References

Chapter 1

1. Aagaard, P, Andersen, JL, Dyhre-Poulsen, P, Leffers, A-M, Wagner, A, Magnusson, SP, Halk-jaer-Kristensen, J, and Simonsen, EB. A mechanism for increased contractile strength of human pennate muscle in response to strength training: changes in muscle architecture. *J Physiol* 534:613-623, 2001.

2. Ackland, DC, Lin, YC, and Pandy, MG. Sensitivity of model predictions of muscle function to changes in moment arms and muscle-tendon properties: a Monte-Carlo analysis. *J Biomech* 45:1463-1471, 2012.

3. Andersen, LL, and Aagaard, P. Influence of maximal muscle strength and intrinsic muscle contractile properties on contractile rate of force development. *Eur J Appl Physiol* 96:46-52, 2006.

4. Andersen, LL, Andersen, JL, Zebis, MK, and Aagaard, P. Early and late rate of force development: differential adaptive responses to resistance training? *Scand J Med Sci Sports* 20:e162-169, 2010.

5. Arnold, EM, Hamner, SR, Seth, A, Millard, M, and Delp, SL. How muscle fiber lengths and velocities affect muscle force generation as humans walk and run at different speeds. *J Exp Biol* 216:2150-2160, 2013.

6. Askew, GN, and Marsh, RL. Optimal shortening velocity (V/Vmax) of skeletal muscle during cyclical contractions: length-force effects and velocity-dependent activation and deactivation. *J Exp Biol* 201:1527-1540, 1998.

7. Avogadro, P, Chaux, C, Bourdin, M, Dalleau, G, and Belli, A. The use of treadmill ergometers for extensive calculation of external work and leg stiffness during running. *Eur J Appl Physiol* 92:182-185, 2004.

8. Azizi, E, Brainerd, EL, and Roberts, TJ. Variable gearing in pennate muscles. *Proc Natl Acad Sci* 105:1745-1750, 2008.

9. Azizi, E, and Roberts, TJ. Geared up to stretch: pennate muscle behavior during active lengthening. *J Exp Biol* 217:376-381, 2014.

10. Barclay, CJ, Woledge, RC, and Curtin, NA. Inferring crossbridge properties from skeletal muscle energetics. *Prog Biophys Mol Biol* 102:53-71, 2010.

11. Baxter, JR, and Piazza, SJ. Plantar flexor moment arm and muscle volume predict torque-generating capacity in young men. *J Appl Physiol (1985)* 116:538-544, 2014.

12. Belli, A, Kyröläinen, H, and Komi, PV. Moment and power of lower limb joints in running. *Int J Sports Med* 23:136-141, 2002.

13. Benford, J, Hughes, J, Waldron, M, and Theis, N. Concentric versus eccentric training: effect on muscle strength, regional morphology, and architecture. *Transl Sports Med* 4:46-55, 2021.

14. Biewener, AA. Locomotion as an emergent property of muscle contractile dynamics. *J Exp Biol* 219:285-294, 2016.

15. Bloemink, MJ, Melkani, GC, Bernstein, SI, and Geeves, MA. The relay/converter interface influences hydrolysis of ATP by skeletal muscle myosin II. *J Biol Chem* 291:1763-1773, 2016.

16. Bottinelli, R, Canepari, M, Pellegrino, MA, and Reggiani, C. Force-velocity properties of human skeletal muscle fibres: myosin heavy chain isoform and temperature dependence. *J Physiol* 495:573-586, 1996.

17. Bottinelli, R, Pellegrino, MA, Canepari, M, Rossi, R, and Reggiani, C. Specific contributions of various muscle fibre types to human muscle performance: an in vitro study. *J Electromyogr Kinesiol* 9:87-95, 1999.

18. Brainerd, EL, and Azizi, E. Muscle fiber angle, segment bulging and architectural gear ratio in segmented musculature. *J Exp Biol* 208:3249-3261, 2005.

19. Burghardt, TP, Hu, JY, and Ajtai, K. Myosin dynamics on the millisecond time scale. *Biophys Chem* 131:15-28, 2007.

20. Cannon, DT, Bimson, WE, Hampson, SA, Bowen, TS, Murgatroyd, SR, Marwood, S, Kemp, GJ, and Rossiter, HB. Skeletal muscle ATP turnover by 31P magnetic resonance spectroscopy during moderate and heavy bilateral knee extension. *J Physiol* 592:5287-5300, 2014.

21. Cavagna, GA, Legramandi, MA, and La Torre, A. Running backwards: soft landing–hard takeoff, a less efficient rebound. *Proc Biol Sci* 278:339-346, 2010.

22. Cavagna, GA, Legramandi, MA, and Peyré-Tartaruga, LA. Old men running: mechanical work and elastic bounce. *Proc Biol Sci* 275:411-418, 2008.

23. Cavagna, GA, Zamboni, A, Faraggiana, T, and Margaria, R. Jumping on the moon: power output at different gravity values. *Aerosp Med* 43:408-414, 1972.

24. Charles, J, Kissane, R, Hoehfurtner, T, and Bates, KT. From fibre to function: are we accurately representing muscle architecture and performance? *Biol Rev* 97:1640-1676, 2022.

25. Coggan, AR. Use of stable isotopes to study carbohydrate and fat metabolism at the whole-body level. *Proc Nutr Soc* 58:953-961, 1999.

26. Comfort, P, Dos'Santos, T, Jones, PA, McMahon, JJ, Suchomel, TJ, Bazyler, C, and Stone, MH. Normalization of early isometric force production as a percentage of peak force during multijoint isometric assessment. *Int J Sports Physiol Perform* 15:478-482, 2019.

27. Comfort, P, Fletcher, C, and McMahon, JJ. Determination of optimal load during the power clean in collegiate athletes. *J Strength Cond Res* 26:2962-2969, 2012.

28. Comfort, P, Haff, GG, Suchomel, TJ, Soriano, MA, Pierce, KC, Hornsby, WG, Haff, EE, Sommerfield, LM, Chavda, S, Morris, SJ, Fry, AC, and Stone, MH. National strength and conditioning association position statement on weightlifting for sports performance. *J Strength Cond Res* 37:1163-1190, 2023.

29. Comfort, P, McMahon, JJ, and Fletcher, C. No kinetic differences during variations of the power clean in inexperienced female collegiate athletes. *J Strength Cond Res* 27:363-368 2013.

30. Cormie, P, McBride, JM, and McCaulley, GO. Validation of power measurement techniques in dynamic lower body resistance exercises. *J Appl Biomech* 23:103-118, 2007.

31. Cormie, P, McBride, JM, and McCaulley, GO. Power-time, force-time, and velocity-time curve analysis during the jump squat: impact of load. *J Appl Biomech* 24:112-120, 2008.

32. Cormie, P, McCaulley, GO, and McBride, JM. Power versus strength-power jump squat training: influence on the load-power relationship. *Med Sci Sports Exerc* 39:996-1003, 2007.

33. Cormie, P, McCaulley, GO, Triplett, NT, and McBride, JM. Optimal loading for maximal power output during lower-body resistance exercises. *Med Sci Sports Exerc* 39:340-349, 2007.

34. Cormie, P, McGuigan, MR, and Newton, RU. Adaptations in athletic performance after ballistic power versus strength training. *Med Sci Sports Exerc* 42:1582-1598, 2010.

35. Cormie, P, McGuigan, MR, and Newton, RU. Influence of strength on magnitude and mechanisms of adaptation to power training. *Med Sci Sports Exerc* 42:1566-1581, 2010.

36. Cormie, P, McGuigan, MR, and Newton, RU. Influence of training status on power absorption & production during lower body stretch-shorten cycle movements. *J Strength Cond Res* 24:1, 2010.

37. Cormie, P, McGuigan, MR, and Newton, RU. Developing maximal neuromuscular power: part 1—biological basis of maximal power production. *Sports Med* 41:17-38, 2011.

38. Cornachione, AS, Leite, F, Bagni, MA, and Rassier, DE. The increase in non-cross-bridge forces after stretch of activated striated muscle is related to titin isoforms. *Am J Physiol Cell Physiol* 310:C19-26, 2016.

39. Croce, R, Miller, J, Chamberlin, K, Filipovic, D, and Smith, W. Wavelet analysis of quadriceps power spectra and amplitude under varying levels of contraction intensity and velocity. *Muscle Nerve* 50:844-853, 2014.

40. Davies, CT, and Young, K. Effects of external loading on short term power output in children and young male adults. *Eur J Appl Physiol Occup Physiol* 52:351-354, 1984.

41. Del Vecchio, A, Casolo, A, Negro, F, Scorcelletti, M, Bazzucchi, I, Enoka, R, Felici, F, and Farina, D. The increase in muscle force after 4 weeks of strength training is mediated by adaptations in motor unit recruitment and rate coding. *J Physiol* 597:1873-1887, 2019.

42. Del Vecchio, A, Negro, F, Falla, D, Bazzucchi, I, Farina, D, and Felici, F. Higher muscle fiber conduction velocity and early rate of torque development in chronically strength trained individuals. *J Appl Physiol (1985)* 125:1218-1226, 2018.

43. Del Vecchio, A, Negro, F, Holobar, A, Casolo, A, Folland, JP, Felici, F, and Farina, D. You are as fast as your motor neurons: speed of recruitment and maximal discharge of motor neurons determine the maximal rate of force development in humans. *J Physiol* 597:2445-2456, 2019.

44. Deschenes, MR, Judelson, DA, Kraemer, WJ, Meskaitis, VJ, Volek, JS, Nindl, BC, Harman, FS, and Deaver, DR. Effects of resistance training on neuromuscular junction morphology. *Muscle Nerve* 23:1576-1581, 2000.

45. Desmedt, JE and Godaux, E. Ballistic contractions in man: characteristic recruitment pattern of single motor units of the tibialis anterior muscle. *J Physiol* 264:673-693, 1977.

46. di Prampero, PE, and Ferretti, G. The energetics of anaerobic muscle metabolism: a reappraisal of older and recent concepts. *Respir Physiol* 118:103-115, 1999.

47. Dick, TJM, and Wakeling, JM. Shifting gears: dynamic muscle shape changes and force-velocity behavior in the medial gastrocnemius. *J Appl Physiol (1985)* 123:1433-1442, 2017.

48. Diederichs, F. From cycling between coupled reactions to the cross-bridge cycle: mechanical power output as an integral part of energy metabolism. *Metabolites* 2:667-700, 2012.

49. Domire, ZJ, and Challis, JH. Maximum height and minimum time vertical jumping. *J Biomech* 48:2865-2870, 2015.

50. Findley, T, Chaudhry, H, and Dhar, S. Transmission of muscle force to fascia during exercise. *J Bodyw Mov Ther* 19:119-123, 2015.

51. Finni, T, Ikegawa, S, Lepola, V, and Komi, PV. Comparison of force-velocity relationships of vastus lateralis muscle in isokinetic and in stretch-shortening cycle exercises. *Acta Physiol Scand* 177:483-491, 2003.

52. Fischer, G, Storniolo, JL, and Peyré-Tartaruga, LA. Effects of fatigue on running mechanics: spring-mass behavior in recreational runners after 60 seconds of countermovement jumps. *J Appl Biomech* 31:445-451, 2015.

53. Fitts, RH, McDonald, KS, and Schluter, JM. The determinants of skeletal muscle force and power: their adaptability with changes in activity pattern. *J Biomech* 24 Suppl 1:111-122, 1991.

54. Fitts, RH, and Widrick, JJ. Muscle mechanics: adaptations with exercise-training. *Exerc Sport Sci Rev* 24:427-473, 1996.

55. Flores, FJ, Sedano, S, and Redondo, JC. Optimal load and power spectrum during jerk and back jerk in competitive weightlifters. *J Strength Cond Res* 31:809-816, 2017.

56. Flores, FJ, Sedano, S, and Redondo, JC. Optimal load and power spectrum during snatch and clean: differences between international and national weightlifters. *Int J Perform Anal Sport* 17:521-533, 2017.

57. Folland, JP, Buckthorpe, MW, and Hannah, R. Human capacity for explosive force production: neural and contractile determinants. *Scand J Med Sci Sports* 24:894-906, 2014.

58. Folland, JP, and Williams, AG. The adaptations to strength training: morphological and neurological contributions to increased strength. *Sports Med* 37:145-168, 2007.

59. Garhammer, J. Power production by Olympic weightlifters. *Med Sci Sports Exerc* 12:54-60, 1980.

60. Garhammer, J. A review of power output studies of Olympic and powerlifting: methodology, performance prediction, and evaluation tests. *J Strength Cond Res* 7:76-89, 1993.

61. Gastin, PB. Energy system interaction and relative contribution during maximal exercise. *Sports Med* 31:725-741, 2001.

62. Giroux, C, Rabita, G, Chollet, D, and Guilhem, G. Optimal balance between force and velocity differs among world-class athletes. *J Appl Biomech* 32:59-68, 2016.

63. Glancy, B, Barstow, T, and Willis, WT. Linear relation between time constant of oxygen uptake kinetics, total creatine, and mitochondrial content in vitro. *Am J Physiol Cell Physiol* 294:C79-C87, 2008.

64. Hadi, GK, Akku SH, and Harbili, E. Three-dimensional kinematic analysis of the snatch technique for lifting different barbell weights. *J Strength Cond Res* 26:1568-1576, 2012.

65. Haff, GG, and Nimphius, S. Training principles for power. *Strength Cond J* 34:2-12 2012.

66. Haff, GG, Whitley, A, McCoy, LB, O'Bryant, HS, Kilgore, JL, Haff, EE, Pierce, K, and Stone, MH. Effects of different set configurations on barbell velocity and displacement during a clean pull. *J Strength Cond Res* 17:95-103, 2003.

67. Hamner, SR, and Delp, SL. Muscle contributions to fore-aft and vertical body mass center accelerations over a range of running speeds. *J Biomech* 46:780-787, 2013.

68. Harridge, SD, Bottinelli, R, Canepari, M, Pellegrino, M, Reggiani, C, Esbjörnsson, M, Balsom, PD, and Saltin, B. Sprint training, in vitro and in vivo muscle function, and myosin heavy chain expression. *J Appl Physiol (1985)* 84:442-449, 1998.

69. Harridge, SD, Bottinelli, R, Canepari, M, Pellegrino, MA, Reggiani, C, Esbjörnsson, M, and Saltin, B. Whole-muscle and single-fibre contractile properties and myosin heavy chain isoforms in humans. *Pflugers Arch* 432:913-920, 1996.

70. Harris, NK, Cronin, JB, Hopkins, WG, and Hansen, KT. Squat jump training at maximal power loads vs. heavy loads: effect on sprint ability. *J Strength Cond Res* 22:1742-1749, 2008.

71. Hashizume, S, Iwanuma, S, Akagi, R, Kanehisa, H, Kawakami, Y, and Yanai, T. The contraction-induced increase in Achilles tendon moment arm: a three-dimensional study. *J Biomech* 47:3226-3231, 2014.

72. Hawley, JA, and Leckey, JJ. Carbohydrate dependence during prolonged, intense endurance exercise. *Sports Med* 45 Suppl 1:S5-S12, 2015.

73. Heise, GD, Smith, JD, and Martin, PE. Lower extremity mechanical work during stance phase of running partially explains interindividual variability of metabolic power. *Eur J Appl Physiol* 111:1777-1785, 2011.

74. Herbert, RD, Moseley, AM, Butler, JE, and Gandevia, SC. Change in length of relaxed muscle fascicles and tendons with knee and ankle movement in humans. *J Physiol* 539:637-645, 2002.

75. Hintzy, F, Mourot, L, Perrey, S, and Tordi, N. Effect of endurance training on different mechanical efficiency indices during submaximal cycling in subjects unaccustomed to cycling. *Can J Appl Physiol* 30:520-528, 2005.

76. Hori, N, Newton, RU, Andrews, WA, Kawamori, N, McGuigan, MR, and Nosaka, K. Comparison of four different methods to measure power output during the hang power clean and the weighted jump squat. *J Strength Cond Res* 21:314-320, 2007.

77. Hori, N, Newton, RU, Andrews, WA, Kawamori, N, McGuigan, MR, and Nosaka, K. Does Performance of hang power clean differentiate performance of jumping, sprinting, and changing of direction? *J Strength Cond Res* 22:412-418 2008.

78. Hunter, SK, Thompson, MW, Ruell, PA, Harmer, AR, Thom, JM, Gwinn, TH, and Adams, RD. Human skeletal sarcoplasmic reticulum Ca^{2+} uptake and muscle function with aging and strength training. *J Appl Physiol (1985)* 86:1858-1865, 1999.

79. Jiménez-Reyes, P, Samozino, P, Cuadrado-Peñafiel, V, Conceição, F, González-Badillo, JJ, and Morin, JB. Effect of countermovement on power-force-velocity profile. *Eur J Appl Physiol* 114:2281-2288, 2014.

80. Kaneko, M, Fuchimoto, T, Toji, H, and Suei, K. Training effect of different loads on the force-velocity relationship and mechanical power output in human muscle. *Scand J Med Sci Sports* 5:50-55, 1983.

81. Karatzaferi, C, Chinn, MK, and Cooke, R. The force exerted by a muscle cross-bridge depends directly on the strength of the actomyosin bond. *Biophys J* 87:2532-2544, 2004.

82. Kawamori, N, Crum, AJ, Blumert, PA, Kulik, JR, Childers, JT, Wood, JA, Stone, MH, and Haff, GG. Influence of different relative intensities on power output during the hang power clean: identification of the optimal load. *J Strength Cond Res* 19:698-708, 2005.

83. Kilduff, LP, Bevan, H, Owen, N, Kingsley, MI, Bunce, P, Bennett, M, and Cunningham, D. Optimal loading for peak power output during the hang power clean in professional rugby players. *Int J Sports Physiol Perform* 2:260-269, 2007.

84. Kipp, K, Harris, C, and Sabick, M. Correlations between internal and external power outputs during weightlifting exercise. *J Strength Cond Res* 27:1025-1030, 2013.

85. Kirby, TJ, McBride, JM, Haines, TL, and Dayne, AM. Relative net vertical impulse determines jumping performance. *J Appl Biomech* 27:207-214, 2011.

86. Kitamura, K, Tokunaga, M, Iwane, AH, and Yanagida, T. A single myosin head moves along an actin filament with regular steps of 5.3 nanometres. *Nature* 397:129-134, 1999.

87. Knudson, DV. Correcting the use of the term "power" in the strength and conditioning literature. *J Strength Cond Res* 23:1902-1908, 2009.

88. Krylow, AM, and Sandercock, TG. Dynamic force responses of muscle involving eccentric contraction. *J Biomech* 30:27-33, 1997.

89. Kyröläinen, H, and Komi, PV. Differences in mechanical efficiency between power- and endurance-trained athletes while jumping. *Eur J Appl Physiol Occup Physiol* 70:36-44, 1995.

90. Kyröläinen, H, Komi, PV, and Belli, A. Mechanical efficiency in athletes during running. *Scand J Med Sci Sports* 5:200-208, 1995.

91. Lake, JP, Lauder, MA, and Smith, NA. Barbell kinematics should not be used to estimate power output applied to the barbell-and-body system center of mass during lower-body resistance exercise. *J Strength Cond Res* 26:1302-1307, 2012.

92. Loturco, I, Kobal, R, Maldonado, T, Piazzi, AF, Bottino, A, Kitamura, K, Abad, CCC, Pereira, LA, and Nakamura, FY. Jump squat is more related to sprinting and jumping abilities than Olympic push press. *Int J Sports Med* 38:604-612, 2017.

93. Loturco, I, Nakamura, FY, Artioli, GG, Kobal, R, Kitamura, K, Cal Abad, CC, Cruz, IF, Romano, F, Pereira, LA, and Franchini, E. Strength and power qualities are highly associated with punching impact in elite amateur boxers. *J Strength Cond Res* 30:109-116, 2016.

94. Loturco, I, Pereira, LA, Freitas, TT, Bishop, C, Pareja-Blanco, F, and McGuigan, MR. Maximum strength, relative strength, and strength deficit: relationships with performance and differences between elite sprinters and professional rugby union players. *Int J Sports Physiol Perform* 16:1148-1153, 2020.

95. Loturco, I, Pereira, LA, Kobal, R, Maldonado, T, Piazzi, AF, Bottino, A, Kitamura, K, Cal Abad, CC, de Arruda, M, and Nakamura, FY. Improving sprint performance in soccer: effectiveness of jump squat and Olympic push press exercises. *PLoS One* 11:e0153958, 2016.

96. Loturco, I, Suchomel, T, Bishop, C, Kobal, R, Pereira, LA, and McGuigan, M. 1RM measures or maximum bar-power output: which is more related to sport performance? *Int J Sports Physiol Perform* 14:33-37, 2018.

97. Loturco, I, Suchomel, T, James, LP, Bishop, C, Abad, CCC, Pereira, LA, and McGuigan, MR. Selective influences of maximum dynamic strength and bar-power output on team sports performance: a comprehensive study of four different disciplines. *Front Physiol* 9:1820, 2018.

98. Luhtanen, P, and Komi, PV. Mechanical energy states during running. *Eur J Appl Physiol Occup Physiol* 38:41-48, 1978.

99. Luhtanen, P, and Komi, PV. Force-, power-, and elasticity-velocity relationships in walking, running, and jumping. *Eur J Appl Physiol Occup Physiol* 44:279-289, 1980.

100. Maffiuletti, NA, Aagaard, P, Blazevich, AJ, Folland, J, Tillin, N, and Duchateau, J. Rate of force development: physiological and methodological considerations. *Eur J Appl Physiol* 116:1091-1116, 2016.

101. Makaruk, H, Starzak, M, Suchecki, B, Czaplicki, M, and Stojiljković, N. The effects of assisted and resisted plyometric training programs on vertical jump performance in adults: a systematic review and meta-analysis. *J Sports Sci Med* 19:347-357, 2020.

102. 1Mansson, A, Rassier, D, and Tsiavaliaris, G. Poorly understood aspects of striated muscle contraction. *Biomed Res Int* 2015:245154, 2015.

103. Markovic, G, and Jaric, S. Positive and negative loading and mechanical output in maximum vertical jumping. *Med Sci Sports Exerc* 39:1757-1764, 2007.

104. Martin, PE, Heise, GD, and Morgan, DW. Interrelationships between mechanical power, energy transfers, and walking and running economy. *Med Sci Sports Exerc* 25:508-515, 1993.

105. McBride, JM, Haines, TL, and Kirby, TJ. Effect of loading on peak power of the bar, body, and system during power cleans, squats, and jump squats. *J Sports Sci* 29:1215-1221, 2011.

106. McBride, JM, Kirby, TJ, Haines, TL, and Skinner, J. Relationship between relative net vertical impulse and jump height in jump squats performed to various squat depths and with various loads. *Int J Sports Physiol Perform* 5:484-496, 2010.

107. McBride, JM, and Snyder, JG. Mechanical efficiency and force–time curve variation during repetitive jumping in trained and untrained jumpers. *Eur J Appl Physiol* 112:3469-3477, 2012.

108. Meechan, D, McMahon, JJ, Suchomel, TJ, and Comfort, P. A comparison of kinetic and kinematic variables during the pull from the knee and hang pull, across loads. *J Strength Cond Res* 34:1819-1829, 2020.

109. Meechan, D, Suchomel, TJ, McMahon, JJ, and Comfort, P. A comparison of kinetic and kinematic variables during the midthigh pull and countermovement shrug, across loads. *J Strength Cond Res* 34:1830-1841, 2020.

110. Methenitis, SK, Zaras, ND, Spengos, KM, Stasinaki, AN, Karampatsos, GP, Georgiadis, GV, and Terzis, GD. Role of muscle morphology in jumping, sprinting, and throwing performance in participants with different power training duration experience. *J Strength Cond Res* 30:807-817, 2016.

111. Miller, MS, Bedrin, NG, Ades, PA, Palmer, BM, and Toth, MJ. Molecular determinants of force production in human skeletal muscle fibers: effects of myosin isoform expression and cross-sectional area. *Am J Physiol Cell Physiol* 308:C473-C484, 2015.

112. Miller, MS, Bedrin, NG, Callahan, DM, Previs, MJ, Jennings, ME, 2nd, Ades, PA, Maughan, DW, Palmer, BM, and Toth, MJ. Age-related slowing of myosin actin cross-bridge kinetics is sex specific and predicts decrements in whole skeletal muscle performance in humans. *J Appl Physiol (1985)* 115:1004-1014, 2013.

113. Morel, B, Rouffet, DM, Saboul, D, Rota, S, Clémençon, M, and Hautier, CA. Peak torque and rate of torque development influence on repeated maximal exercise performance: contractile and neural contributions. *PLoS One* 10:e0119719, 2015.

114. Nardello, F, Ardigò, LP, and Minetti, AE. Measured and predicted mechanical internal work in human locomotion. *Hum Mov Sci* 30:90-104, 2011.

115. Newton, RU, Häkkinen, K, Häkkinen, A, McCormick, M, Volek, J, and Kraemer, WJ. Mixed-methods resistance training increases power and strength of young and older men. *Med Sci Sports Exerc* 34:1367-1375, 2002.

116. Newton, RU, and Kraemer, WJ. Developing explosive muscular power: implications for a mixed methods training strategy. *Strength Cond J* 16:20-31, 1994.

117. O'Brien, TD, Reeves, ND, Baltzopoulos, V, Jones, DA, and Maganaris, CN. Strong relationships exist between muscle volume, joint power and whole-body external mechanical power in adults and children. *Exp Physiol* 94:731-738, 2009.

118. Pennington, J, Laubach, L, De Marco, G, and Linderman, JON. Determining the optimal load for maximal power output for the power clean and snatch in collegiate male football players. *J Exercise Physiol Online* 13:10-19, 2010.

119. Plas, RL, Degens, H, Meijer, JP, de Wit, GM, Philippens, IH, Bobbert, MF, and Jaspers, RT. Muscle contractile properties as an explanation of the higher mean power output in marmosets than humans during jumping. *J Exp Biol* 218:2166-2173, 2015.

120. Proske, U. Muscle tenderness from exercise: mechanisms? *J Physiol* 564:1, 2005.

121. Proske, U, and Allen, TJ. Damage to skeletal muscle from eccentric exercise. *Exerc Sport Sci Rev* 33:98-104, 2005.

122. Rassier, DE, MacIntosh, BR, and Herzog, W. Length dependence of active force production in skeletal muscle. *J Appl Physiol (1985)* 86:1445-1457, 1999.

123. Rubenson, J, Lloyd, DG, Heliams, DB, Besier, TF, and Fournier, PA. Adaptations for economical bipedal running: the effect of limb structure on three-dimensional joint mechanics. *J R Soc Interface* 8:740-755, 2010.

124. Sasaki, K, Neptune, RR, and Kautz, SA. The relationships between muscle, external, internal and joint mechanical work during normal walking. *J Exp Biol* 212:738-744, 2009.

125. Schache, AG, Brown, NA, and Pandy, MG. Modulation of work and power by the human lower-limb joints with increasing steady-state locomotion speed. *J Exp Biol* 218:2472-2481, 2015.

126. Scott, CB. Contribution of blood lactate to the energy expenditure of weight training. *J Strength Cond Res* 20:404-411, 2006.

127. Seebacher, F, Tallis, JA, and James, RS. The cost of muscle power production: muscle oxygen consumption per unit work increases at low temperatures in Xenopus laevis. *J Exp Biol* 217:1940-1945, 2014.

128. Shen, ZH, and Seipel, JE. A fundamental mechanism of legged locomotion with hip torque and leg damping. *Bioinspir Biomim* 7:046010, 2012.

129. Snow, DH, Harris, RC, and Gash, SP. Metabolic response of equine muscle to intermittent maximal exercise. *J Appl Physiol (1985)* 58:1689-1697, 1985.

130. Søgaard, K, Gandevia, SC, Todd, G, Petersen, NT, and Taylor, JL. The effect of sustained low-intensity contractions on supraspinal fatigue in human elbow flexor muscles. *J Physiol* 573:511-523, 2006.

131. Soriano, MA, Jiménez-Reyes, P, Rhea, MR, and Marin, PJ. The optimal load for maximal power production during lower-body resistance exercises: a meta-analysis. *Sports Med* 45:1191-1205, 2015.

132. Suchomel, TJ, Beckham, GK, and Wright, GA. Lower body kinetics during the jump shrug: impact of load. *J Trainol* 2:19-22, 2013.

133. Suchomel, TJ, Beckham, GK, and Wright, GA. The impact of load on lower body performance variables during the hang power clean. *Sports Biomech* 13:87-95, 2014.

134. Suchomel, TJ, Beckham, GK, and Wright, GA. The effect of various loads on the force-time characteristics of the hang high pull. *J Strength Cond Res* 29:1295-1301, 2015.

135. Suchomel, TJ, Comfort, P, and Lake, JP. Enhancing the force-velocity profile of athletes using weightlifting derivatives. *Strength Cond J* 39:10-20, 2017.

136. Suchomel, TJ, Nimphius, S, Bellon, CR, and Stone, MH. The importance of muscular strength: training considerations. *Sports Med* 48:765-785, 2018.

137. Suchomel, TJ, Nimphius, S, and Stone, MH. the importance of muscular strength in athletic performance. *Sports Med* 46:1419-1449, 2016.

138. Suchomel, TJ, Wright, GA, Kernozek, TW, and Kline, DE. Kinetic comparison of the power development between power clean variations. *J Strength Cond Res* 28:350-360, 2014.

139. Suzuki, M, Fujita, H, and Ishiwata, Si. A new muscle contractile system composed of a thick filament lattice and a single actin filament. *Biophys J* 89:321-328, 2005.

140. Taboga, P, Lazzer, S, Fessehatsion, R, Agosti, F, Sartorio, A, and di Prampero, PE. Energetics and mechanics of running men: the influence of body mass. *Eur J Appl Physiol* 112:4027-4033, 2012.

141. Takei, S, Hirayama, K, and Okada, J. Is the optimal load for maximal power output during hang power cleans submaximal? *Int J Sports Physiol Perform* 15:18-24, 2020.

142. Takei, S, Hirayama, K, and Okada, J. Comparison of the power output between the hang power clean and hang high pull across a wide range of loads in weightlifters. *J Strength Cond Res* 35:S84-S88, 2021.

143. Toji, H, and Kaneko, M. Effect of multiple-load training on the force-velocity relationship. *J Strength Cond Res* 18:792-795, 2004.

144. Toji, H, Suei, K, and Kaneko, M. Effects of combined training loads on relations among force, velocity, and power development. *Can J Appl Physiol* 22:328-336, 1997.

145. Trappe, S, Godard, M, Gallagher, P, Carroll, C, Rowden, G, and Porter, D. Resistance training improves single muscle fiber contractile function in older women. *Am J Physiol Cell Physiol* 281:C398-C406, 2001.

146. Turner, AN, Comfort, P, McMahon, J, Bishop, C, Chavda, S, Read, P, Mundy, P, and Lake, J. Developing powerful athletes part 2: practical applications. *Strength Cond J* 43:23-31, 2020.

147. Turner, AN, Comfort, P, McMahon, J, Bishop, C, Chavda, S, Read, P, Mundy, P, and Lake, J. Developing powerful athletes, part 1: mechanical underpinnings. *Strength Cond J* 42:30-39, 2020.

148. Van Cutsem, M, Duchateau, J, and Hainaut, K. Changes in single motor unit behaviour contribute to the increase in contraction speed after dynamic training in humans. *J Physiol* 513 Pt 1:295-305, 1998.

149. Waterman-Storer, CM. The cytoskeleton of skeletal muscle: is it affected by exercise? A brief review. *Med Sci Sports Exerc* 23:1240-1249, 1991.

150. Willems, PA, Cavagna, GA, and Heglund, NC. External, internal and total work in human locomotion. *J Exp Biol* 198:379-393, 1995.

151. Williams, PE, and Goldspink, G. Longitudinal growth of striated muscle fibres. *J Cell Sci* 9:751-767, 1971.

152. Willis, WT, Jackman, MR, Messer, JI, Kuzmiak-Glancy, S, and Glancy, B. A simple hydraulic analog model of oxidative phosphorylation. *Med Sci Sports Exerc* 48:990-1000, 2016.

153. Winter, EM, Abt, G, Brookes, FBC, Challis, JH, Fowler, NE, Knudson, DV, Knuttgen, HG, Kraemer, WJ, Lane, AM, Mechelen, WV, Morton, RH, Newton, RU, Williams, C, and Yeadon, MR. Misuse of "power" and other mechanical terms in sport and exercise science research. *J Strength Cond Res* 30:292-300, 2016.

Chapter 2

1. Agar-Newman, DJ, and Klimstra, MD. Efficacy of horizontal jumping tasks as a method for talent identification of female rugby players. *J Strength Cond Res* 29:737-743, 2015.

2. Baker, D, and Newton, RU. Methods to increase the effectiveness of maximal power training for the upper body. *Strength Cond J* 27:24-32, 2005.

3. Balsalobre-Fernández, C, Glaister, M, and Lockey, RA. The validity and reliability of an iPhone app for measuring vertical jump performance. *J Sports Sci* 33:1574-1579, 2015.

4. Bosco, C, Luhtanen, P, and Komi, PV. A simple method for measurement of mechanical power in jumping. *Eur J Appl Physiol Occup Physiol* 50:273-282, 1983.

5. Cárdenas, DV, Díaz, RC, Mons, V, Badilla, PV, Pichon, A, Aguilar, DC, Albuquerque, MR, da Silva Santos, JF, and Valenzuela, TH. Physical and physiological profile in youth elite Chilean wrestlers. *Archives of Budo*, 2019.

6. Chia, M, and Aziz, AR. Modelling maximal oxygen uptake in athletes: allometric scaling versus ratio-scaling in relation to body mass. *Ann Acad Med Singap* 37:300-306, 2008.

7. Comfort, P, Haff, GG, Suchomel, TJ, Soriano, MA, Pierce, KC, Hornsby, WG, Haff, EE, Sommerfield, LM, Chavda, S, Morris, SJ, Fry, AC, and Stone, MH. National Strength and Conditioning Association position statement on weightlifting for sports performance. *J Strength Cond Res* 37:1163-1190, 2023.

8. Comyns, TM, Flanagan, EP, Fleming, S, Fitzgerald, E, and Harper, DJ. Inter-day reliability and usefulness of reactive strength index derived from 2 maximal rebound jump tests. *Int J Sports Physiol Perform* 14:1200-1204, 2019.

9. Cormack, SJ, Newton, RU, McGuigan, MR, and Doyle, TL. Reliability of measures obtained during single and repeated countermovement jumps. *Int J Sports Physiol Perform* 3:131-144, 2008.

10. Cormie, P, McBride, JM, and McCaulley, GO. Validation of power measurement techniques in dynamic lower body resistance exercises. *J Appl Biomech* 23:103-118, 2007.

11. Cormie, P, McBride, JM, and McCaulley, GO. Power-time, force-time, and velocity-time curve analysis during the jump squat: impact of load. *J Appl Biomech* 24:112-120, 2008.

12. Cormie, P, McCaulley, GO, Triplett, NT, and McBride, JM. Optimal loading for maximal power output during lower-body resistance exercises. *Med Sci Sports Exerc* 39:340-349, 2007.

13. Crewther, BT, Kilduff, LP, Cook, CJ, Cunningham, DJ, Bunce, PJ, Bracken, RM, and Gaviglio, CM. Scaling strength and power for body mass differences in rugby union players. *J Sports Med Phys Fitness* 52:27-32, 2012.

14. Crewther, BT, Kilduff, LP, Cunningham, DJ, Cook, C, Owen, N, and Yang, GZ. Validating two systems for estimating force and power. *Int J Sports Med* 32:254-258, 2011.

15. Crewther, BT, McGuigan, MR, and Gill, ND. The ratio and allometric scaling of speed, power, and strength in elite male rugby union players. *J Strength Cond Res* 25:1968-1975, 2011.

16. Cronin, J, and Sleivert, G. Challenges in understanding the influence of maximal power training on improving athletic performance. *Sports Medicine* 35:213-234, 2005.

17. Dugan, EL, Doyle, TL, Humphries, B, Hasson, CJ, and Newton, RU. Determining the optimal load for jump squats: a review of methods and calculations. *J Strength Cond Res* 18:668-674, 2004.

18. Escobar Álvarez, JA, Fuentes García, JP, Da Conceição, FA, and Jiménez-Reyes, P. Individualized training based on force–velocity profiling during jumping in ballet dancers. *Int J Sports Physiol Perform* 15:788-794, 2020.

19. Flanagan, EP, and Comyns, TM. The use of contact time and the reactive strength index to optimize fast stretch-shortening cycle training. *Strength Cond J* 30:32-38, 2008.

20. Freeston, JL, Carter, T, Whitaker, G, Nicholls, O, and Rooney, KB. Strength and power correlates of throwing velocity on subelite male cricket players. *J Strength Cond Res* 30:1646-1651, 2016.

21. García-Ramos, A, Pérez-Castilla, A, and Jaric, S. Optimisation of applied loads when using the two-point method for assessing the force-velocity relationship during vertical jumps. *Sports Biomech* 20:274-289, 2021.

22. Garhammer, J. A review of power output studies of Olympic and powerlifting: methodology, performance prediction, and evaluation tests. *J Strength Cond Res* 7:76-89, 1993.

23. Haff, GG, and Nimphius, S. Training principles for power. *Strength Cond J* 34:2-12 2012.

24. Harman, EA, Rosenstein, MT, Frykman, PN, Rosenstein, RM, and Kraemer, WJ. Estimation of human power output from vertical jump. *J Strength Cond Res* 5:116-120, 1991.

25. Harry, JR, Krzyszkowski, J, Chowning, LD, and Kipp, K. Phase-specific force and time predictors of standing long jump distance. *J Appl Biomech* 37:400-407, 2021.

26. Hasson, CJ, Dugan, EL, Doyle, TLA, Humphries, B, and Newton, RU. Neuromechanical strategies employed to increase jump height during the initiation of the squat jump. *J Electromyogr Kinesiol* 14:515-521, 2004.

27. Hicks, DS, Drummond, C, and Williams, KJ. Measurement agreement between Samozino's method and force plate force-velocity profiles during barbell and hexbar countermovement jumps. *J Strength Cond Res* 36:3290-3300, 2022.

28. Hopkins, WG. How to interpret changes in an athletic performance test. *Sportscience* 8:1-7, 2004.

29. Hopkins, WG, Schabort, EJ, and Hawley, JA. Reliability of power in physical performance tests. *Sports Med* 31:211-234, 2001.

30. Hori, N, Newton, RU, Andrews, WA, Kawamori, N, McGuigan, MR, and Nosaka, K. Comparison of four different methods to measure power output during the hang power clean and the weighted jump squat. *J Strength Cond Res* 21:314-320, 2007.

31. Hori, N, Newton, RU, Kawamori, N, McGuigan, MR, Kraemer, WJ, and Nosaka, K. Reliability of performance measurements derived from ground reaction force data during countermovement jump and the influence of sampling frequency. *J Strength Cond Res* 23:874-882, 2009.

32. Hori, N, Newton, RU, Nosaka, K, and McGuigan, MR. Comparison of different methods of determining power output in weightlifting exercises. *Strength Cond J* 28:34-40, 2006.

33. Jaric, S. Role of body size in the relation between muscle strength and movement performance. *Exerc Sport Sci Rev* 31:8-12, 2003.

34. Jiménez-Reyes, P, Samozino, P, Pareja-Blanco, F, Conceição, F, Cuadrado-Peñafiel, V, González-Badillo, JJ, and Morin, J-B. Validity of a simple method for measuring force-velocity-power profile in countermovement jump. *Int J Sports Physiol Perform* 12:36-43, 2017.

35. Kirby, TJ, McBride, JM, Haines, TL, and Dayne, AM. Relative net vertical impulse determines jumping performance. *J Appl Biomech* 27:207-214, 2011.

36. Knudson, DV. Correcting the use of the term "power" in the strength and conditioning literature. *J Strength Cond Res* 23:1902-1908, 2009.

37. Krishnan, A, Sharma, D, Bhatt, M, Dixit, A, and Pradeep, P. Comparison between standing broad jump test and Wingate test for assessing lower limb anaerobic power in elite sportsmen. *Med J Armed Forces India* 73:140-145, 2017.

38. Kumar, A, Singh, RK, Apte, VV, and Kolekar, A. Comparison between seated medicine ball throw test and Wingate test for assessing upper body peak power in elite power sports players. *Indian J Physiol Pharmacol* 64:286-291, 2021.

39. Lake, JP, Lauder, MA, and Smith, NA. Barbell kinematics should not be used to estimate power output applied to the barbell-and-body system center of mass during lower-body resistance exercise. *J Strength Cond Res* 26:1302-1307 2012.

40. Linthorne, NP. The correlation between jump height and mechanical power in a countermovement jump is artificially inflated. *Sports Biomech* 20:3-21, 2021.

41. Mann, JB, Bird, M, Signorile, JF, Brechue, WF, and Mayhew, JL. Prediction of anaerobic power from standing long jump in NCAA Division IA football players. *J Strength Cond Res* 35:1542-1546, 2021.

42. Marovic, I, Janicijevic, D, Knežević, OM, Garcia-Ramos, A, Prebeg, G, and Mirkov, DM. Potential use of the medicine ball throw test to reveal the upper-body maximal capacities to produce force, velocity, and power. *Proc Inst Mech Eng P J Sport Eng Technol*, 2022. [e-pub ahead of print].

43. Maulder, P, and Cronin, J. Horizontal and vertical jump assessment: reliability, symmetry, discriminative and predictive ability. *Phys Ther Sport* 6:74-82, 2005.

44. McBride, JM, Haines, TL, and Kirby, TJ. Effect of loading on peak power of the bar, body, and system during power cleans, squats, and jump squats. *J Sports Sci* 29:1215-1221, 2011.

45. McBride, JM, Kirby, TJ, Haines, TL, and Skinner, J. Relationship between relative net vertical impulse and jump height in jump squats performed to various squat depths and with various loads. *Int J Sports Physiol Perform* 5:484-496, 2010.

46. McBurnie, AJ, Allen, KP, Garry, M, Martin, M, Thomas, DS, Jones, PA, Comfort, P, and McMahon, JJ. The benefits and limitations of predicting one repetition maximum using the load-velocity relationship. *Strength Cond J* 41:28-40, 2019.

47. McClymont, D and Hore, A. Use of the reactive strength index (RSI) as an indicator of plyometric training conditions. In *Science and Football V: The Proceedings of the Fifth World Congress on Sports Science and Football*. Reilly, T, Cabri, J, and Araújo, D, eds. London: Routledge, 408-416, 2003.

48. McGuigan, MR, Doyle, TL, Newton, M, Edwards, DJ, Nimphius, S, and Newton, RU. Eccentric utilization ratio: effect of sport and phase of training. *J Strength Cond Res* 20:992-995, 2006.

49. McLellan, CP, Lovell, DI, and Gass, GC. The role of rate of force development on vertical jump performance. *J Strength Cond Res* 25:379-385, 2011.

50. McMahon, JJ, Jones, PA, Badby, AJ, Ripley, NJ, and Comfort, P. The eccentric utilization ratio is influenced by between-jump differences in propulsion displacement. *J Strength Cond Res* 35:e107-e108, 2020.

51. McMahon, JJ, Lake, JP, Dos'Santos, T, Jones, P, Thomasson, M, and Comfort, P. Counter-movement jump standards in rugby league: what is a "good" performance? *J Strength Cond Res* 36:1691-1698, 2022.

52. McMahon, JJ, Ripley, NJ, and Comfort, P. Force plate-derived countermovement jump normative data and benchmarks for professional rugby league players. *Sensors* 22:8669, 2022.

53. McMahon, JJ, Suchomel, TJ, Lake, JP, and Comfort, P. Understanding the key phases of the countermovement jump force-time curve. *Strength Cond J* 40:96-106, 2018.

54. McMaster, DT, Gill, N, Cronin, J, and McGuigan, M. A brief review of strength and ballistic assessment methodologies in sport. *Sports Med* 44:603-623, 2014.

55. Moir, GL, Gollie, JM, Davis, SE, Guers, JJ, and Witmer, CA. The effects of load on system and lower-body joint kinetics during jump squats. *Sports Biomech* 11:492-506, 2012.

56. Nevill, AM, Bate, S, and Holder, RL. Modeling physiological and anthropometric variables known to vary with body size and other confounding variables. *Am J Phys Anthropol* 128(Suppl 41):141-153, 2005.

57. Nevill, AM, Ramsbottom, R, and Williams, C. Scaling physiological measurements for individuals of different body size. *Eur J Appl Physiol Occup Physiol* 65:110-117, 1992.

58. Nevill, AM, Stewart, AD, Olds, T, and Holder, R. Are adult physiques geometrically similar? The dangers of allometric scaling using body mass power laws. *Am J Phys Anthropol* 124:177-182, 2004.

59. Newton, RU, Häkkinen, K, Häkkinen, A, McCormick, M, Volek, J, and Kraemer, WJ. Mixed-methods resistance training increases power and strength of young and older men. *Med Sci Sports Exerc* 34:1367-1375, 2002.

60. Nimphius, S, McGuigan, MR, and Newton, RU. Relationship between strength, power, speed, and change of direction performance of female softball players. *J Strength Cond Res* 24:885-895, 2010.

61. Nimphius, S, McGuigan, MR, and Newton, RU. Changes in muscle architecture and performance during a competitive season in female softball players. *J Strength Cond Res* 26:2655-2666, 2012.

62. Nuzzo, JL, McBride, JM, Cormie, P, and McCaulley, GO. Relationship between countermovement jump performance and multijoint isometric and dynamic tests of strength. *J Strength Cond Res* 22:699-707, 2008.

63. Owen, NJ, Watkins, J, Kilduff, LP, Bevan, HR, and Bennett, MA. Development of a criterion method to determine peak mechanical power output in a countermovement jump. *J Strength Cond Res* 28:1552-1558, 2014.

64. Petronijevic, MS, Garcia Ramos, A, Mirkov, DM, Jaric, S, Valdevit, Z, and Knezevic, OM. Self-preferred initial position could be a viable alternative to the standard squat jump testing procedure. *J Strength Cond Res* 32:3267-3275, 2018.

65. Samozino, P, Morin, J-B, Hintzy, F, and Belli, A. A simple method for measuring force, velocity and power output during squat jump. *Journal of Biomechanics* 41:2940-2945, 2008.

66. Samozino, P, Rivière, JR, Jimenez-Reyes, P, Cross, MR, and Morin, J-B. Is the concept, method, or measurement to blame for testing error? An illustration using the force-velocity-power profile. *Int J Sports Physiol Perform* 17:1760-1768, 2022.

67. Sánchez-Sixto, A, Harrison, A, and Floría, P. Importance of countermovement depth in stretching and shortening cycle analysis. *Revista Internacional de Medicina y Ciencias de la Actividad Física y del Deporte* 19:33-44, 2019.

68. Sayers, SP, Harackiewicz, DV, Harman, EA, Frykman, PN, and Rosenstein, MT. Cross-validation of three jump power equations. *Med Sci Sports Exerc* 31:572-577, 1999.

69. Scherrer, D, Barker, L, and Harry, J. Influence of takeoff and landing displacement strategies on standing long jump performance. *Int J Strength Cond* 2, 2022.

70. Sheppard, JM and Doyle, TL. Increasing compliance to instructions in the squat jump. *J Strength Cond Res* 22:648-651, 2008.

71. Stone, MH, Stone, ME, and Sands, WA. Champaign, Illinois: Human Kinetics, 2007.

72. Stratford, C, Dos'Santos, T, and McMahon, JJ. The 10/5 repeated jumps test: are 10 repetitions and three trials necessary? *Biomechanics* 1:1-14, 2021.

73. Street, G, McMillan, S, Board, W, Rasmussen, M, and Heneghan, JM. Sources of error in determining countermovement jump height with the impulse method. *J Appl Biomech* 17:43-54, 2001.

74. Suchomel, TJ, McMahon, JJ, and Lake, JP. Combined assessment methods. In *Performance Assessment in Strength and Conditioning.* Comfort, P, Jones, PA, and McMahon, JJ, eds. London: Routledge, 275-290, 2018.

75. Suchomel, TJ, Nimphius, S, and Stone, MH. The importance of muscular strength in athletic performance. *Sports Med* 46:1419-1449, 2016.

76. Suchomel, TJ, Nimphius, S, and Stone, MH. Scaling isometric mid-thigh pull maximum strength in division I athletes: are we meeting the assumptions? *Sports Biomech*, 2018. [e-pub ahead of print].

77. Tessier, JF, Basset, FA, Simoneau, M, and Teasdale, N. Lower-limb power cannot be estimated accurately from vertical jump tests. *J Hum Kinet* 38:5-13, 2013.

78. Thornton, HR, Delaney, JA, Duthie, GM, and Dascombe, BJ. Developing athlete monitoring systems in team sports: data analysis and visualization. *Int J Sports Physiol Perform* 14:698-705, 2019.

79. Trunt, A, Reed, CA, and MacFadden, LN. Assessing the validity of an instrumented medicine ball for measuring throw speed. *Sports Engineering* 26:20, 2023.

80. Turner, AN, Jones, B, Stewart, P, Bishop, C, Parmar, N, Chavda, S, and Read, P. Total score of athleticism: holistic athlete profiling to enhance decision-making. *Strength Cond J* 41:91-101, 2019.

81. van den Tillaar, R, and Marques, MC. Reliability of seated and standing throwing velocity using differently weighted medicine balls. *J Strength Cond Res* 27:1234-1238, 2013.

82. Vanderburgh, PM, Sharp, M, and Nindl, B. Nonparallel slopes using analysis of covariance for body size adjustment may reflect inappropriate modeling. *Meas Phys Educ Exerc Sci* 2:127-135, 1998.

83. Wakai, M, and Linthorne, NP. Optimum take-off angle in the standing long jump. *Human Movement Science* 24:81-96, 2005.

84. Wilson, GJ, Newton, RU, Murphy, AJ, and Humphries, BJ. The optimal training load for the development of dynamic athletic performance. *Med Sci Sports Exerc* 25:1279-1286, 1993.

85. Winter, EM, Abt, G, Brookes, FBC, Challis, JH, Fowler, NE, Knudson, DV, Knuttgen, HG, Kraemer, WJ, Lane, AM, Mechelen, WV, Morton, RH, Newton, RU, Williams, C, and Yeadon, MR. Misuse of "power" and other mechanical terms in sport and exercise science research. *J Strength Cond Res* 30:292-300, 2016.

86. Zoeller, RF, Ryan, ED, Gordish-Dressman, H, Price, TB, Seip, RL, Angelopoulos, TJ, Moyna, NM, Gordon, PM, Thompson, PD, and Hoffman, EP. Allometric scaling of biceps strength before and after resistance training in men. *Med Sci Sports Exerc* 39:1013-1019, 2007.

87. Zoeller, RF, Ryan, ED, Gordish-Dressman, H, Price, TB, Seip, RL, Angelopoulos, TJ, Moyna, NM, Gordon, PM, Thompson, PD, and Hoffman, EP. Allometric scaling of isometric biceps strength in adult females and the effect of body mass index. *Eur J Appl Physiol* 104:701-710, 2008.

88. Zushi, A, Yoshida, T, Zushi, K, Kariyama, Y, and Ogata, M. Characteristics of three lower limb joint kinetics affecting rebound jump performance. *PLoS One* 17:e0268339, 2022.

Chapter 3

1. Aagaard, P, Simonsen, EB, Andersen, JL, Magnusson, P, and Dyhre-Poulsen, P. Increased rate of force development and neural drive of human skeletal muscle following resistance training. *J Appl Physiol* 93:1318-1326, 2002.

2. Aagaard, P, Simonsen, EB, Andersen, JL, Magnusson, P, and Dyhre-Poulsen, P. Neural adaptation to resistance training: changes in evoked V-wave and H-reflex responses. *J Appl Physiol* 92:2309-2318, 2002.

3. Aagaard, P, Simonsen, EB, Trolle, M, Bangsbo, J, and Klausen, K. Effects of different strength training regimes on moment and power generation during dynamic knee extensions. *Eur J Appl Physiol* 69:382-386, 1994.

4. Baker, D. Comparison of upper-body strength and power between professional and college-aged rugby league players. *J Strength Cond Res* 15:30-35, 2001.

5. Baker, D. A series of studies on the training of high-intensity muscle power in rugby league football players. *J Strength Cond Res* 15:198-209, 2001.

6. Banister, EW, Carter, JB, and Zarkadas, PC. Training theory and taper: validation in triathlon athletes. *Eur J Appl Physiol Occup Physiol* 79:182-191, 1999.

7. Barker, M, Wyatt, TJ, Johnson, RL, Stone, MH, O'Bryant, HS, Poe, C, and Kent, M. Performance factors, physiological assessment, physical characteristic, and football playing ability. *J Strength Cond Res* 7:224-233, 1993.

8. Bartolomei, S, Hoffman, JR, Merni, F, and Stout, JR. A comparison of traditional and block periodized strength training programs in trained athletes. *J Strength Cond Res* 28:990-997, 2014.

9. Bompa, TO, and Buzzichelli, CA. Periodization as planning and programming of sport training. In *Periodization Training for Sports*. 3rd ed. Champaign, IL: Human Kinetics, 87-98, 2015.

10. Bompa, TO, and Haff, GG. *Periodization: Theory and Methodology of Training*. 5th ed. Champaign, IL: Human Kinetics, 1-424, 2009.

11. Bondarchuk, AP. Track and field training. *Legkaya Atletika* 12:8-9, 1986.

12. Bondarchuk, AP. Constructing a training system. *Track Tech* 102:254-269, 1988.

13. Bondarchuk, AP. The role and sequence of using different training-load intensities. *Fit Sports Rev Inter* 29:202-204, 1994.

14. Bosquet, L, Montpetit, J, Arvisais, D, and Mujika, I. Effects of tapering on performance: a meta-analysis. *Med Sci Sports Exerc* 39:1358-1365, 2007.

15. Bruin, G, Kuipers, H, Keizer, HA, and Vander Vusse, GJ. Adaptation and overtraining in horses subjected to increasing training loads. *J Appl Physiol* 76:1908-1913, 1994.

16. Buckner, SL, Jessee, MB, Mouser, JG, Dankel, SJ, Mattocks, KT, Bell, ZW, Abe, T, and Loenneke, JP. The basics of training for muscle size and strength: a brief review on the theory. *Med Sci Sports Exerc* 52:645-653, 2020.

17. Chiu, LZF, and Barnes, JL. The fitness-fatigue model revisited: implications for planning short- and long-term training. *Strength Cond J* 25:42-51, 2003.

18. Comfort, P, Haff, GG, Suchomel, TJ, Soriano, MA, Pierce, KC, Hornsby, WG, Haff, EE, Sommerfield, LM, Chavda, S, Morris, SJ, Fry, AC, and Stone, MH. National strength and conditioning association position statement on weightlifting for sports performance. *J Strength Cond Res* 37:1163-1190, 2023.

19. Cormie, P, McGuigan, MR, and Newton, RU. Adaptations in athletic performance following ballistic power vs. strength training. *Med Sci Sports Exerc* 42:1582-1598, 2010.

20. Cormie, P, McGuigan, MR, and Newton, RU. Developing maximal neuromuscular power: part 2—training considerations for improving maximal power production. *Sports Med* 41:125-146, 2011.

21. Cormier, P, Freitas, TT, Loturco, I, Turner, A, Virgile, A, Haff, GG, Blazevich, AJ, Agar-Newman, D, Henneberry, M, Baker, DG, McGuigan, M, Alcaraz, PE, and Bishop, C. Within session exercise sequencing during programming for complex training: historical perspectives, terminology, and training considerations. *Sports Med* 52:2371-2389, 2022.

22. Counsilman, JE, and Counsilman, BE. Advanced theories in planning of training. In *The New Science of Swimming*. 2nd ed. Englewood Cliffs, NJ: Prentice Hall, 229-255, 1994.

23. Coyne, J, and French, D. Concurrent technical and non-technical training considerations. In *A Cross-Sectional Performance Analysis and Projection of the UFC Athlete*. French, D, ed. Las Vegas, NV: UFC Performance Institue, 156-160, 2021.

24. Cronin, JB, McNair, PJ, and Marshall, RN. The role of maximal strength and load on initial power production. *Med Sci Sports Exerc* 32:1763-1769, 2000.

25. Cunanan, AJ, DeWeese, BH, Wagle, JP, Carroll, KM, Sausaman, R, Hornsby, WG, 3rd, Haff, GG, Triplett, NT, Pierce, KC, and Stone, MH. The General adaptation syndrome: a foundation for the concept of periodization. *Sports Med* 48:787-797, 2018.

26. DeBeliso, M, Harris, C, Spitzer-Gibson, T, and Adams, KJ. A comparison of periodised and fixed repetition training protocol on strength in older adults. *J Sci Med Sport* 8:190-199, 2005.

27. DeWeese, BH, Hornsby, G, Stone, M, and Stone, MH. The training process: planning for strength–power training in track and field. Part 1: theoretical aspects. *J Sport Health Sci* 4:308-317, 2015.

28. DeWeese, BH, Hornsby, G, Stone, M, and Stone, MH. The training process: planning for strength–power training in track and field. Part 2: practical and applied aspects. *J Sport Health Sci* 4:318-324, 2015.

29. Elbadry, N, Hamza, A, Pietraszewski, P, Alexe, DI, and Lupu, G. Effect of the French contrast method on explosive strength and kinematic parameters of the triple jump among female college athletes. *J Hum Kinet* 69:225-230, 2019.

30. Fleck, SJ, and Kraemer, WJ. Periodized training. In *The Ultimate Training System: Periodization Breakthrough*. New York, NY: Advanced Research Press, 17-22, 1996.

31. Fleck, SJ, and Kraemer, WJ. Advanced training strategies. In *Designing Resistance Training Programs*. 4th ed. Champaign, IL: Human Kinetics, 257-296, 2014.

32. Foster, C. Monitoring training in athletes with reference to overtraining syndrome. *Med Sci Sports Exerc* 30:1164-1168, 1998.

33. Francis, C. *The Structure of Training for Speed*. CharlieFrancis.Com, 1-72, 2008.

34. Fry, AC. The role of training intensity in resistance exercise overtraining and overreaching. In *Overtraining in Sport*. Kreider, RB, Fry, AC, O'Toole, ML, eds. Champaign, IL: Human Kinetics,107-127, 1998.

35. Garcia-Pallares, J, Garcia-Fernandez, M, Sanchez-Medina, L, and Izquierdo, M. Performance changes in world-class kayakers following two different training periodization models. *Eur J Appl Physiol* 110:99-107, 2010.

36. Gorostiaga, EM, Navarro-Amezqueta, I, Calbet, JA, Hellsten, Y, Cusso, R, Guerrero, M, Granados, C, Gonzalez-Izal, M, Ibanez, J, and Izquierdo, M. Energy metabolism during repeated sets of leg press exercise leading to failure or not. *PLoS One* 7:e40621, 2012.

37. Haff, GG. Periodization of training. In *Conditioning for Strength and Human Performance*. 2nd ed. Brown, LE, and Chandler J, eds. Philadelphia, PA: Wolters Kluwer, Lippincott, Williams & Wilkins, 326-345, 2012.

38. Haff, GG. Periodization. In *Essentials of Strength Training and Conditioning*. 4th ed. Haff, GG, and Triplett, NT, eds. Champaign, IL: Human Kinetics, 583-604, 2016.

39. Haff, GG. Isometric and dynamic testing. In *Performance Assessments for Strength and Conditioning Coaches*. Comfort, P, Jones, PA, McMahon, JJ, eds. Oxon, United Kingdom: Taylor Francis Books, 168-194, 2019.

40. Haff, GG. Periodization strategies for youth development. In *Strength and Conditioning for the Young Athlete: Science and Application*. 2nd ed. Lloyd, R, and Oliver, JL, eds. London, England: Routledge, 281-299, 2019.

41. Haff, GG. The essentials of periodisation. In *Strength and Conditioning for Sports Performance*. 2nd ed. Jeffreys, I, and Moody, J, eds. Abingdon, Oxon: Routledge, 394-444, 2021.

42. Haff, GG. Peaking. In *High-Performance Training for Sports*. 2nd ed. Joyce, D, and Lewindon, D, eds. Champaign, IL: Human Kinetics, 330-343, 2022.

43. Haff, GG. Periodization and programming of individual sports. In *NSCA'S Essentials of Sport Science*. French, D, and Torres Ronda, L, eds. Champaign, IL: Human Kinetics, 27-42, 2022.

44. Haff, GG, Burgess, S, and Stone, MH. Cluster training: theoretical and practical applications for the strength and conditioning professional. *Prof Strength Cond* 12:12-17, 2008.

45. Haff, GG, Carlock, JM, Hartman, MJ, Kilgore, JL, Kawamori, N, Jackson, JR, Morris, RT, Sands, WA, and Stone, MH. Force-time curve characteristics of dynamic and isometric muscle actions of elite women Olympic weightlifters. *J Strength Cond Res* 19:741-748, 2005.

46. Haff, GG, and Haff, EE. Resistance training program design. In *Essentials of Periodization*. 2nd ed. Malek, MH, and Coburn, JW, eds. Champaign, IL: Human Kinetics, 359-401, 2012.

47. Haff, GG, and Haff, EE. Training integration and periodization. In *Strength and Conditioning Program Design*. Hoffman, J, ed. Champaign, IL: Human Kinetics, 209-254, 2012.

48. Haff, GG, and Harden, M. Cluster Sets: scientific background and practical applications. In *Advanced Strength and Conditioning: An Evidence-Based Approach*. 2nd ed. Turner, A, and Comfort, P, eds. London: Routledge Taylor Francis, 213-232, 2022.

49. Haff, GG, Hobbs, RT, Haff, EE, Sands, WA, Pierce, KC, and Stone, MH. Cluster training: a novel method for introducing training program variation. *Strength Cond J* 30:67-76, 2008.

50. Haff, GG, and Nimphius, S. Training principles for power. *Strength Cond J* 34:2-12, 2012.

51. Haff, GG, Ruben, RP, Lider, J, Twine, C, and Cormie, P. A comparison of methods for determining the rate of force development during isometric midthigh clean pulls. *J Strength Cond Res* 29:386-395, 2015.

52. Haff, GG, Stone, MH, O'Bryant, HS, Harman, E, Dinan, CN, Johnson, R, and Han, KH. Force-time dependent characteristics of dynamic and isometric muscle actions. *J Strength Cond Res* 11:269-272, 1997.

53. Haff, GG, Whitley, A, and Potteiger, JA. A brief review: explosive exercises and sports performance. *Strength Cond J* 23:13-20, 2001.

54. Hardee, JP, Travis Triplett, N, Utter, AC, Zwetsloot, KA, and McBride, JM. Effect of interrepetition rest on power output in the power clean. *J Strength Cond Res* 26: 883-889, 2012.

55. Harre, D, Harre, D, and Barsch, J. The formation of the standard of athletic performance. In *Principles of Sports Training: Introduction to the Theory and Methods of Training*. Muskegon, MI: Ultimate Athlete Concepts, 70-112, 2012.

56. Harris, GR, Stone, MH, O'Bryant, HS, Proulx, CM, and Johnson, RL. Short-term performance effects of high power, high force, or combined weight-training methods. *J Strength Cond Res* 14:14-20, 2000.

57. Harris NK, Cronin JB, Hopkins WG, and Hansen KT. Squat jump training at maximal power loads vs. heavy loads: effect on sprint ability. *J Strength Cond Res* 22:1742-1749, 2008.

58. Hartmann, H, Wirth, K, Keiner, M, Mickel, C, Sander, A, and Szilvas, E. Short-term periodization models: effects on strength and speed-strength performance. *Sports Med* 45:1373-1386, 2015.

59. Hernandez-Preciado, JA, Baz, E, Balsalobre-Fernandez, C, Marchante, D, and Santos-Concejero, J. Potentiation effects of the French contrast method on vertical jumping ability. *J Strength Cond Res* 32:1909-1914, 2018.

60. Hornsby, WG, Gentles, JA, MacDonald, CJ, Mizuguchi, S, Ramsey, MW, and Stone, MH. Maximum strength, rate of force development, jump height, and peak power alterations in weightlifters across five months of training. *Sports* 5:78, 2017.

61. Howatson, G, Brandon, R, and Hunter, AM. The response to and recovery from maximum strength and power training in elite track and field athletes. *Int J Sports Physiol Perform* 11:356-362, 2015.

62. Imbach, F, Sutton-Charani N, Montmain J, Candau R, and Perrey S. The Use of Fitness-Fatigue Models for Sport Performance Modelling: Conceptual Issues and Contributions from Machine-Learning. *Sports Med Open* 8: 29, 2022.

63. Ishida, A, Travis, SK, and Stone, MH. Short-term periodized programming may improve strength, power, jump kinetics, and sprint efficiency in soccer. *J Funct Morphol Kinesiol* 6:45, 2021.

64. Issurin, V. Block periodization versus traditional training theory: a review. *J Sports Med Phys Fitness* 48:65-75, 2008.

65. Issurin, V. *Block Periodization: Breakthrough in Sports Training*. Muskegon, MI: Ultimate Athlete Concepts, 1-213, 2008.

66. Issurin, V. Microcycles, mesocycles, and training stages. In *Block Periodization: Breakthrough in Sports Training*. Muskegon, MI: Ultimate Athlete Concepts, 78-127, 2008.

67. Issurin, V. Periodization training from ancient precursors to structured block models. *Kinesiology* 46:3-9, 2014.

68. Issurin, VB. New horizons for the methodology and physiology of training periodization. *Sports Med* 40:189-206, 2010.

69. Izquierdo, M, Ibanez, J, Gonzalez-Badillo, JJ, Ratamess, NA, Kraemer, WJ, Häkkinen, K, Bonnabau, H, Granados, C, French, DN, and Gorostiaga, EM. Detraining and tapering effects on hormonal responses and strength performance. *J Strength Cond Res* 21:768-775, 2007.

70. Jeffreys, I. Quadrennial planning for the high school athlete. *Strength Cond J* 30:74-83, 2008.

71. Jovanović, M. Planning. In *Strength Training Manual: The Agile Periodization Approach: Volume 2*. Belgrade, Serbia: Complementary Training, 9-63, 2019.

72. Kaneko, M, Fuchimoto, T, Toji, H, and Suei ,K. Training effect of different loads on the force-velocity relationship and mechanical power output in human muscle. *Scand J Sports Sci* 5:50-55, 1983.

73. Kataoka, R, Vasenina, E, Loenneke, J, and Buckner, SL. Periodization: variation in the definition and discrepancies in study design. *Sports Med* 51:625-651, 2021.

74. Kawamori, N, and Haff, GG. The optimal training load for the development of muscular power. *J Strength Cond Res* 18:675-684, 2004.

75. Keiner, M, Sander, A, Wirth, K, Caruso, O, Immesberger, P, and Zawieja, M. Strength performance in youth: trainability of adolescents and children in the back and front squats. *J Strength Cond Res* 27:357-362, 2013.

76. Kirby, TJ, Erickson, T, and McBride, JM. Model for progression of strength, power, and speed training. *Strength Cond J* 32:86-90, 2010.

77. Kraemer, WJ, and Fleck, SJ. Periodization of resistance training. In *Optimizing Strength Training*. Champaign, IL: Human Kinetics, 1-26, 2007.

78. Kraemer, WJ, Hatfield, DL, and Fleck, SJ. Types of muscle training. In: *Strength Training*. Brown, LE, ed. Champaign, IL: Human Kinetics, 45-72, 2007.

79. Kraska, JM, Ramsey, MW, Haff, GG, Fethke, N, Sands, WA, Stone, ME, and Stone, MH. Relationship between strength characteristics and unweighted and weighted vertical jump height. *Int J Sports Physiol Perform* 4:461-473, 2009.

80. Kubo, T, Hirayama, K, Nakamura, N, and Higuchi, M. Influence of different loads on force-time characteristics during back squats. *J Sports Sci Med* 17:617-622, 2018.

81. Kurz, T. Cycles in sports training. In *Science of Sports Training*. 2nd ed. Island Pond, VT: Stadion Publishing Company, Inc., 51-98, 2001.

82. Lawton, TW, Cronin, JB, and Lindsell, RP. Effect of interrepetition rest intervals on weight training repetition power output. *J Strength Cond Res* 20:172-176, 2006.

83. Loturco, I, Dello Iacono, A, Nakamura, FY, Freitas, TT, Boullosa, D, Valenzuela, PL, Pereira, LA, and McGuigan, MR. The optimum power load: a simple and powerful tool for testing and training. *Int J Sports Physiol Perform* 17:151-159, 2022.

84. Lovell, DI, Cuneo, R, and Gass, GC. The effect of strength training and short-term detraining on maximum force and the rate of force development of older men. *Eur J Appl Physiol* 109:429-435, 2010.

85. Maffiuletti, NA, Aagaard, P, Blazevich, AJ, Folland, J, Tillin, N, and Duchateau, J. Rate of force development: physiological and methodological considerations. *Eur J Appl Physiol* 116:1091-1116, 2016.

86. Marshall, J, Bishop, C, Turner, A, and Haff, GG. Optimal training sequences to develop lower body force, velocity, power, and jump height: a systematic review with meta-analysis. *Sports Med* 51:1245-1271, 2021.

87. Matveyev, LP. *Fundamentals of Sports Training*. Moscow: Fizkultua i Sport, 1-311, 1977.

88. McBride, JM, Triplett-McBride, T, Davie, A, and Newton, RU. A comparison of strength and power characteristics between power lifters, Olympic lifters, and sprinters. *J Strength Cond Res* 13:58-66, 1999.

89. McBride, JM, Triplett-McBride, T, Davie, A, and Newton, RU. The effect of heavy- vs. light-load jump squats on the development of strength, power, and speed. *J Strength Cond Res* 16:75-82, 2002.

90. McMaster, DT, Gill, N, Cronin, J, and McGuigan, M. The development, retention and decay rates of strength and power in elite rugby union, rugby league and American football: a systematic review. *Sports Med* 43:367-384, 2013.

91. Minetti, AE. On the mechanical power of joint extensions as affected by the change in muscle force (or cross-sectional area), ceteris paribus. *Eur J Appl Physiol* 86:363-369, 2002.

92. Moss, BM, Refsnes, PE, Abildgaard, A, Nicolaysen, K, and Jensen, J. Effects of maximal effort strength training with different loads on dynamic strength, cross-sectional area, load-power and load-velocity relationships. *Eur J Appl Physiol* 75:193-199, 1997.

93. Mujika, I, Halson, S, Burke, L, Balagué, G, and Farrow, D. An integrated, multifactorial approach to periodization for optimal performance in individual and team sports. *Int J Sports Physiol Perform* 13:538-561, 2018.

94. Mujika, I, and Padilla, S. Detraining: loss of training-induced physiological and performance adaptations. Part I: short term insufficient training stimulus. *Sports Med* 30:79-87, 2000.

95. Mujika, I, and Padilla, S. Detraining: loss of training-induced physiological and performance adaptations. Part II: Long term insufficient training stimulus. *Sports Med* 30:145-154, 2000.

96. Mujika, I, and Padilla, S. Scientific bases for precompetition tapering strategies. *Med Sci Sports Exerc* 35:1182-1187, 2003.

97. Munroe, L, and Haff, GG. Sprint cycling. In *Routledge Handbook of Strength and Conditioning*. Turner, A, ed. New York: Routledge, 506-525, 2018.

98. Nádori, L. Theoretical and methodological basis of training planning. In *Theoretical and Methodological Basis of Training Planning With Special Considerations Within a Microcycle*. Nádori, L, and Granek, I, eds. Lincoln, NE: NSCA, 1-25, 1989.

99. Nagatani, T, Haff, GG, Guppy, SN, and Kendall, KL. Practical application of traditional and cluster set configurations within a resistance training program. *Strength Cond J* 44:87-101, 2022.

100. Nagatani, T, Kendall, KL, Guppy, SN, and Haff, GG. Using cluster set configurations within a resistance training programme. *Prof Strength Cond* 65:7-17, 2022.

101. Newton, RU, and Kraemer, WJ. Developing explosive muscular power: implications for a mixed methods training strategy. *Strength Cond J* 16:20-31, 1994.

102. Olbrect, J. *The Science of Winning: Planning, Periodizing, and Optimizing Swim Training*. Luton, England: Swimshop, 1-282, 2000.

103. Painter, K, Haff, G, Ramsey, M, McBride, J, Triplett, T, Sands, W, Lamont, H, Stone, M, and Stone, M. Strength gains: block versus daily undulating periodization weight training among track and field athletes. *Int J Sports Physiol Perform* 7:161-169, 2012.

104. Plisk, SS, and Stone, MH. Periodization strategies. *Strength Cond J* 25:19-37, 2003.

105. Rhea, MR, Ball, SD, Phillips, WT, and Burkett, LN. A comparison of linear and daily undulating periodized programs with equated volume and intensity for strength. *J Strength Cond Res* 16:250-255, 2002.

106. Roll, F, and Omer, J. Football: Tulane football winter program. *Strength Cond J* 9:34-38, 1987.

107. Rowbottom, DG. Periodization of training. In *Exercise and Sport Science*. Garrett, WE, and Kirkendall DT, eds. Philadelphia, PA: Lippincott Williams and Wilkins, 499-512, 2000.

108. Ruben, RM, Molinari, MA, Bibbee, CA, Childress, MA, Harman, MS, Reed, KP, and Haff, GG. The acute effects of an ascending squat protocol on performance during horizontal plyometric jumps. *J Strength Cond Res* 24:358-369, 2010.

109. Seitz, L, Saez de Villarreal, E, and Haff, GG. The temporal profile of postactivation potentiation is related to strength level. *J Strength Cond Res* 28:706-715, 2014.

110. Seitz, LB, and Haff, GG. Factors modulating post-activation potentiation of jump, sprint, throw and upper-body ballistic performances: a systematic review with meta-analysis. *Sports Med* 46:231-240, 2016.

111. Selye, H. The birth of the G.A.S. In *The stress of life*. New York: McGraw-Hill, 25-47, 1956.

112. Sheppard, J, and Triplett, NT. Program design for resistance training. In *Essentials of Strength Training and Conditioning*. 4th ed. Haff, GG, Triplett, N, eds. Champaign, IL: Human Kinetics, 439-470, 2016.

113. Siff, MC. Organisation of training. In *Supertraining*. 6th ed. Denver, CO: Supertraining Institute, 311-390, 2003.

114. Smith, DJ. A framework for understanding the training process leading to elite performance. *Sports Med* 33:1103-1126, 2003.

115. Soriano, MA, Jimenez-Reyes, P, Rhea, MR, and Marin, PJ. The optimal load for maximal power production during lower-body resistance exercises: a meta-analysis. *Sports Med* 45:1191-1205, 2015.

116. Soriano, MA, Suchomel, TJ, and Marín, PJ. The optimal load for maximal power production during upper-body resistance exercises: a meta-analysis. *Sports Med* 47:757-768, 2017.

117. Stone, MH, Hornsby, WG, Haff, GG, Fry, AC, Suarez, DG, Liu, J, Gonzalez-Rave, JM, and Pierce, KC. Periodization and block periodization in sports: emphasis on strength-power training—a provocative and challenging narrative. *J Strength Cond Res* 35:2351-2371, 2021.

118. Stone, MH, Moir, G, Glaister, M, and Sanders, R. How much strength is necessary? *Physical Therapy in Sport* 3:88-96, 2002.

119. Stone, MH, O'Bryant, H, and Garhammer, J. A hypothetical model for strength training. *J Sports Med* 21:342-351, 1981.

120. Stone, MH, Stone, ME, and Sands, WA. *Principles and Practice of Resistance Training*. Champaign, IL: Human Kinetics, 1-376, 2007.

121. Stone, MH, Suchomel, TJ, Hornsby, WG, Wagle, JP, and Cunanan, AJ. *Strength and Conditioning in Sports: From Science to Practice.* New York: Routledge, 221-251, 2023.

122. Stults-Kolehmainen, MA, Bartholomew, JB, and Sinha, R. Chronic psychological stress impairs recovery of muscular function and somatic sensations over a 96-hour period. *J Strength Cond Res* 28:2007-2017, 2014.

123. Suarez, DG, Mizuguchi, S, Hornsby, WG, Cunanan, AJ, Marsh, DJ, and Stone, MH. Phase-specific changes in rate of force development and muscle morphology throughout a block periodized training cycle in weightlifters. *Sports* 7:129, 2019.

124. Suchomel, TJ, Comfort, P, and Lake, JP. Enhancing the force–velocity profile of athletes using weightlifting derivatives. *Strength Cond J* 39:10-20, 2017.

125. Suchomel, TJ, Nimphius, S, Bellon, CR, and Stone, MH. The importance of muscular strength: training considerations. *Sports Med* 48:765-785, 2018.

126. Suchomel, TJ, Nimphius, S, and Stone, MH. The importance of muscular strength in athletic performance. *Sports Med* 46:1419-1449, 2016.

127. Suchomel, TJ, Wagle, JP, Douglas, J, Taber, CB, Harden, M, Haff, GG, and Stone, MH. Implementing eccentric resistance training—part 1: a brief review of existing methods. *J Funct Morphol Kinesiol* 4:38, 2019.

128. Suchomel, TJ, Wagle, JP, Douglas, J, Taber, CB, Harden, M, Haff, GG, and Stone, MH. Implementing eccentric resistance training—part 2: practical recommendations. *J Funct Morphol Kinesiol* 4:55, 2019.

129. Sukop, J, and Nelson, R. Effect of isometric training on the force-time characteristics of muscle contraction. In *Biomechanics IV.* Nelson, RC, and Morehouse, CA, eds. Baltimore, MD: University Park Press, 440-447, 1974.

130. Thibaudeau, C. The science of strength. In *Theory and Application of Modern Strength and Power Methods.* Grand Rapids MI: F. Lepine Publishing, 9-40, 2006.

131. Thorstensson, A, Grimby, G, and Karlsson, J. Force-velocity relations and fiber composition in human knee extensor muscles. *J Appl Physiol* 40:12-16, 1976.

132. Toji, H, and Kaneko, M. Effect of multiple-load training on the force-velocity relationship. *J Strength Cond Res* 18:792-795, 2004.

133. Toji, H, Suei, K, and Kaneko, M. Effects of combined training programs on force-velocity relation and power output in human muscle. *Jpn J Phys Fitness Sports Med* 44:439-445, 1995.

134. Travis, SK, Mujika, I, Gentles, JA, Stone, MH, and Bazyler, CD. Tapering and peaking maximal strength for powerlifting performance: a review. *Sports* 8:125, 2020.

135. Tufano, JJ, Conlon, JA, Nimphius, S, Brown, LE, Seitz, LB, Williamson, BD, and Haff, GG. Maintenance of velocity and power with cluster sets during high-volume back squats. *Int J Sports Physiol Perform* 11:885-892, 2016.

136. Verkhoshansky, Y. Organization of the training process. *New Stud Athl* 13:21-31, 1998.

137. Verkhoshansky, Y, and Siff, MC. *Supertraining: Expanded Version.* 6th ed. Rome, Italy: Verkhoshansky, 1-577, 2009.

138. Verkhoshansky, Y, and Verkhoshansky, N. Organization of special strength training in the training process and the block training system. In *Special Strength Training Manual for Coaches.* Rome, Italy: Verkhoshansky SSTM, 117-144, 2011.

139. Verkhoshansky, YU. *Programming and Organization of Training.* Moscow: Fizkultura i Sport, 1985.

140. Verkhoshansky, YU. Theory and methodology of sport preparation: block training system for top-level athletes. *Teoria i Practica Physicheskoj Culturi* 4:2-14, 2007.

141. Verkhoshansky, YV. Regularities of the Process of attaining sport mastery. In *Programming and Organization of Training.* Livonia, MI: Sportivny Press, 18-81, 1988.

142. Viitasalo, JT, and Komi, PV. Rate of force development, muscle structure and fatigue. In *Biomechanics VII-A: Proceedings of the 7th International Congress of Biomechanics.* Morecki, A, Kazimirz, F, Kedzior, K, and Wit, A, eds. Baltimore, MD: University Park Press, 136-141, 1981.

143. Wilson, GJ, Newton, RU, Murphy, AJ, and Humphries, BJ. The optimal training load for the development of dynamic athletic performance. *Med Sci Sports Exerc* 25:1279-1286, 1993.

144. Yakovlev, NN. Biochemistry of sport in the Soviet Union: beginning, development, and present status. *Med Sci Sports* 7:237-247, 1975.

145. Zamparo, P, Minetti, AE, and di Prampero, PE. Interplay among the changes of muscle strength, cross-sectional area and maximal explosive power: theory and facts. *Eur J Appl Physiol* 88:193-202, 2002.

146. Zatsiorsky, VM. Basic concepts of training theory. In *Science and Practice of Strength Training*. Champaign, IL: Human Kinetics, 3-19, 1995.

147. Zatsiorsky, VM, Kraemer, WJ, and Fry, AC. *Science and Practice of Strength Training*. 3rd ed. Champaign, IL: Human Kinetics, 1-344, 2021.

148. Zemkova, E, Poor, O, and Pecho, J. peak rate of force development and isometric maximum strength of back muscles are associated with power performance during load-lifting tasks. *Am J Mens Health* 13:1557988319828622, 2019.

Chapter 4

1. Arampatzis, A, Degens, H, Baltzopoulos, V, and Rittweger, J. Why do older sprinters reach the finish line later? *Exerc Sport Sci Rev* 39:18-22, 2011.

2. Baechle, TR, and Westcott, W. *Fitness Professional's Guide to Strength Training Older Adults*. 2nd ed. Champaign, IL: Human Kinetics, 2018.

3. Bean, JF, Kiely, DK, Herman, S, Leveille, SG, Mizer, K, Frontera, WR, and Fielding, RA. The relationship between leg power and physical performance in mobility-limited older people. *J Am Geriatr Soc* 50:461-467, 2002.

4. Behm, DG, and Sale, DG. Intended rather than actual movement velocity determines velocity-specific training response. *J Appl Physiol (1985)* 74:359-368, 1993.

5. Behm, DG, Young, JD, Whitten, JHD, Reid, JC, Quigley, PJ, Low, J, Li, Y, Lima, CD, Hodgson, DD, Chaouachi, A, Prieske, O, and Granacher, U. Effectiveness of traditional strength vs. power training on muscle strength, power and speed with youth: a systematic review and meta-analysis. *Front Physiol* 8:423, 2017.

6. Behringer, M, Vom Heede, A, Matthews, M, and Mester, J. Effects of strength training on motor performance skills in children and adolescents: a meta-analysis. *Pediatr Exerc Sci* 23:186-206, 2011.

7. Beunen, G, Malina, RM. Growth and physical performance relative to the timing of the adolescent spurt. *Exerc Sport Sci Rev* 16:503-540, 1988.

8. Beunen, G, Ostyn, M, Simons, J, Renson, R, Claessens, AL, Vanden Eynde, B, Lefevre, J, Vanreusel, B, Malina, RM, and van't Hof, MA. Development and tracking in fitness components: Leuven longtudinal study on lifestyle, fitness and health. *Int J Sports Med* 18 (Suppl 3):S171-S178, 1997.

9. Branta, C, Haubenstricker, J, and Seefeldt, V. Age changes in motor skills during childhood and adolescence. *Exerc Sport Sci Rev* 12:467-520, 1984.

10. Caserotti, P, Aagaard, P, Simonsen, EB, and Puggaard, L. Contraction-specific differences in maximal muscle power during stretch-shortening cycle movements in elderly males and females. *Eur J Appl Physiol* 84:206-212, 2001.

11. Chaouachi, A, Hammami, R, Kaabi, S, Chamari, K, Drinkwater, EJ, and Behm, DG. Olympic weightlifting and plyometric training with children provides similar or greater performance improvements than traditional resistance training. *J Strength Cond Res* 28:1483-1496, 2014.

12. Cohen, D, Voss, C, Taylor, M, Delextrat, A, Ogunleye, A, and Sandercock, G. Ten-year secular changes in muscular fitness in English children. *Acta Paediatr* 100:e175-e177, 2011.

13. Cormie, P, McGuigan, MR, and Newton, RU. Developing maximal neuromuscular power: part 2—training considerations for improving maximal power production. *Sports Med* 41:125-146, 2011.

14. Cuoco, A, Callahan, DM, Sayers, S, Frontera, WR, Bean, J, and Fielding, RA. Impact of muscle power and force on gait speed in disabled older men and women. *J Gerontol A Biol Sci Med Sci* 59:1200-1206, 2004.

15. Dalziel, WM, Neal, RJ, and Watts, MC. A comparison of peak power in the shoulder press and shoulder throw. *J Sci Med Sport* 5:229-235, 2002.

16. de Vos, NJ, Singh, NA, Ross, DA, Stavrinos, TM, Orr, R, and Fiatarone Singh, MA. Effect of power-training intensity on the contribution of force and velocity to peak power in older adults. *J Aging Phys Act* 16:393-407, 2008.

17. de Vos, NJ, Singh, NA, Ross, DA, Stavrinos, TM, Orr, R, and Fiatarone Singh, MA. Optimal load for increasing muscle power during explosive resistance training in older adults. *J Gerontol A Biol Sci Med Sci* 60:638-647, 2005.

18. Dotan, R, Mitchell, C, Cohen, R, Klentrou, P, Gabriel, D, and Falk, B. Child-adult differences in muscle activation—a review. *Pediatr Exerc Sci* 24:2-21, 2012.

19. Drey, M, Sieber, CC, Degens, H, McPhee, J, Korhonen, MT, Muller, K, Ganse, B, and Rittweger, J. Relation between muscle mass, motor units and type of training in master athletes. *Clin Physiol Funct Imaging* 36:70-76, 2016.

20. Du, K, Goates, S, Arensberg, MB, Pereira, S, and Gaillard, T. Prevalence of sarcopenia and sarcopenic obesity vary with race/ethnicity and advancing age. *Divers Equal Health Care* 14:175-183, 2018.

21. Earles, DR, Judge, JO, and Gunnarsson, OT. Velocity training induces power-specific adaptations in highly functioning older adults. *Arch Phys Med Rehabil* 82:872-878, 2001.

22. El Hadouchi, M, Kiers, H, de Vries, R, Veenhof, C, and van Dieen, J. Effectiveness of power training compared to strength training in older adults: a systematic review and meta-analysis. *Eur Rev Aging Phys Act* 19:18, 2022.

23. Faigenbaum, AD, Farrell, A, Fabiano, M, Radler, T, Naclerio, F, Ratamess, NA, Kang, J, and Myer, GD. Effects of integrative neuromuscular training on fitness performance in children. *Pediatr Exerc Sci* 23:573-584, 2011.

24. Faigenbaum, AD, Farrell, AC, Fabiano, M, Radler, TA, Naclerio, F, Ratamess, NA, Kang, J, and Myer, GD. Effects of detraining on fitness performance in 7-year-old children. *J Strength Cond Res* 27:323-330; 2013.

25. Faigenbaum, AD, Lloyd, RS, MacDonald, J, and Myer, GD. Citius, Altius, Fortius: beneficial effects of resistance training for young athletes: narrative review. *Br J Sports Med* 50:3-7, 2016.

26. Faigenbaum, AD, Lloyd, RS, and Oliver JL. *ACSM Essentials of Youth Fitness.* Champaign, IL: Human Kinetics; 2019.

27. Fernandes, JFT, Lamb, KL, Norris, JP, Moran, J, Drury, B, Borges, NR, and Twist, C. Aging and recovery after resistance-exercise-induced muscle damage: current evidence and implications for future research. *J Aging Phys Act* 29:544-551, 2021.

28. Fielding, RA, LeBrasseur, NK, Cuoco, A, Bean, J, Mizer, K, and Fiatarone Singh, MA. High-velocity resistance training increases skeletal muscle peak power in older women. *J Am Geriatr Soc* 50:655-662, 2002.

29. Foldvari, M, Clark, M, Laviolette, LC, Bernstein, MA, Kaliton, D, Castaneda, C, Pu, CT, Hausdorff, JM, Fielding, RA, and Singh, MA. Association of muscle power with functional status in community-dwelling elderly women. *J Gerontol A Biol Sci Med Sci* 55:M192-M199, 2000.

30. Gorostiaga, EM, Izquierdo, M, Ruesta, M, Iribarren, J, Gonzalez-Badillo, JJ, and Ibanez, J. Strength training effects on physical performance and serum hormones in young soccer players. *Eur J Appl Physiol* 91:698-707, 2004.

31. Granacher, U, Lesinski, M, Busch, D, Muehlbauer, T, Prieske, O, Puta, C, Gollhofer, A, and Behm, DG. Effects of resistance training in youth athletes on muscular fitness and athletic performance: a conceptual model for long-term athlete development. *Front Physiol* 7:164; 2016.

32. Haff, GG, and Nimphius, S. Training principles for power. *Strength Cond J* 34:2-12; 2012.

33. Hafsteinsson, A. Prevalence of sarcopenia in community-dwelling habitués of day-care and social services at three nursing homes in the Greater Reykjavik area. University of Iceland; 2023.

34. Hakkinen, K, Kraemer, WJ, Newton, RU, and Alen, M. Changes in electromyographic activity, muscle fibre and force production characteristics during heavy resistance/power strength training in middle-aged and older men and women. *Acta Physiol Scand* 171:51-62, 2001.

35. Harries, SK, Lubans, DR, and Callister, R. Resistance training to improve power and sports performance in adolescent athletes: a systematic review and meta-analysis. *J Sci Med Sport* 15:532-540; 2012.

36. Hazell, T, Kenno, K, Jakobi, J. Functional benefit of power training for older adults. *J Aging Phys Act* 15:349-359, 2007.

37. Hinman, JD, Peters, A, Cabral, H, Rosene, DL, Hollander, W, Rasband, MN, and Abraham, CR. Age-related molecular reorganization at the node of Ranvier. *J Comp Neurol* 495:351-362, 2006.

38. HURUSA. 4 power training methods for older adults 2022. https://hurusa.com/power-training-for-older-adults-how-to-train-for-power/.

39. Izquierdo, M, Merchant, RA, Morley, JE, Anker, SD, Aprahamian, I, Arai, H, Aubertin-Leheudre, M, Bernabei, R, Cadore, EL, Cesari, M, Chen, LK, de Souto Barreto, P, Duque, G, Ferrucci, L, Fielding, RA, Garcia-Hermoso, A, Gutierrez-Robledo, LM, Harridge, SDR, Kirk, B, Kritchevsky, S, Landi, F, Lazarus, N, Martin, FC, Marzetti, E, Pahor, M, Ramirez-Velez, R, Rodriguez-Manas, L, Rolland, Y, Ruiz, JG, Theou, O, Villareal, DT, Waters, DL, Won Won, C, Woo, J, Vellas, B, and Fiatarone Singh, M. International exercise recommendations in older adults (ICFSR): expert consensus guidelines. *J Nutr Health Aging* 25:824-853; 2021.

40. Jankelowitz, SK, McNulty, PA, and Burke, D. Changes in measures of motor axon excitability with age. *Clin Neurophysiol* 118:1397-1404, 2007.

41. Keiner, M, Sander, A, Wirth, K, Caruso, O, Immesberger, P, and Zawieja, M. Strength performance in youth: trainability of adolescents and children in the back and front squats. *J Strength Cond Res* 27:357-362, 2013.

42. Komi, PV. Stretch-shortening cycle: a powerful model to study normal and fatigued muscle. *J Biomech* 33:1197-1206, 2000.

43. Kowalchuk, K, and Butcher, S. Eccentric overload flywheel training in older adults. *J Funct Morphol Kinesiol* 4:61, 2019.

44. Kumar, NTA, Radnor, JM, Oliver, JL, Lloyd, RS, Pedley, JS, Wong, MA, and Dobbs, IJ. The influence of maturity status on drop jump kinetics in male youth. *J Strength Cond Res* 38:38-46, 2024.

45. le Gall, F, Carling, C, Williams, M, and Reilly, T. Anthropometric and fitness characteristics of international, professional and amateur male graduate soccer players from an elite youth academy. *J Sci Med Sport* 13:90-95, 2010.

46. Lesinski, M, Herz, M, Schmelcher, A, and Granacher, U. Effects of resistance training on physical fitness in healthy children and adolescents: an umbrella review. *Sports Med* 50:1901-1928, 2020.

47. Lesinski, M, Prieske, O, and Granacher, U. Effects and dose–response relationships of resistance training on physical performance in youth athletes: a systematic review and meta-analysis. *Br J Sports Med* 50:781-795, 2016.

48. Lexell, J. Ageing and human muscle: observations from Sweden. *Can J Appl Physiol* 18:2-18, 1993.

49. Linkul, R. Strength training for the older client—a blueprint for program design. *Personal Training Quarterly* 5.1, 2017.

50. Lloyd, R, Radnor, J, De Ste Croix, M, Cronin, J, and Oliver, J. Changes in sprint and jump performances after traditional, plyometric, and combined resistance training in male youth pre- and post-peak height velocity. *J Strength Cond Res* 30:1239-1247, 2016.

51. Lloyd, RS, Cronin, JB, Faigenbaum, AD, Haff, GG, Howard, R, Kraemer, WJ, Micheli, LJ, Myer, GD, and Oliver, JL. National Strength and Conditioning Association position statement on long-term athletic development. *J Strength Cond Res* 30:1491-1509, 2016.

52. Lloyd, RS, Dobbs, IJ, Wong, MA, Moore, IS, and Oliver, JL. Effects of training frequency during a 6-month neuromuscular training intervention on movement competency, strength, and power in male youth. *Sports Health* 14:57-68, 2022.

53. Lloyd, RS, Faigenbaum, A, Stone, M, Oliver, J, Jeffreys, I, Moody, J, Brewer, C, Pierce, K, McCambridge, T, Howard, R, Herrington, L, Hainline, B, Micheli, L, Jaques, R, Kraemer, W, McBride, M, Best, T, Chu, D, Alvar, B, and Myer, G. Position statement on youth resistance training: the 2014 International Consensus. *Br J Sports Med* 48:498-505, 2014.

54. Lloyd, RS, and Oliver, JL. The youth physical development model: a new approach to long-term athletic development. *Strength Cond J* 34:61-72, 2012.

55. Lloyd, RS, Oliver, JL, Faigenbaum, AD, Howard, R, De Ste Croix, MB, Williams, CA, Best, TM, Alvar, BA, Micheli, LJ, Thomas, DP, Hatfield, DL, Cronin, JB, and Myer, GD. Long-term athletic development, part 2: barriers to success and potential solutions. *J Strength Cond Res* 29:1451-1464; 2015.

56. Lloyd, RS, Oliver, JL, Faigenbaum, AD, Myer, GD, and De Ste Croix, MB. Chronological age vs. biological maturation: implications for exercise programming in youth. *J Strength Cond Res* 28:1454-1464, 2014.

57. Lloyd, RS, Oliver, JL, Hughes, MG, and Williams, CA. Age-related differences in the neural regulation of stretch-shortening cycle activities in male youths during maximal and sub-maximal hopping. *J Electromyogr Kinesiol* 22:37-43; 2012.

58. Lloyd, RS, Oliver, JL, Hughes, MG, and Williams, CA. The effects of 4-weeks of plyometric training on reactive strength index and leg stiffness in male youths. *J Strength Cond Res* 26:2812-2819, 2012.

59. Lloyd, RS, Oliver, JL, Hughes, MG, and Williams, CA. The influence of chronological age on periods of accelerated adaptation of stretch-shortening cycle performance in pre and postpubescent boys. *J Strength Cond Res* 25:1889-1897, 2011.

60. Marques, MC, Izquiredo, M, and Pereira, A. High-speed resistance training in elderly peopl: a new approach toward counteracting age-related functional capacity loss. *Strength Cond J* 35:23-29, 2013.

61. Marsh, AP, Miller, ME, Rejeski, WJ, Hutton, SL, and Kritchevsky, SB. Lower extremity muscle function after strength or power training in older adults. *J Aging Phys Act* 17:416-443; 2009.

62. Meylan, CM, Cronin, JB, Oliver, JL, Hopkins, WG, and Contreras, B. The effect of maturation on adaptations to strength training and detraining in 11-15-year-olds. *Scand J Med Sci Sports* 24:e156-e164, 2014.

63. Meylan, CM, Cronin, JB, Oliver, JL, Hughes, MG, and Manson, S. An evidence-based model of power development in youth soccer. *Int J Sports Sci Coach* 9:1241-1264, 2014.

64. Miszko, TA, Cress, ME, Slade, JM, Covey, CJ, Agrawal, SK, and Doerr, CE. Effect of strength and power training on physical function in community-dwelling older adults. *J Gerontol A Biol Sci Med Sci* 58:171-175, 2003.

65. Moeskops, S, Oliver, J, Read, P, Cronin, J, Myer, G, Moore, I, and Lloyd, R. The influence of biological maturity on dynamic force–time variables and vaulting performance in young female gymnasts. *J Sci Sport Exerc* 2:319-329, 2020.

66. Moeskops, S, Oliver, JL, Read, PJ, Haff, GG, Myer, GD, and Lloyd, RS. Effects of a 10-month neuromuscular training program on strength, power, speed, and vault performance in young female gymnasts. *Med Sci Sports Exerc* 54:861-871, 2022.

67. Moeskops, S, Pedley, JS, Oliver, JL, and Lloyd, RS. The influence of competitive level on stretch-shortening cycle function in young female gymnasts. *Sports (Basel)* 10:107, 2022.

68. Moody, JA, Naclerio, F, Green, P, and Lloyd, RS. Motor skill development in youths. In Lloyd, RS, and Oliver, JL, eds. *Strength and Conditioning for Young Athletes: Science and Application.* Oxon, England: Routledge, 49-65, 2013.

69. Moran, J, Sandercock, G, Rumpf, MC, and Parry, DA. Variation in responses to sprint training in male youth athletes: a meta-analysis. *Int J Sports Med* 38:1-11, 2017.

70. Morris, SJ, Oliver, JL, Pedley, JS, Haff, GG, Lloyd, RS. Taking a long-term approach to the development of weightlifting ability in young athletes. *Strength Cond J* 42:71-90; 2020.

71. Myer, G, Sugimoto, D, Thomas, S, and Hewett, T. The influence of age on the effectiveness of neuromuscular training to reduce anterior cruciate ligament injuries in female athletes: a meta analysis. *Am J Sports Med* 41:203-215, 2013.

72. Myer, GD, Lloyd, RS, Brent, JL, and Faigenbaum, AD. how young is "too young" to start training? *ACSMs Health Fit J* 17:14-23, 2013.

73. Newton, RU, Hakkinen, K, Hakkinen, A, McCormick, M, Volek, J, and Kraemer, WJ. Mixed-methods resistance training increases power and strength of young and older men. *Med Sci Sports Exerc* 34:1367-1375, 2002.

74. Nogueira, W, Gentil, P, Mello, SN, Oliveira, RJ, Bezerra, AJ, and Bottaro, M. Effects of power training on muscle thickness of older men. *Int J Sports Med* 30:200-204, 2009.

75. Pedley, JS, DiCesare, CA, Lloyd, RS, Oliver, JL, Ford, KR, Hewett, TE, and Myer, GD. Maturity alters drop vertical jump landing force-time profiles but not performance outcomes in adolescent females. *Scand J Med Sci Sports* 31:2055-2063, 2021.

76. Peitz, M, Behringer, M, and Granacher, U. A systematic review on the effects of resistance and plyometric training on physical fitness in youth—what do comparative studies tell us? *PLoS One* 13:e0205525, 2018.

77. Pereira, A, Izquierdo, M, Silva, AJ, Costa, AM, Bastos, E, Gonzalez-Badillo, JJ, and Marques, MC. Effects of high-speed power training on functional capacity and muscle performance in older women. *Exp Gerontol* 47:250-255, 2012.

78. Pescatello, LS, Arena, R, Riebe, D, and Thompson, PD. *ACSM's Guidelines for Exercise Testing and Prescription*. 9th ed. Philadelphia, PA: Lippincott, Williams, and Wilkins, 2014.

79. Petrella, JK, Kim, JS, Tuggle, SC, and Bamman, MM. Contributions of force and velocity to improved power with progressive resistance training in young and older adults. *Eur J Appl Physiol* 99:343-351, 2007.

80. Pichardo, AW, Oliver, JL, Harrison, CB, Maulder, PS, Lloyd, RS, and Kandoi. R. The influence of maturity offset, strength, and movement competency on motor skill performance in adolescent males. *Sports (Basel)* 7:168, 2019.

81. Piirainen, JM, Cronin, NJ, Avela, J, and Linnamo, V. Effects of plyometric and pneumatic explosive strength training on neuromuscular function and dynamic balance control in 60-70 year old males. *J Electromyogr Kinesiol* 24:246-252, 2014.

82. Porter, MM. Power training for older adults. *Appl Physiol Nutr Metab* 31:87-94, 2006.

83. Porter, MM, Vandervoort, AA, Lexell, J. Aging of human muscle: structure, function and adaptability. *Scand J Med Sci Sports* 5:129-142, 1995.

84. Quatman, CE, Ford, KR, Myer, GD, and Hewett, TE. Maturation leads to gender differences in landing force and vertical jump performance: a longitudinal study. *Am J Sports Med* 34:806-813, 2006.

85. Radnor, JM, Moeskops, S, Morris, SJ, Mathews, TA, Kumar, NTA, Pullen, BJ, Meyers, RW, Pedley, JS, Gould, ZI, Oliver, JL, and Lloyd, RS. Developing athletic motor skill competencies in youth. *Strength Cond J* 42:54-70, 2020.

86. Radnor, JM, Oliver, JL, Waugh, CM, Myer, GD, and Lloyd, RS. Influence of muscle architecture on maximal rebounding in young boys. *J Strength Cond Res* 35:3378-3385, 2021.

87. Radnor, JM, Oliver, JL, Waugh, CM, Myer, GD, and Lloyd, RS. Muscle architecture and maturation influence sprint and jump ability in young boys: a multistudy approach. *J Strength Cond Res* 36:2741-2751, 2022.

88. Radnor, JM, Oliver, JL, Waugh, CM, Myer, GD, Moore, IS, and Lloyd, RS. The influence of growth and maturation on stretch-shortening cycle function in youth. *Sports Med* 48:57-71, 2018.

89. Reid, KF, and Fielding, RA. Skeletal muscle power: a critical determinant of physical functioning in older adults. *Exerc Sport Sci Rev* 40:4-12, 2012.

90. Reid, KF, Martin, KI, Doros, G, Clark, DJ, Hau, C, Patten, C, Phillips, EM, Frontera, WR, and Fielding, RA. Comparative effects of light or heavy resistance power training for improving lower extremity power and physical performance in mobility-limited older adults. *J Gerontol A Biol Sci Med Sci* 70:374-380, 2015.

91. Runhaar, J, Collard, DC, Singh, A, Kemper, HC, van Mechelen, W, Chinapaw, M. Motor fitness in Dutch youth: differences over a 26-year period (1980-2006). *J Sci Med Sport* 13:323-328, 2010.

92. Sander, A, Keiner, M, Wirth, K, and Schmidtbleicher, D. Influence of a 2-year strength training programme on power performance in elite youth soccer players. *Eur J Sport Sci* 13:445-451, 2013.

93. Sayers, SP, Bean, J, Cuoco, A, LeBrasseur, NK, Jette, A, and Fielding, RA. Changes in function and disability after resistance training: does velocity matter? A pilot study. *Am J Phys Med Rehabil* 82:605-613, 2003.

94. Sayers SP, Gibson K. A comparison of high-speed power training and traditional slow-speed resistance training in older men and women. *J Strength Cond Res* 24:3369-3380, 2010.

95. Shaibi, GQ, Cruz, ML, Ball, GD, Weigensberg, MJ, Salem, GJ, Crespo, NC, and Goran, MI. Effects of resistance training on insulin sensitivity in overweight Latino adolescent males. *Med Sci Sports Exerc* 38:1208-1215, 2006.

96. Shiekhy, J. Phyio Network2022. https://www.physio-network.com/blog/dose-strength-training-older-adults/#:~:text=Strength%20training%20is%20vital%20for,hard"%20to%20"hard.

97. Skelton, DA, Greig, CA, Davies, JM, and Young, A. Strength, power and related functional ability of healthy people aged 65-89 years. *Age Ageing* 23:371-377, 1994.

98. Skelton, DA, Kennedy, J, and Rutherford, OM. Explosive power and asymmetry in leg muscle function in frequent fallers and non-fallers aged over 65. *Age Ageing* 31:119-125, 2002.

99. Slimani, M, Paravlic, A, and Granacher, U. A meta-analysis to determine strength training related dose-response relationships for lower-limb muscle power development in young athletes. *Front Physiol* 9:1155, 2018.

100. Sommerfield, LM, Harrison, CB, Whatman, CS, and Maulder, PS. Relationship between strength, athletic performance, and movement skill in adolescent girls. *J Strength Cond Res* 36:674-679, 2022.

101. Stone, MH, O'Bryant, HS, McCoy, L, Coglianese, R, Lehmkuhl, M, and Schilling, B. Power and maximum strength relationships during performance of dynamic and static weighted jumps. *J Strength Cond Res* 17:140-147, 2003.

102. Tonson, A, Ratel, S, Le Fur, Y, Cozzone, P, and Bendahan, D. Effect of maturation on the relationship between muscle size and force production. *Med Sci Sports Exerc* 40: 918-925, 2008.

103. Tremblay, MS, Gray, CE, Akinroye, K, Harrington, DM, Katzmarzyk, PT, Lambert, EV, Liukkonen, J, Maddison, R, Ocansey, RT, Onywera, VO, Prista, A, Reilly, JJ, Rodriguez, Martinez, MP, Sarmiento, Duenas, OL, Standage, M, and Tomkinson, G. Physical activity of children: a global matrix of grades comparing 15 countries. *J Phys Act Health* 11(Suppl 1):S113-S125, 2014.

104. Tschopp, M, Sattelmayer, MK, and Hilfiker, R. Is power training or conventional resistance training better for function in elderly persons? a meta-analysis. *Age Ageing* 40:549-556, 2011.

105. Tudorascu, I, Sfredel, V, Riza, AL, Danciulescu Miulescu, R, Ianosi, SL, and Danoiu, S. Motor unit changes in normal aging: a brief review. *Rom J Morphol Embryol* 55:1295-1301, 2014.

106. Ward, RE, Boudreau, RM, Caserotti, P, Harris, TB, Zivkovic, S, Goodpaster, BH, Satterfield, S, Kritchevsky, S, Schwartz, AV, Vinik, AI, Cauley, JA, Newman, AB, and Strotmeyer, ES. Health ABCs. Sensory and motor peripheral nerve function and longitudinal changes in quadriceps strength. *J Gerontol A Biol Sci Med Sci* 70:464-470, 2015.

107. Wong, P, Chamari, K, and Wisloff, U. Effects of 12-week on-field combined strength and power training on physical performance among U-14 young soccer players. *J Strength Cond Res* 24:644-652, 2010.

108. Wuebben, J. Barbells vs dumbbells: what's better for your workout? Onnit, 2020 (updated May 15, 2020). https://www.onnit.com/academy/barbells-vs-dumbbells/.

Chapter 5

1. Anderson, CE, Sforza, GA, and Sigg, JA. The effects of combining elastic and free weight resistance on strength and power in athletes. *J Strength Cond Res* 22:567-574, 2008.

2. Argus, CK, Gill, ND, Keogh, JW, and Hopkins WG. Assessing the variation in the load that produces maximal upper-body power. *J Strength Cond Res* 28:240-244, 2014.

3. Baker, D. A series of studies on the training of high-intensity muscle power in rugby league football players. *J Strength Cond Res* 15:198-209, 2001.

4. Baker, D, Nance, S, and Moore, M. The load that maximizes the average mechanical power output during explosive bench press throws in highly trained athletes. *J Strength Cond Res* 15:20-24, 2001.

5. Baker, D, and Newton, RU. Methods to increase the effectiveness of maximal power training for the upper body. *Strength Cond J* 27:24-32, 2005.

6. Bartolomei, S, Hoffman, JR, Merni, F, and Stout, JR. A comparison of traditional and block periodized strength training programs in trained athletes. *J Strength Cond Res* 28:990-997, 2014.

7. Bellar, DM, Muller, MD, Barkley, JE, Kim, CH, Ida, K, Ryan, EJ, Bliss, MV, and Glickman, EL. The effects of combined elastic- and free-weight tension vs. free-weight tension on one-repetition maximum strength in the bench press. *J Strength Cond Res* 25:459-463, 2011.

8. Bevan, HR, Bunce, PJ, Owen, NJ, Bennett, MA, Cook, CJ, Cunningham, DJ, Newton, RU, and Kilduff, LP. Optimal loading for the development of peak power output in professional rugby players. *J Strength Cond Res* 24:43-47, 2010.

9. Bouhlel, E, Chelly, MS, Tabka, Z, and Shephard, R. Relationships between maximal anaerobic power of the arms and legs and javelin performance. *J Sports Med Phys Fitness* 47:141-146, 2007.

10. Calatayud, J, Borreani, S, Colado, JC, Martin, F, Tella, V, and Andersen, LL. Bench press and push-up at comparable levels of muscle activity results in similar strength gains. *J Strength Cond Res* 29:246-253, 2015.

11. Chelly, MS, Hermassi, S, Aouadi, R, and Shephard, RJ. Effects of 8-week in-season plyometric training on upper and lower limb performance of elite adolescent handball players. *J Strength Cond Res* 28:1401-1410, 2014.

12. Chelly, MS, Hermassi, S, and Shephard, RJ. Relationships between power and strength of the upper and lower limb muscles and throwing velocity in male handball players. *J Strength Cond Res* 24:1480-1487, 2010.

13. Comstock, BA, Solomon-Hill, G, Flanagan, SD, Earp, JE, Luk, HY, Dobbins, KA, Dunn-Lewis, C, Fragala, MS, Ho, JY, Hatfield, DL, Vingren, JL, Denegar, CR, Volek, JS, Kupchak, BR, Maresh, CM, and Kraemer, WJ. Validity of the Myotest in measuring force and power production in the squat and bench press. *J Strength Cond Res* 25:2293-2297, 2011.

14. Cormie, P, McGuigan, MR, and Newton, RU. Developing maximal neuromuscular power: part 1—biological basis of maximal power production. *Sports Med* 41:17-38, 2011.

15. Dines, JS, Bedi, A, Williams, PN, Dodson, CC, Ellenbecker, TS, Altchek, DW, Windler, G, and Dines, DM. Tennis injuries: epidemiology, pathophysiology, and treatment. *J Am Acad Orthop Surg* 23:181-189, 2015.

16. Dugdale, JH, Hunter, AM, Di Virgilio, TG, Macgregor, LJ, and Hamilton, DL. Influence of the "Slingshot" bench press training aid on bench press kinematics and neuromuscular activity in competitive powerlifters. *J Strength Cond Res* 33:327-336, 2019.

17. Durall, CJ, Udermann, BE, Johansen, DR, Gibson, B, Reineke, DM, and Reuteman, P. The effects of preseason trunk muscle training on low-back pain occurrence in women collegiate gymnasts. *J Strength Cond Res* 23:86-92, 2009.

18. Earp, JE, and Kraemer, WJ. Medicine ball training implications for rotational power sports. *Strength Cond J* 32:20-25, 2010.

19. Falvo, MJ, Schilling, BK, and Weiss, LW. Techniques and considerations for determining iso-inertial upper-body power. *Sports Biomech* 5:293-311, 2015.

20. Garcia-López, D, Hernández-Sánchez, S, Martín, E, Marín, PJ, Zarzosa, F, and Herrero, AJ. Free-weight augmentation with elastic bands improves bench press kinematics in professional rugby players. *J Strength Cond Res.* 30:2493-2499, 2016.

21. Ghigiarelli, JJ, Nagle, EF, Gross, FL, Robertson, RJ, Irrgang, JJ, and Myslinski, T. The effects of a 7-week heavy elastic band and weight chain program on upper-body strength and upper-body power in a sample of division 1-AA football players. *J Strength Cond Res* 23:756-764, 2009.

22. Goto, K, and Morishima, T. Compression garment promotes muscular strength recovery after resistance exercise. *Med Sci Sports Exerc* 46:2265-2270, 2014.

23. Haff, GG, and Nimphius, S. Training principles for power. *Strength & Conditioning Journal* 34:2-12, 2012.

24. Hooper, DR, Dulkis, LL, Secola, PJ, Holtzum, G, Harper, SP, Kalkowski, RJ, Comstock, BA, Szivak, TK, Flanagan, SD, Looney, DP, DuPont, WH, Maresh, CM, Volek, JS, Culley, KP, and Kraemer, WJ. The roles of an upper body compression garment on athletic performances. *J Strength Cond Res* 29:2655-2660, 2015.

25. Jancosko, JJ, and Kazanjian, JE. Shoulder injuries in the throwing athlete. *Phys Sportsmed* 40:84-90, 2012.

26. Jones, MT. Effect of compensatory acceleration training in combination with accommodating resistance on upper body strength in collegiate athletes. *Open Access J Sports Med* 5:183-189, 2014.

27. Joy, JM, Lowery, RP, Oliveira de Souza, E, and Wilson, JM. Elastic bands as a component of periodized resistance training. *J Strength Cond Res,* 30:2100-2106, 2016.

28. Kennedy, DJ, Visco, CJ, and Press, J. Current concepts for shoulder training in the overhead athlete. *Curr Sports Med Rep* 8:154-160, 2009.

29. Kibler, WB, Press, J, and Sciascia, A. The role of core stability in athletic function. *Sports Med* 36:189-198, 2006.

30. Kraemer, WJ, Flanagan, SD, Comstock, BA, Fragala, MS, Earp, JE, Dunn-Lewis, C, Ho, JY, Thomas, GA, Solomon-Hill, G, Penwell, ZR, Powell, MD, Wolf, MR, Volek, JS, Denegar, CR, and Maresh, CM. Effects of a whole body compression garment on markers of recovery after a heavy resistance workout in men and women. *J Strength Cond Res* 24:804-814, 2010.

31. Martínez-Cava, A, Morán-Navarro, R, Hernández-Belmonte, A, Courel-Ibáñez, J, Conesa-Ros, E, González-Badillo, JJ, and Pallarés, JG. Range of motion and sticking region effects on the bench press load-velocity relationship. *J Sports Sci Med.* 18(4):645-652, 2019.

32. Martorelli, SS, Martorelli, AS, Pereira MC, Rocha-Junior, VA, Tan, JG, Alvarenga, JG, Brown, LE, and Bottaro, M. Graduated compression sleeves: effects on metabolic removal and neuromuscular performance. *J Strength Cond Res* 29:1273-1278, 2015.

33. Mayhew, JL, Johns, RA, and Ware, JS. Changes in absolute upper body power following resistance training in college males. *J Appl Sport Science Res* 18:516-520, 1997.

34. McGill, SM. Low back stability: from formal description to issues for performance and rehabilitation. *Exerc Sport Sci Rev* 29:26-31, 2001.

35. McGill, SM, Childs, A, and Liebenson, C. Endurance times for low back stabilization exercises: clinical targets for testing and training from a normal database. *Arch Phys Med Rehabil* 80:941-944, 1999.

36. Newton, RU, Kraemer, WJ, Hakkinen, K, Humphries, BJ, and Murphy, AJ. Kinematics, kinetics and muscle activation during explosive upper body movements. *J Appl Biomech* 12:31-43, 1996.

37. Newton, RU, Murphy, AJ, Humphries, BJ, Wilson, GJ, Kraemer, WJ, and Hakkinen, K. Influence of load and stretch shortening cycle on the kinematics, kinetics and muscle activation that occurs during explosive upper-body movements. *Eur J Appl Physiol Occup Physiol* 75:333-342, 1997.

38. Orange, ST, Metcalfe, JW, Liefeith, A, Marshall, P, Madden, LA, Fewster, CR, and Vince, RV. Validity and reliability of a wearable inertial sensor to measure velocity and power in the back squat and bench press. *J Strength Cond Res* 33:2398-2408, 2019.

39. Rivière, M, Louit, L, Strokosch, A, and Seitz, LB. Variable resistance training promotes greater strength and power adaptations than traditional resistance training in elite youth rugby league players. *J Strength Cond Res* 31:947-55, 2017.

40. Rucci, JA, and Tomporowski, PD. Three types of kinematic feedback and the execution of the hang power clean. *J Strength Cond Res* 24:771-778, 2010.

41. Saeterbakken, AH, Andersen, V, van den Tillaar, R, Joly, F, Stien, N, Pedersen, H, Shaw, MP, and Solstad, TEJ. The effects of ten weeks resistance training on sticking region in chest-press exercises. *PLoS One* 15:e0235555, 2020.

42. Sayers, MGL, and Bishop, S. Reliability of a new medicine ball throw power test. *J Strength Cond Res* 33:311-315, 2017.

43. Shinkle J, Nesser, TW, Demchak, TJ, and McMannus, DM. Effect of core strength on the measure of power in the extremities. *J Strength Cond Res* 26:373-380, 2012.

44. Shoepe, TC, Ramirez, DA, Rovetti, RJ, Kohler, DR, and Almstedt, HC. The effects of 24 weeks of resistance training with simultaneous elastic and free weight loading on muscular performance of novice lifters. *J Hum Kinet* 29:93-106, 2011.

45. Suchomel, TJ, Techmanski, BD, Kissick, CR, and Comfort, P. Reliability, validity, and comparison of barbell velocity measurement devices during the jump shrug and hang high pull. *J Funct Morphol Kinesiol* 8:35, 2023.

46. Tillaar, RV, Saeterbakken, AH, and Ettema, G. Is the occurrence of the sticking region the result of diminishing potentiation in bench press? *J Sports Sci* 30:591-599, 2012.

47. Ye, X, Beck, TW, Stock, MS, Fahs, CA, Kim, D, Loenneke, JP, Thiebaud, RS, Defreitas, JM, Rossow, LM, Bemben, DA, and Bemben, MG. Acute effects of wearing an elastic, supportive device on bench press performance in young, resistance-trained males. *Gazzetta Med Italiana* 173:91-102, 2014.

Chapter 6

1. Bachero-Mena, B, and González-Badillo, J. Effects of resisted sprint training on acceleration with three different loads accounting for 5, 12.5, and 20% of body mass. *J Strength Cond Res* 28:2954-2960, 2014.

2. Baker, D. Acute and long-term power responses to power training: observations on the training of an elite power athlete. *Strength Cond J* 23:47-56, 2001.

3. Baker, D. Comparison of upper-body strength and power between professional and college-aged rugby league players. *J Strength Cond Res* 15:30-35, 2001.

4. Baker, D, and Newton, R. Change in power output across a high-repetition set of bench throws and jump squats in highly trained athletes. *J Strength Cond Res* 21:1007-1011, 2007.

5. Baker, D, Nance, S, and Moore, M. The load that maximizes the average mechanical power output during jump squats in power-trained athletes. *J Strength Cond Res* 15:92-97, 2001.

6. Cormie, P, Deane, R, and McBride, J. Methodological concerns for determining power output in the jump squat. *J Strength Cond Res* 21:424-430, 2007.

7. de Villarreal, ESS, González-Badillo, JJ, and Izquierdo, M. Low and moderate plyometric training frequency produces greater jumping and sprinting gains compared with high frequency. *J Strength Cond Res* 22:715-725, 2008.

8. Dos'Santos, T, Thomas, C, McBurnie, A, Comfort, P, and Jones, PA. Biomechanical determinants of performance and injury risk during cutting: a performance-injury conflict? *Sports Med* 51:1983-1998, 2021.

9. Fleck, SJ, and Kraemer, WJ. *Designing Resistance Training Programs. 4th ed.* Champaign, IL: Human Kinetics, 2014.

10. Kawamori, N, and Haff, GG. The optimal training load for the development of muscular power. *J Strength Cond Res* 18:675-684, 2004.

11. Komi, PV, Nicol, C, and Avela, J. The stretch-shortening cycle: a model to study naturally occurring neuromuscular fatigue. *Sports Med* 36:977-999, 2006.

12. Newton, RU, and Kraemer, WJ. Developing explosive muscular power: implications for a mixed methods training strategy. *Strength Cond J* 16:20-31, 1994.

13. Potach, DH, and Chu, DA. Program design and technique for plyometic training. In *Essentials of Strength Training and Conditioning*. 4th ed. Haff, GG, and Triplett, NT, eds. Champaign, IL: Human Kinetics, 471-520, 2016.

14. Sanchez, D. What is the kinetic chain? 2019. Accessed November 8, 2023. www.acefitness.org/fitness-certifications/ace-answers/exam-preparation-blog/2929/what-is-the-kinetic-chain/.

15. Simmons, L. *Westside Barbell Book of Methods*. Westside Barbell, 2007.

16. Stone, MH. Position statement and literature review: explosive exercises and training. *Strength Cond J* 15:7-15, 1993.

17. Swinton, PA, Stewart, AD, Keogh, JW, Agouris, I, and Lloyd, R. Kinematic and kinetic analysis of maximal velocity deadlifts performed with and without the inclusion of chain resistance. *J Strength Cond Res* 25:3163-3174, 2011.

Chapter 7

1. Filipa, A, Byrnes, R, Paterno, MV, Myer, GD, and Hewett, TE. Neuromuscular training improves performance on the star excursion balance test in young female athletes. *J Orthop Sports Phys Ther* 40:551-558, 2010.

2. French, D. Adaptations to anaerobic training programs. In *Essentials of Strength Training and Conditioning*. 4th ed. Haff, G, and Triplett, N, eds. Champaign, IL: Human Kinetics, 87-114, 2021.

3. Hibbs, A, Thompson, K, French, D, Wrigley, A, and Spears, I. Optimizing performance by improving core stability and core strength. *Sports Med* 38:995-1008, 2008.

4. Hoshikawa, Y, Iida, T, Muramatsu, M, Ii, N, Nakajima, Y, Chumank, K, and Kanehisa, H. Effects of stabilization training on trunk muscularity and physical performances in youth soccer players. *J Strength Cond Res* 27:3142-3149, 2013.

5. Imai, A, Kaneoka, K, Okubo, Y, and Shiraki, H. Comparison of the immediate effect of different types of trunk exercise on the star excursion balance test in male adolescent soccer players. *Int J Sports Phys Ther* 9:429-435, 2014.

6. Imai, A, Kaneoka, K, Okubo, Y, and Shiraki, H. Effects of two types of trunk exercises on balance and athletic performance in youth soccer players. *Int J Sports Phys Ther* 9:47-57, 2014.

7. Lee, BC, and McGill, SM. Effect of long-term isometric training on core/torso stiffness. *J Strength Cond Res* 29:1515-1526, 2015.

8. Leetun, D, Ireland, M, Willson, J, Ballantyne, B, and McClay, I. Core stability measures as risk factors for lower extremity injury in athletes. *Med Sci Sports Exerc* 36:926-934, 2004.

9. Manchado, C, García-Ruiz, J, Cortell-Tormo, JM, and Tortosa-Martínez, J. Effect of core training on male handball players' throwing velocity. *J Hum Kinet* 56:177-185, 2017.

10. McGill, S. Core training: evidence translating to better performance and injury prevention. *Strength Cond J* 32:33-47, 2010.

11. McGill, SM. *Low Back Disorders. Evidence-Based Prevention and Rehabilitation*. 2nd ed. Champaign, IL: Human Kinetics, 230-241, 2007.

12. Nesser, TW, and Lee, WL. The relationship between core strength and performance in Division I female soccer players. *J Exerc Physiol Online* [serial online]. 12(2):21-28, 2009. www.asep.org/asep/asep/JEPonlineApril2009.html. Accessed April 1, 2023.

13. Nesser, TW, Huxel, KC, Tincher, JL, and Okado, T. The relationship between core stability and performance in Division I football players. *J Strength Cond Res* 22:1750-1754, 2008.

14. Prieske, O, Muehlbauer, T, Borde, R, Gube, M, Bruhn, S, Behm, DG, and Granacher, U. Neuromuscular and athletic performance following core strength training in elite youth soccer: role of instability. *Scand J Med Sci in Sports* 26:48-56, 2016.

15. Reed, CA, Ford, KR, Myer, GD, and Hewett, TE. The effects of isolated and integrated "core stability" training on athletic performance measures: a systematic review. *Sports Med* 42:697-706, 2012.

16. Saeterbakken, AH, Van den Tillaar, R, and Seiler, S. Effect of core stability training on throwing velocity in female handball players. *J Strength Cond Res* 25:712-718, 2011.

17. Sandrey, M, and Mitzel, J. Improvement in dynamic balance and core endurance after a 6-week core-stability-training program in high school track and field athletes. *J Sport Rehab* 22:264-271, 2013.

18. Sato, K, and Mokha, M. Does core strength training influence running kinetics, lower-extremity stability, and 5000-m performance in runners? *J Strength Cond Res* 23:133-140, 2009.

19. Sharma, A, Geovinson, SG, and Singh Sandhu, J. Effects of a nine-week core strengthening exercise program on vertical jump performances and static balance in volleyball players with trunk instability. *J Sports Med Phys Fitness* 52:606-15, 2012.

20. Sharrock, C, Cropper, J, Mostad, J, Johnson, M, and Malone, T. A pilot study of core stability and athletic performance: is there a relationship? *Int J Sports Phys Ther* 6:63-67, 2011.

21. Stanton, R, Reaburn, PR, and Humphries, B. The effect of short-term Swiss ball training on core stability and running economy. *J Strength Cond Res* 18:522-528, 2004.

22. Tvrdy, D. Examining the connection between training the core and performance. *NSCA Coach* 8:42-46, 2021.

Chapter 8

1. Baker, D, and Nance, S. The relationship between running speed and measures of strength and power in professional rugby league players. *J Strength Cond Res* 13:230-235, 1999.

2. Canavan, PK, Garrett, GE, and Armstrong, LE. Kinematic and kinetic relationships between an Olympic-style lift and the vertical jump. *J Strength Cond Res* 10:127-130, 1996.

3. Carlock, JM, Smith, SL, Hartman, MJ, Morris, RT, Ciroslan, DA, Pierce, KC, Newton, RU, Harman, EA, Sands, WA, and Stone, MH. The relationship between vertical jump power estimates and weightlifting ability: a field-test approach. *J Strength Cond Res* 18:534-539, 2004.

4. Channell, BT, and Barfield, JP. Effect of Olympic and traditional resistance training on vertical jump improvement in high school Boys. *J Strength Cond Res* 22:1522-1527, 2008.

5. Comfort, P, Fletcher, C, and McMahon, JJ. Determination of optimal load during the power clean in collegiate athletes. *J Strength Cond Res* 26:2962-2969, 2012.

6. Comfort, P, Haff, GG, Suchomel, TJ, Soriano, MA, Pierce, KC, Hornsby, WG, Haff, EE, Sommerfield, LM, Chavda, S, Morris, SJ, Fry, AC, and Stone, MH. National Strength and Conditioning Association position statement on weightlifting for sports performance. *J Strength Cond Res* 37:1163-1190, 2023.

7. Cormie, P, McCaulley, GO, Triplett, NT, and McBride, JM. Optimal loading for maximal power output during lower-body resistance exercises. *Med Sci Sports Exerc* 39:340-349, 2007.

8. Cormie, P, McGuigan, MR, and Newton, RU. Developing maximal neuromuscular power: part 1—biological basis of maximal power production. *Sports Med* 41:17-38, 2011.

9. Cormie, P, McGuigan, MR, and Newton, RU. Developing maximal neuromuscular power: part 2—training considerations for improving maximal power production. *Sports Medicine* 41:125-146, 2011.

10. Garhammer, J. Power production by Olympic weightlifters. *Med Sci Sports Exerc* 12:54-60, 1980.

11. Garhammer, J. Energy flow during Olympic weight lifting. *Med Sci Sports Exerc* 14:353-360, 1982.

12. Garhammer, J. A comparison of maximal power outputs between elite male and female weight-lifters in competition. *Int J Sports Biomech* 3:3-11, 1991.

13. Garhammer, J. A review of power output studies of Olympic and powerlifting: methodology, performance prediction, and evaluation tests. *J Strength Cond Res* 7:76-89, 1993.

14. Garhammer, J, and Gregor, R. Propulsion forces as a function of intensity for weightlifting and vertical jumping. *J Strength Cond Res* 6:129-134, 1992.

15. Hori, N, Newton, RU, Andrews, WA, Kawamori, N, McGuigan, MR, and Nosaka, K. Does performance of hang power clean differentiate performance of jumping, sprinting, and changing of direction? *J Strength Cond Res* 22:412-418, 2008.

16. Hori, N, Newton, RU, Nosaka, K, and Stone, MH. Weightlifting exercises enhance athletic performance that requires high-load speed strength. *Strength Cond J* 27:50-55, 2005.

17. Kawamori, N, Crum, AJ, Blumert, PA, Kulik, JR, Childers, JT, Wood, JA, Stone, MH, and Haff, GG. Influence of different relative intensities on power output during the hang power clean: identification of the optimal load. *J Strength Cond Res* 19:698-708, 2005.

18. Kilduff, LP, Bevan, H, Owen, N, Kingsley, MI, Bunce, P, Bennett, M, and Cunningham, D. Optimal loading for peak power output during the hang power clean in professional rugby players. *Int J Sports Physiol Perform* 2:260-269, 2007.

19. Soriano, MA, Jimenez-Reyes, P, Rhea, MR, and Marin, PJ. the optimal load for maximal power production during lower-body resistance exercises: a meta-analysis. *Sports Med* 45:1191-1205, 2015.

20. Soriano, MA, Suchomel, TJ, and Comfort, P. Weightlifting overhead pressing derivatives: a review of the literature. *Sports Med* 49:867-885, 2019.

21. Storey, AG, and Smith, H. Unique aspects of competitive weightlifting. *Sports Med* 42:769-790, 2012.

22. Suchomel, T, Comfort, P, and Stone, M. Weightlifting pulling derivatives: rationale for implementation and application. *Sports Med* 45:823-839, 2015.

23. Suchomel, TJ, Comfort, P, and Lake, JP. Enhancing the force-velocity profile of athletes using weightlifting derivatives. *Strength Cond J* 39:10-20, 2017.

24. Tricoli, V, Lamas, L, Carnevale, R, and Ugrinowitsch, C. Short-term effects on lower-body functional power development: weightlifting vs.vertical jump training programs. *J Strength Cond Res* 19:433-437, 2005.

Chapter 9

1. Aboodarda, S, Page, P, and Behm, D. Eccentric and concentric jumping performance during augmented jumps with elastic resistance: a meta-analysis. *Int J Sports Phys Ther* 10:839-849, 2015.

2. Adams, K, O'Shea, J, O'Shea, K, and Climstein, M. The effects of six weeks of squat, plyometric and squat-plyometric training on power production. *J Appl Sport Sci Res* 6:36-41, 1992.

3. Anderson, C, Sforzo, G, and Sigg, J. The effects of combining elastic and free weight resistance on strength and power in athletes. *J Strength Cond Res* 22:567-574, 2008.

4. Argus, C, Gill, N, Keogh, J, Blazevich, A, and Hopkins, W. Kinetic and training comparisons between assisted, resisted, and free countermovement jumps. *J Strength Cond Res* 25:2219-2227, 2011.

5. Baker, D. A series of studies on the training of high intensity muscle power in rugby league football players. *J Strength Cond Res* 15:198-209, 2001.

6. Baker, D, and Nance, S. The relationship between strength and power in professional rugby league players. *J Strength Cond Res* 13:224-229, 1999.

7. Baker, D, and Newton, R. Methods to increase the effectiveness of maximal power training for the upper body. *J Strength Cond Res* 27:24-32, 2005.

8. Baker, D, and Newton, R. Effect of kinetically altering a repetition via the use of chain resistance on velocity during the bench press. *J Strength Cond Res* 23:1941-1946, 2009.

9. Behm, D, and Sale, D. Intended rather than actual movement velocity determines velocity-specific training responses. *J Appl Physiol* 74:359-368, 1993.

10. Bellar, D, Muller, M, Barkley, J, Kim, C, Ida, K, Ryan, E, Bliss, M, and Glickman, E. The effects of combined elastic- and free-weight tension vs. free-weight tension on one-repetition maximum strength in the bench press. *J Strength Cond Res* 25:459-463, 2011.

11. Berning, J, Coker, C, and Adams, K. Using chains for strength and conditioning. *Strength and Cond J* 26:80-84, 2004.

12. Blazevich, A, Gill, N, Bronks, R, and Newton, R. Training-specific muscle architecture adaptation after 5-wk training in athletes. *Med Sci Sports Exerc* 35:2013-2022, 2003.

13. Brandenburg, J, and Docherty, D. The effect of accentuated eccentric loading on strength, muscle hypertrophy, and neural adaptations in trained individuals. *J Strength Cond Res* 16:25-32, 2002.

14. Brandon, R, Howatson, G, Strachan, F, and Hunter, A. Neuromuscular response differences to power vs. strength back squat exercise in elite athletes. *Scand J Med Sci Sport* 25:630-639, 2015.

15. Bright, T, Handford, M, Mundy, P, Lake, J, Theis, N, and Hughes, J. Building a future: a systematic review of the effects of eccentric resistance training on measures of physical performance in youth athletes. *Sports Med* 53:1219-1254, 2023.

16. Burger, T, Boyer-Kendrick, T, and Dolny, D. Complex training compared to a combined weight training and plyometric training program. *J Strength Cond Res* 14:360, 2000.

17. Carlock, J, Smith, S, Hartman, M, Morris, R, Ciroslan, D, Pierce, K, Newton, R, Hartman, E, Sands, W, and Stone, M. The relationship between vertical jump power estimates and weight-lifting ability: a field-test approach. *J Strength Cond Res* 18:534-539, 2004.

18. Chatzopoulos, D, Michailidis, C, Giannakos, A, Alexiou, K, Patikas, D, Antonopoulos, C, and Kotzamanidis, C. Postactivation potentiation effects after heavy resistance exercise on running speed. *J Strength Cond Res* 21:1278-1281, 2007.

19. Chiu, L, Fry, A, Schilling, B, Johnson, E, and Weiss, L. Neuromuscular fatigue and potentiation following two successive high intensity resistance exercise sessions. *Eur J Appl Physiol Occup Physiol* 92:385-392, 2004.

20. Chiu, L, Fry, A, Weiss, L, Schilling, B, Brown, L, and Smith, S. Postactivation potentiation response in athletic and recreationally trained individuals. *J Strength Cond Res* 17:671-677, 2003.

21. Clark, R, Bryant, A, and Humphries, B. A comparison of force curve profiles between the bench press and ballistic bench throws. *J Strength Cond Res* 22:1755-1759, 2008.

22. Cormie, P, McGuigan, M, and Newton, R. Influence of strength on magnitude and mechanisms of adaptation to power training. *Med Sci Sports Exerc* 42:1566-1581, 2010.

23. Cormie, P, McGuigan, M, and Newton, R. Developing maximal neuromuscular power—part I: biological basis of maximal power production. *Sports Med* 41:17-38, 2011.

24. Cormie, P, McGuigan, M, and Newton, R. Developing maximal neuromuscular power—part II: training considerations for improved maximal power production. *Sports Med* 41:125-146, 2011.

25. Cormier, P, Freitas, T, Rubio-Arias, J, and Alcaraz, P. Complex and contrast training: does strength and power training sequence affect performance-based adaptations in team sports? A systematic review and meta-analysis. *J Strength Cond Res* 34:1461-1479, 2020.

26. Cormier, P, Freitas, T, Loturco, I, Turner, A, Virgile, A, Haff, G, Blazevich, A, Agar-Newman, D, Henneberry, M, Baker, D, McGuigan, M, Alcaraz, P, and Bishop, C. Within session exercise sequencing during programming for complex training: historical perspectives, terminology, and training considerations. *Sport Med* 52:2371-2389, 2022.

27. Cronin, J, McNair, P, and Marshall, R. The effects of bungee weight training on muscle function and functional performance. *J Sport Sci* 21:59-71, 2003.

28. Cronin, J, McNair, P, and Marshall, R. Force–velocity analysis of strength-training techniques and load: implications for training strategy and research. *J Strength Cond Res* 17:148-155, 2003.

29. Dapena, J. The high jump. In *Biomechanics in Sport: Performance Enhancement and Injury Prevention*. Zatsiorsky, V, ed. Oxford, UK: Blackwell Science, 284-311, 2000.

30. de Villarreal, E, Izquierdo, M, and Gonzalez-Badillo, J. Enhancing jumping performance after combined vs. maximal power, heavy-resistance, and plyometric training alone. *J Strength Cond Res* 25:3274-3281, 2011.

31. Docherty, D, and Hodgson, M. The application of postactivation potentiation to elite sport. *Int J Sports Physiol Perf* 2:439-444, 2007.

32. Ebben, W. Complex training: a brief review. *J Sport Sci Med* 1:42-46, 2002.

33. Ebben, W, and Jensen, R. Electromyographic and kinematic analysis of traditional, chain, and elastic band squats. *J Strength Cond Res* 16:547-550, 2002.

34. Ebben, W, and Watts, P. A review of combined weight training and plyometric training modes: complex training. *Strength and Cond J* 20:18-27, 1998.

35. Elliot, B, Wilson, G, and Kerr, G. A biomechanical analysis of the sticking region in the bench press. *Med Sci Sports Exerc* 21:450-462, 1989.

36. Evans, A, Hodgkins, T, Durham, M, Berning, J, and Adams, K. The acute effects of 5RM bench press on power output. *Med Sci Sports Exerc* 32:S311, 2000.

37. Faigenbaum, A, O'Connell, J, La Rosa, R, and Westcott, W. Effects of strength training and complex training on upper-body strength and endurance development in children. *J Strength Cond Res* 13:424, 1999.

38. Fatourous, I, Jamurtas, A, Leontsini, D, Taxildaris, K, Aggelousis, N, Kostopoulos, N, and Buckenmeyer, P. Evaluation of plyometric exercise training, weight training, and their combination on vertical jump and leg strength. *J Strength Cond Res* 14:470-476, 2000.

39. Flanagan, E, and Comyns, T. The use of contact time and the reactive strength index to optimize fast stretch-shortening cycle training. *Strength and Cond J* 30:33-38, 2008.

40. Fleck, S, and Kraemer, W. *Designing Resistance Training Programs.* Champaign, IL: Human Kinetics, 2004.

41. Folland, J, and Williams, A. The adaptations to strength training: morphological and neurological contributions to increased strength. *Sports Med* 37:145-168, 2007.

42. French, D, Kraemer, W, and Cooke, C. Changes in dynamic exercise performance following a sequence of preconditioning isometric muscle actions. *J Strength Cond Res* 17:678-685, 2003.

43. Friedmann-Bette, B, Bauer, T, Kinscherf, R, Vorwald, S, Klute, K, Bischoff, D, Müller, H, Weber, M, Metz, J, Kauczor, H, Bärtsch, P, and Billeter, R. Effects of strength training with eccentric overload on muscle adaptation in male athletes. *Sports Med* 108:821-836, 2010.

44. Frost, D, Cronin, J, and Newton, R. A biomechanical evaluation of resistance: fundamental concepts for training and sports performance. *Sports Med* 40:303-326, 2010.

45. García-Ramos, A, Padial, P, Haff, G, Argüelles-Cienfuegos, J, García-Ramos, M, Conde-Pipó, J, and Feriche, B. Effect of different interrepetition rest periods on barbell velocity loss during the ballistic bench press exercise. *J Strength Cond Res* 29:2388-2396, 2015.

46. Garhammer, J. A review of power output studies of Olympic and powerlifting: methodology, performance prediction, and evaluation tests. *J Strength Cond Res* 7:76-89, 1993.

47. Gilbert, G, Lees, A, and Graham-Smith, P. Temporal profile of post-tetanic potentiation of muscle force characteristics after repeated maximal exercise. *J Sport Sci* 19:6, 2001.

48. Gonzalez-Badillo, J, and Sanchez-Medina, L. Movement velocity as a measure of loading intensity in resistance training. *Int J Sports Med* 31:347-352, 2010.

49. Gonzalo-Skok, O, Tous-Fajardo, J, Moras, G, Arjol-Serrano, J, and Mendez-Villanueva, A. A repeated power training enhances fatigue resistance while reducing intraset fluctuations. *J Strength Cond Res* 33:2711-2721, 2019.

50. Gourgoulis, V, Aggeloussis, N, Kasimatis, P, Mavromatis, G, and Garas, A. Effect of a submaximal half-squats warm-up program on vertical jumping ability. *J Strength Cond Res* 17:342-344, 2003.

51. Gullich, A, and Schmidtbleicher, D. MVC-induced short-term potentiation of explosive force. *N Stud Athlet* 11:67-81, 1996.

52. Guppy, S, Nagatani, T, Poon, W, Kendall, K, Lake, J, and Haff, G. The stability of the deadlift three repetition maximum. *Int J Sport Sci Coaching*, 2023. [e-pub ahead of print]. https://doi.org/10.1177/17479541231174316.

53. Guppy, S, Nagatani, T, Poon, W, Kendall, K, Lake, J, and Haff, G. Changes in deadlift six repetition maximum, countermovement jump performance, barbell velocity, and perceived exertion over the duration of a microcycle. *Int J Sport Sci Coaching*, 2023. [e-pub ahead of print]. https://doi.org/10.1177/17479541231172569.

54. Haff, G, Burgess, S, and Stone, M. Cluster training: theoretical and practical applications for the strength and conditioning professional. *Prof Strength Cond* 12:12-16, 2008.

55. Haff, G, Whitley, A, McCoy, L, O'Bryant, H, Kilgore, J, Haff, E, Pierce, K, and Stone, M. Effects of different set configurations on barbell velocity and displacement during clean pull. *J Strength Cond Res* 17:95-103, 2003.

56. Hamada, T, Sale, D, MacDougall, J, and Tarnopolsky, MA. Interaction of fibre type, potentiation and fatigue in human knee extensor muscles. *Acta Physiol Scand* 178:165-173, 2003.

57. Hodgson, M, Docherty, D, and Robbins, D. Post-activation potentiation: underlying physiology and implications for motor performance. *Sports Med* 35:585-595, 2005.

58. Hori, N, Newton, R, Nosaka, K, and Stone, M. Weightlifting exercises enhance athletic performance that requires high-load speed strength. *Strength and Cond J* 27:50-55, 2005.

59. Israetel, M, McBride, J, Nuzzo, J, Skinner, J, and Dayne, A. Kinetic and kinematic differences between squats performed with and without elastic bands. *J Strength Cond Res* 24:190-194, 2010.

60. Jandacka, D, and Beremlijski, P. Determination of strength exercise intensities based on the load-power-velocity relationship. *J Hum Kinetics* 28:33-44, 2011.

61. Janusevicius, D, Snieckus, A, Skurvydas, A, Silinaskas, V, Trinkunas, E, Cadefau, J, and Kamandulis, S. Effects of high velocity elastic band versus heavy resistance training on hamstring strength, activation, and sprint running performance. *J Sports Sci Med* 16:239-246, 2017.

62. Jarić, S, Ropret, R, and Ilić, D. Role of agonist and antagonist muscle strength in performance of rapid movements. *Eur J Appl Physiol Occup Physiol* 71:464-468, 1995.

63. Jeffreys, I. A review of post activation potentiation and its application in strength and conditioning. *Prof Strength Cond* 12:17-25, 2008.

64. Jidovtseff, B, Quievre, J, Hanon, C, and Crielaard, J. Inertial muscular profiles allow a more accurate training load definition. *Sci and Sports* 24:91-96, 2009.

65. Joy, J, Lowery, P, Oliveira De Souza, E, and Wilson, J. Elastic bands as a component of periodized resistance training. *J Strength Cond Res* 30:2100-2106, 2016.

66. Kaneko, M, Fuchimoto, T, Toji, H, and Suei, K. Training effects of different loads on the force-velocity relationship and mechanical power output in human muscle. *Scand J Sport Sci* 5:50-55, 1983.

67. Kawamori, N, and Haff, G. The optimal training load for the development of muscular power. *J Strength Cond Res* 18:675-684, 2004.

68. Kilduff, L, Bevan, H, Kingsley, M, Owen, N, Bennett, M, Bunce, P, Hore, A, Maw, J, and Cunningham, D. Postactivation potentiation in professional rugby players: optimal recovery. *J Strength Cond Res* 21:1134-1138, 2007.

69. Kirby, T, McBride, J, Haines, T, and Dayne, A. Relative net vertical impulse determines jumping performance. *J Appl Biomech* 27:207-214, 2011.

70. Knudson, D. Correcting the use of the term "power" in the strength and conditioning literature. *J Strength Cond Res* 23:1902-1908, 2009.

71. Komi, P, and Virmavirta, M. Determinants of successful ski-jumping performance. In *Biomechanics in Sport: Performance Enhancement and Injury Prevention*. Zatsiorsky, V, ed. Oxford, UK: Blackwell Science, 349-362, 2000.

72. Kraemer, W, and Looney, D. Underlying mechanisms and physiology of muscular power. *Strength and Cond J* 34:13-19, 2012.

73. Kulig, K, Andrews, J, and Hay, J. Human strength curves. *Exerc Sport Sci Rev* 12:417-466, 1984.

74. Kuntz, C, Masi, M, and Lorenz, D. Augmenting the bench press with elastic resistance: scientific and practical applications. *Strength and Cond J* 36:96-102, 2014.

75. Lacerte. M, Delateur. B, Alquist. A, and Questad. K. Concentric versus combined concentric-eccentric isokinetic training programs: effect of peak torque on human quadriceps femoris muscle. *Arch Phys Med Rehabil* 73:1059-1062, 1992.

76. Lake, J, Lauder, M, Smith, N, and Shorter, K. A comparison of ballistic and nonballistic lower-body resistance exercise and the methods used to identify their positive lifting phases. *J Appl Biomech* 28:431-437, 2012.

77. Lanka, J. Shot putting. In *Biomechanics in Sport: Performance Enhancement and Injury Prevention*. Zatsiorsky, V, ed. Oxford, UK: Blackwell Science, 435-457, 2000.

78. Lyttle, A, Wilson, G, and Ostrowski, K. Enhancing performance: maximal power versus combined weights and plyometric training. *J Strength Cond Res* 10:173-179, 1996.

79. MacKenzie, S, Lavers, R, and Wallace, B. A biomechanical comparison of the vertical jump, power clean, and jump squat. *J Sport Sci* 1632:1576-1585, 2014.

80. Maio Alves, J, Rebelo, A, Abrantes, C, and Sampaio, J. Short-term effects of complex and contrast training in soccer players' vertical jump, sprint, and agility abilities. *J Strength Cond Res* 24:936-941, 2010.

81. Makaruk, H, Starzak, M, Suchecki, B, Czaplicki, M, and Stojiljkovic, N. The effects of assisted and resisted plyometric training programs on vertical jump performance in adults: a systematic review and meta-analysis. *J Sports Sci Med* 19:347-357, 2020.

82. Markovic, G, and Jaric, S. Positive and negative loading and mechanical output in maximum vertical jumping. *Med Sci Sports Exerc* 39:1757-1764, 2007.

83. Markovic, G, Vuk, S, and Jaric, S. Effects of jump training with negative versus positive loading on jumping mechanics. *Int J Sports Med* 32:365-372, 2011.

84. Marshall, J, Bishop, C, Turner, A, and Haff, G. Optimal training sequences to develop lower body force, velocity, power, and jump height: a systematic review with meta-analysis. *Sports Med* 51:1245-1271, 2021.

85. McBride, JM, Nimphius, S, and Erickson, TM. The acute effects of heavy-load squats and loaded countermovement jumps on sprint performance. *J Strength Cond Res* 19:893-897, 2005.

86. McBride, J, Triplett-McBride, N, Davie, A, and Newton, M. The effect of heavy- vs. light-load jump squats on the development of strength, power, and speed. *J Strength Cond Res* 16:72-82, 2002.

87. McLeod, C, and James, K. Netball. In *Routledge Handbook of Strength and Conditioning*. Turner A, ed. New York: Routledge, 2018.

88. McGill, S, Chaimberg, J, Frost, D, and Fenwick, C. Evidence of a double peak in muscle activation to enhance strike speed and force: an example with elite mixed martial arts fighters. *J Strength Cond Res* 24:348-357, 2010.

89. McMaster, D, Cronin, J, and McGuigan, M. Forms of variable resistance training. *J Strength Cond Res* 31:50-64, 2009.

90. McMaster, D, Cronin, J, and McGuigan, M. Quantification of rubber and chain-based resistance modes. *J Strength Cond Res* 24:2056-2064, 2010.

91. Mero, A, and Komi, P. Force-, EMG-, and elasticity-velocity relationships at submaximal, maximal and supramaximal running speeds in sprinters. *Eur J Appl Physiol Occup Physiol* 55:553-561, 1986.

92. Miller, D. Springboard and platform diving. In *Biomechanics in Sport: Performance Enhancement and Injury Prevention*. Zatsiorsky, V, ed. Oxford, UK: Blackwell Science, 326-348, 2000.

93. Moir, G, Munford, S, Moroski, L, and Davis, S. The effects of ballistic and nonballistic bench press on mechanical variables. *J Strength Cond Res* 32:3333-3339, 2018.

94. Mosey, T. Power endurance and strength training methods of the Australian lightweight men's four. *J Aust Strength Cond* 19:9-19, 2011.

95. Natera, A, Cardinale M, and Keogh J. The effect of high volume power training on repeated high-intensity performance and the assessment of repeat power ability: a systematic review. *Sports Med* 50:1317-1339, 2020.

96. Neelly, K, Terry, J, and Morris, M. A mechanical comparison of linear and double-looped hung supplemental heavy chain resistance to the back squat: a case study. *J Strength Cond Res* 24:278-281, 2010.

97. Newton, R and Kraemer, W. Developing explosive muscular power: implications for a mixed methods training strategy. *Strength and Cond J* 16:20-31, 1994.

98. Newton, R, Kraemer, W, and Hakkinen, K. Effects of ballistic training on preseason preparation of elite volleyball players. *Med Sci Sports Exerc* 31:323-330, 1999.

99. Newton, R, Kraemer, W, Hakkinen, K, Humphries, B, and Murphy, A. Kinematics, kinetics, and muscle activation during explosive upper body movements. *J Appl Biomech* 12:31-43, 1996.

100. Newton, R, Murphy, A, Humphries, B, Wilson, G, Kraemer, W, and Hakkinen, K. Influence of load and stretch shortening cycle on the kinematics, kinetics and muscle activation that occurs during explosive bench press throws. *Eur J Appl Physiol Occup Physiol* 75:333-342, 1997.

101. Paasuke, M, Ereline, J, and Gapeyeva, H. Twitch potentiation capacity of plantar-flexor muscles in endurance and power athletes. *Biol Sport* 15:171-178, 1996.

102. Pereria, M, and Gomes, P. Movement velocity in resistance training. *Sports Med* 33:427-438, 2003.

103. Pipes, T. Variable resistance versus constant resistance strength training in adult males. *Eur J Appl Physiol Occup Physiol* 39:27-35, 1978.

104. Radcliffe, J, and Radcliffe, J. Effects of different warm-up protocols on peak power output during a single response jump task. *Med Sci Sports Exerc* 38:S189, 1999.

105. Rajamohan, G, Kanagasabai, P, Krishnaswamy, S, and Balakrishnan, A. Effect of complex and contrast resistance and plyometric training on selected strength and power parameters. *J Exp Sciences* 1:1-12, 2010.

106. Ramírez, J, Núñez, V, Lancho, C, Poblador, M, and Lancho, J. Velocity based training of lower limb to improve absolute and relative power outputs in concentric phase of half-squat in soccer players. *J Strength Cond Res*, 29:3084-3088, 2015.

107. Rhea, M, Kenn, J, and Dermody, B. Alterations in speed of squat movement and the use of accommodated resistance among college athletes training for power. *J Strength Cond Res* 23:2645-2650, 2009.

108. Robbins, D. Postactivation potentiation and its practical applicability: a brief review. *J Strength Cond Res* 19:453-458, 2005.

109. Roll, F, and Omer, J. Football: Tulane football winter program. *Strength Cond J* 9:34-38, 1987.

110. Sale, D. Postactivation potentiation role in human performance. *Exerc Sport Sci Rev* 30:138-143, 2002.

111. Schaefer, L, and Bittman, F. Are there two forms of isometric muscle action? Results of the experimental study support a distinction between a holding and a pushing isometric muscle function. *Sport Sci Med and Rehab* 9:11, 2017.

112. Seitz, L, Saez de Villarreal, E, and Haff, GG. The temporal profile of postactivation potentiation is related to strength level. *J Strength Cond Res* 28:706-715, 2014.

113. Seitz, LB, and Haff, GG. Application of methods of inducing postactivation potentiation during the preparation of rugby players. *Strength Cond J* 37:40-49, 2015.

114. Seitz, L, Trajano, G, Dal Maso, F, Haff, G, and Blazevich, A. Postactivation potentiation during voluntary contractions after continued knee extensor task-specific practice. *Appl Physiol Nutr Metab* 40:230-237, 2015.

115. Seitz, LB, Trajano, GS, and Haff, GG. The back squat and the power clean elicit different degrees of potentiation. *Int J Sports Physiol Perform* 9:643-649, 2014.

116. Shea, C, Kohl, R, Guadagnoli, M, and Shebilske, W. After-contraction phenomenon: influences on performance and learning. *J Mot Behav* 23:51-62, 1991.

117. Sheppard, J, Dingley, A, Janssen, I, Spratford, W, Chapman, D, and Newton, R. The effect of assisted jumping on vertical jump height in high-performance volleyball players. *J Sci Med Sport* 14:85-89, 2011.

118. Soria-Gila, M, Chirosa, I, Bautista, I, Chirosa, L, and Salvador, B. Effects of variable resistance training on maximal strength: a meta-analysis. *J Strength Cond Res*, 29:3260-3270, 2015.

119. Sotiropoulos, K, Smilios, I, Douda, H, Chritou, M, and Tokmakidis, S. Contrast loading: power output and rest interval effects on neuromuscular performance. *Int J Sports Physiol Perf* 9:567-574, 2014.

120. Stone, M, O'Bryant, H, McCoy, L, Coglianese, R, Lehmkuhl, M, and Schilling, B. Power and maximal strength relationships during performance of dynamic and static weighted jumps. *J Strength Cond Res* 17:140-147, 2003.

121. Stone, M, Sanborn, K, O'Bryant, H, Hartman, M, Stone, M, Prouix, C, Ward, B, and Hruby, J. Maximal strength-power-performance relationships in collegiate throwers. *J Strength Cond Res* 17:739-745, 2003.

122. Stone, M, Sands, W, Pierce, K, Ramsey, M, and Haff, G. Power and power potentiation among strength power athletes: preliminary study. *Int J Sports Physiol Perf* 3:55-67, 2008.

123. Stone, M, Stone, M, and Sands, W. *Principles and Practice of Resistance Training.* Champaign, IL: Human Kinetics, 2007.

124. Suchomel, T, Wagle, J, Douglas, J, Taber, C, Harden, M, Haff, G, and Stone, M. Implementing eccentric resistance training—part 1: a brief review of existing methods. *J Funct Morphol Kinesiol* 24:38, 2019.

125. Swinton, P, Stewart, A, Keogh, J, Agouris, I, and Lloyd, R. Kinematic and kinetic analysis of maximal velocity deadlifts performed with and without the inclusion of chain resistance. *J Strength Cond Res* 25:3163-3174, 2011.

126. Thomas, K, French, D, and Hayes, P. The effects of two plyometric training techniques on muscular power and agility in youth soccer players. *J Strength Cond Res* 23:332-335, 2009.

127. Thomasson, M, and Comfort, P. Occurrence of fatigue during sets of static squat jumps performed at a variety of loads. *J Strength Cond Res* 26:677-683, 2012.

128. Tillin, N, and Bishop, D. Factors modulating post-activation potentiation and its effect on performance of subsequent explosive activities. *Sports Med* 39:147-166, 2009.

129. Tran, T, Coburn, J, Lynn, S, and Brown, L. Effects of assisted jumping on vertical jump parameters. *Cur Sports Med Rep* 11:155-159, 2012.

130. Turner, A. Training for power: principles and practice. *Prof Strength Cond* 14:20-32, 2009.

131. Verkhoshansky, Y, and Tatyan, V. Speed-strength preparation for future champions. *Logkaya Atletika* 2:2-13, 1973.

132. Verkhoshansky, Y, and Verkhoshansky, N. *Special Strength Training: Manual for Coaches*. Rome, Italy: Verkhoshansky SSTM, 2011.

133. Wagle, J, Taber, C, Cunanan, A, Bingham, G, Carroll, K, DeWeese, B, Sato, K, and Stone, M. Accentuated eccentric loading for training and performance: a review. *Sports Med* 47:2473-2495, 2017.

134. Wallace, B, Winchester, J, and McGuigan, M. Effects of elastic bands on force and power characteristics during the back squat exercise. *J Strength Cond Res* 20:268-272, 2006.

135. Wilson, G. Disinhibition of the neural system: uses in programming, training and competition. *Strength Cond Coach* 3:3-5, 1995.

136. Wilson, G, Murphy, A, and Walshe, A. Performance benefits from weight and plyometric training: effects of initial strength level. *Coaching Sport Sci J* 2:3-8, 1997.

137. Wilson, G, Newton, R, Murphy, A, and Humphries, B. The optimal training load for the development of dynamic athletic performance. *Med Sci Sports Exerc* 23:1279-1286, 1993.

138. Wilson, J, and Kritz, M. Practical guidelines and considerations for the use of elastic bands in strength and conditioning. *Strength and Cond J* 36:1-9, 2014.

139. Yetter, M, and Moir, GL. The acute effects of heavy back and front squats on speed during forty-meter sprint trials. *J Strength Cond Res* 22:159-165, 2008.

140. Young, W, Jenner, A, and Griffiths, K. Acute enhancement of power performance from heavy load squats. *J Strength Cond Res* 12:82-84, 1998.

141. Zatsiorsky, V. Studies of motion and motor abilities of sportsmen. In *Biomechanics IV*. Nelson, R, and Morehouse, C, eds. Baltimore: University Park Press, 273-275, 1974.

142. Zatsiorsky, V, and Kraemer, W. *Science and Practice of Strength Training*. Champaign, IL: Human Kinetics, 1995.

143. Zepeda, P, and Gonzalez, J. Complex training: three weeks pre-season conditioning in Division I female basketball players. *J Strength Cond Res* 14:372, 2000.

Chapter 10

1. Argus, CK, Gill, ND, Keogh, JW, McGuigan, MR, and Hopkins, WG. Effects of two contrast training programs on jump performance in rugby union players during a competition phase. *Int J Sports Physiol Perform* 7:68-75, 2012.

2. Baker, DG, and Newton, RU. Comparison of lower body strength, power, acceleration, speed, agility, and sprint momentum to describe and compare playing rank among professional rugby league players. *J Strength Cond Res* 22:153-158, 2008.

3. Cuthbert, M, Haff, GG, Arent, SM, Ripley, N, McMahon, JJ, Evans, M, and Comfort, P. Effects of variations in resistance training frequency on strength development in well-trained populations and implications for in-season athlete training: a systematic review and meta-analysis. *Sports Med* 51:1962-1982, 2021.

4. Haff, GG, and Nimphius, S. Training principles for power. *Strength and Cond J* 34:2-12 2012.

5. Haischer, MH, Krzyszkowski, J, Roche, S, and Kipp, K. Impulse-based dynamic strength index: considering time-dependent force expression. *J Strength Cond Res* 5:1177-2118, 2021.

6. Harrison, PW, James, LP, McGuigan, MR, Jenkins, DG, and Kelly, VG. Resistance priming to enhance neuromuscular performance in sport: evidence, potential mechanisms and directions for future research. *Sports Med* 49:1499-1514, 2019.

7. Mason, B, McKune, A, Pumpa, K, and Ball, N. The use of acute exercise interventions as game day priming strategies to improve physical performance and athlete readiness in team-sport athletes: a systematic review. *Sports Med* 50:1943-1962, 2020.

8. McMahon, JJ, Lake, JP, Ripley, NJ, and Comfort, P. Vertical jump testing in rugby league: a rationale for calculating take-off momentum. *J Appl Biomech* 36:370-374, 2020.

9. Newton, RU, Håkkinen, K, Håkkinen, A, McCormick, M, Volek, J, and Kraemer, WJ. Mixed-methods resistance training increases power and strength of young and older men. *Med Sci Sports Exerc* 34:1367-1375, 2002.

10. Newton, RU, and Kraemer, WJ. Developing explosive muscular power: implications for a mixed methods training strategy. *Strength and Cond J* 16:20-31, 1994.

11. Ripley, NJ, Cuthbert, M, Comfort, P, and McMahon, JJ. Effect of additional Nordic hamstring exercise or sprint training on the modifiable risk factors of hamstring strain injuries and performance. *PLoS One* 18:e0281966, 2023.

12. Seitz, LB, Reyes, A, Tran, TT, de Villarreal, ES, and Haff, GG. Increases in lower-body strength transfer positively to sprint performance: a systematic review with meta-analysis. *Sports Med* 44:1693-1702, 2014.

13. Sheppard, JM, Chapman, DW, and Taylor, K. An evaluation of a strength qualities assessment method for the lower body. *J Aust Strength Cond* 19:4-10, 2011.

14. Thomas, C, Dos'Santos, T, and Jones, PA. A comparison of dynamic strength index between team-sport athletes. *Sports* 5:71, 2017.

Chapter 11

1. Aagaard, P, and Andersen, JL. Effects of strength training on endurance capacity in top-level endurance athletes. *Scand J Med Sci Sports* 20(Suppl 2):39-47, 2010.

2. Beattie, K, Kenny, IC, Lyons, M, and Carson, BP. The effect of strength training on performance in endurance athletes. *Sports Med* 44:845-865, 2014.

3. Behm, DG, Wahl, MJ, Button, DC, Power, KE, and Anderson, KG. Relationship between hockey skating speed and selected performance measures. *J Strength Cond Res* 19:326-331, 2005.

4. Bullock, N, Martin, DT, Ross, A, Rosemond, D, Holland, T, and Marino, FE. Characteristics of the start in women's World Cup skeleton. *Sports Biomech* 7:351-360, 2008.

5. Calderbank, JA, Comfort, P, and McMahon, JJ. Association of jumping ability and maximum strength with dive distance in swimmers. *Int J Sports Physiol Perform* 16:296-303, 2020.

6. Colomar, J, Corbi, F, Brich, Q, and Baiget, E. Determinant physical factors of tennis serve velocity: a brief review. *Int J Sports Physiol Perform* 17:1159-1169, 2022.

7. Coyne, JOC, Tran, TT, Secomb, JL, Lundgren, LE, Farley, ORL, Newton, RU, and Sheppard, JM. Maximal strength training improves surfboard sprint and endurance paddling performance in competitive and recreational surfers. *J Strength Cond Res* 31:244-253, 2017.

8. Crow, JF, Buttifant, D, Kearny, SG, and Hrysomallis, C. Low load exercises targeting the gluteal muscle group acutely enhance explosive power output in elite athletes. *J Strength Cond Res* 26:438-442, 2012.

9. de Koning, JJ, Thomas, R, Berger, M, de Groot, G, and van Ingen Schenau, GJ. The start in speed skating: from running to gliding. *Med Sci Sports Exerc* 27:1703-1708, 1995.

10. Delisle-House, P, Chiarlitti, RE, Reid, RE, and Andersen, RE. Predicting on-ice skating using laboratory- and field-based assessments in college ice hockey players. *Int J Sports Physiol Perform* 14:1184-1189, 2019.

11. Ferrier, B, Sheppard, JM, Farley, ORL, Secomb, JL, Parsonage, J, Newton, RU, and Nimphius, S. Scoring analysis of the men's 2014, 2015 and 2016 world championship tour of surfing: the importance of aerial maneuvers in competitive surfing. *J Sports Sci* 36:2189-2195, 2018.

12. Forsyth, JR, de la Harpe, R, Riddiford-Harland, DL, Whitting, JW, and Steele, JR. Analysis of scoring maneuvers performed in elite men's professional surfing competitions. *Int J Sports Physiol Perform* 12:1243-1248, 2017.

13. Gordon, BS, Moir, GL, Davis, SE, Witmer, CA, and Cummings, DM. An investigation into the relationship of flexibility, power and strength to club head speed in male golfers. *J Strength Cond Res* 23:1606-1610, 2009.

14. Harrison, PW, James, LP, McGuigan, MR, Jenkins, DG, and Kelly, VG. Resistance priming to enhance neuromuscular performance in sport: evidence, potential mechanisms and directions for future research. *Sports Med* **49**:1499-1514, 2019.

15. Haug, WB, Drinkwater, EJ, Cicero, NJ, Barthell, JA, and Chapman, DW. The impact of dry-land sprint start training on the short track speed skating start. *J Strength Cond Res* 32:544-548, 2019.

16. Haug, WB, Drinkwater, EJ, Mitchell, LJ, and Chapman, DW. The relationship between start performance and race outcome in elite 500-m short-track speed skating. *Int J Sports Physiol Perform* 10:902-906, 2015.

17. Kilduff, LP, Finn, CV, Baker, JS, Cook, CJ, and West, DJ. Preconditioning strategies to enhance physical performance on the day of competition. *Int J Sports Physiol Perform* 8:677-681, 2013.

18. Lawton, TW, Cronin, JB, and McGuigan, MR. Strength testing and training of rowers: a review. *Sports Med* 41:413-432, 2011.

19. Liebermann, DG, Maitland, ME, and Katz, L. Lower-limb extension power: how well does it predict short distance speed skating performance? *Isokinet Exerc Sci* 10:87-95, 2002.

20. Loturco, I, McGuigan, M, Freitas, TT, Valenzuela, P, Pereira, LA, and Pareja-Blanco, F. *Performance and reference data in the jump squat at different relative loads in elite sprinters, rugby players, and soccer players. Biol Sport 38:219-227, 2021.*

21. McKay, AK, Stellingwerff, TS, Smith, ES, Martin, DT, Mujika, I, Goosey-Tolfrey, VL, Sheppard, JM, and Burke, LM. Defining training and performance caliber: a participant classification framework. *Int J Sports Physiol Perform 17:317-331, 2022.*

22. Nishioka, T, and Okada, J. Influence of strength level on performance enhancement using resistance priming. *J Strength Cond Res* 36:37-46, 2022.

23. Noorbergen, OS, Konings, MJ, Micklewright, D, Elferink-Gemser, MT, and Hettinga, FJ. Pacing behaviour and tactical positioning in 500m and 1000m short-track speed skating. *Int J Sports Physiol Perform* 11:742-748, 2016.

24. Parchmann, CJ, and McBride, JM. Relationship between functional movement screen and athletic performance. *J Strength Cond Res* 25:3378-3384, 2011.

25. Perez-Olea, JI, Valenzuela, PL, Aponte, C, and Izquierdo, M. Relationship between dryland strength and swimming performance: pull-up mechanics as a predictor of swimming speed. *J Strength Cond Res* 32:1637-1642, 2018.

26. Read, PJ, Lloyd, RS, De Ste Croix, M, and Oliver, JL. Relationships between field-based measures of strength and power and golf club head speed. *J Strength Cond Res* 27:2708-2713, 2013.

27. Renaud, PJ, Robbins, SM, Dixon, C, Shell, JR, Turcotte, RA, and Pearsall, DJ. Ice hockey skate starts: a comparison of high and low calibre skaters. *Sports Eng* 10:255-266, 2017.

28. Ronnestad, BR, Kojedal, O, Losnegard, T, Kvamme, B, and Raastad, T. Effect of heavy strength training on muscle thickness, strength, jump performance, and endurance performance in well-trained Nordic Combined athletes. *Eur J Appl Physiol* 112:2341-2352, 2012.

29. Secomb, JL, Farley, ORL, Lundgren, LE, Tran, TT, King, A, Nimphius, S, and Sheppard, JM. Associations between the performance of scoring maneuvers and lower-body strength and power in elite surfers. *Int J Sports Sci Coach* 10:911-918, 2015.

30. Secomb, JL, Dascombe, BJ, and Nimphius, S. Importance of joint-angle-specific hip strength for skating performance in semiprofessional ice hockey athletes. *J Strength Cond Res* 35:2599-2603, 2021.

31. Sheppard, JM, McNamara, P, Osborne, M, Andrews, M, Oliveira Borges, T, Walshe, P, and Chapman, DW. Association between anthropometry and upper-body strength qualities with sprint paddling performance in competitive wave surfers. *J Strength Cond Res* 26:3345-3348, 2012.

32. Weber, AE, Bedi, A, Tibor, LM, Zaltz, I, and Larson, CM. The hyperflexible hip: managing hip pain in the dancer and gymnast. *Sports Health 7:346-358, 2015.*

33. Zanoletti, C, La Torre, A, Merati, G, Rampinini, E, and Imperllizzeri, FM. Relationship between push phase and final race time in skeleton performance. *J Strength Cond Res* 20:579-583, 2006.

Index

Note: The italicized *f* and *t* following page numbers refer to figures and tables, respectively.

About the NSCA

The **National Strength and Conditioning Association (NSCA)** is the world's leading organization in the field of sport conditioning. Drawing on the resources and expertise of the most recognized professionals in strength training and conditioning, sport science, performance research, education, and sports medicine, the NSCA is the world's trusted source of knowledge and training guidelines for coaches and athletes. The NSCA provides the crucial link between the lab and the field.

About the Editor

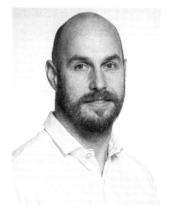

Paul Comfort, PhD, CSCS, *D is a full professor in strength and conditioning at the University of Salford and is an adjunct professor at Edith Cowan University. He is a founder and accredited member of the UK Strength and Conditioning Association (UKSCA) and was a member of the NSCA board of directors from 2000 to 2023. He is a senior associate editor for the *Journal of Strength and Conditioning Research* and sits on the editorial board of numerous other journals. Comfort has presented extensively at conferences around the world, coauthored over 150 peer-reviewed journal articles, and served as the editor of four books.

About the Contributors

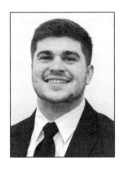

Brandon Burdge, MS, CSCS, is a sport performance coach and personal trainer with experience working with athletes in the high school, collegiate, and professional levels. He is a former director of sport performance for Reach Your Potential Training (RYPT) in New Jersey and strength and conditioning coordinator for Ohio Northern University. His previous stints were with Tufts University, University at Buffalo, the New York Guardians of the XFL, and Montclair State University. He currently teaches history and career research courses at Storm Grove Middle School while coaching athletes and other clients at Vero Fitness in Florida.

Dale W. Chapman, PhD, CSCS, is a senior lecturer in exercise and sport science at Curtin University. He has extensive industry experience as a sport scientist, including being an Australian Olympic team member at four Olympic Games. His research focus is applied sport research that leads to practical solutions to problems that are limiting an athlete's performance. This includes topics such as neuromuscular fatigue, exercise-induced muscle damage, applied physiology of strength and conditioning, and the use and development of microtechnology applications.

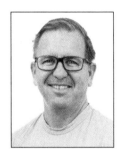

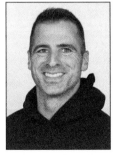

Wil Fleming, USAW LVL 5, is a notable strength and conditioning coach whose expertise has helped numerous athletes to international acclaim, particularly in Olympic weightlifting. He has a history of athletic competition himself and has transitioned that passion into coaching, guiding athletes to national championships and international medals in weightlifting and in track and field. Renowned for his innovative training methodologies and passion for coaching, Fleming is a respected pillar within the performance world. His influence extends beyond the gym through his contributions as an author, speaker, and seminar host, reaching a wide audience that includes aspiring athletes and fellow coaches.

Duncan N. French, PhD, CSCS,*D, RSCC*E, is senior vice president of the UFC Performance Institute, where he is responsible for directing performance services to 650 UFC fighters globally. He has 25 years of experience in elite professional sport and has coached Olympic

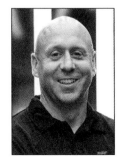

medalists and world record holders. He has been the national strength and conditioning lead for Great Britain Basketball, Great Britain Taekwondo, and Paralympic Swimming. He was the head of strength and conditioning for Newcastle United FC in the English Premier League. He has authored or coauthored over 60 scientific manuscripts and 9 book chapters. In 2014 French received an honorary fellowship from the United Kingdom Strength and Conditioning Association (UKSCA) for his services to strength and conditioning.

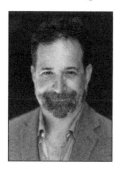

G. Gregory Haff, PhD, CSCS,*D, FNSCA, is the professor of strength and conditioning at Edith Cowan University. A past president of the National Strength and Conditioning Association (NSCA), he is also the author of *Scientific Foundations and Practical Applications of Periodization* and the coeditor of *NSCA's Essentials of Strength and Conditioning.* Haff is a national-level weightlifting coach in both Australia and the United States. He was awarded the NSCA's Impact Award in 2021 in recognition of the impact of his research, teaching and service to the strength and conditioning profession. Additionally, in 2014, the UKSCA recognized him as the Strength and Conditioning Coach of the Year for Education and Research for the impact of his work. He was the 2011 winner of NSCA's William J. Kraemer Sport Scientist of the Year Award.

Dave Hamilton, CSCS, is a director of performance and a strength and conditioning coach. Hamilton has navigated athletic landscapes from aspiring youth athletes to Olympic medal winners and Super Bowl champions. His career has seen him work globally (in the United Kingdom, Qatar, Hong Kong, Canada, and United States), with elite programs such as the British and American Olympic teams (Team GB and Team USA), Penn State, and the Tampa Bay Buccaneers.

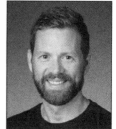

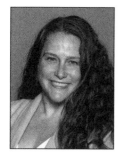

Disa L. Hatfield, PhD, CSCS, is currently a full professor in the department of kinesiology at the University of Rhode Island. Hatfield's research focus is multidisciplinary and focuses on strength and conditioning, athletic performance, nutrition and supplementation, perception of exercise, exercise endocrinology, and nonnutritional ergogenic aids. Hatfield's 70 published research articles and numerous book chapters focus on how these factors interact and are affected by resistance training and exercise across the lifespan. Hatfield has also worked as a strength and conditioning coach in the private sector and as a personal trainer. She is a former World Games competitor, a three-time USAPL national champion powerlifter, a two-time American bench press record holder, and former head coach for the men's Pan American Games powerlifting team.

Paul A. Jones, PhD, MSc, BSc (Hons), CSCS, CSci, FHEA, is a lecturer in sport biomechanics and strength and conditioning at the University of Salford. He has over 23 years of experience in providing strength and conditioning support to athletes and teams—primarily in athletics, football, and rugby—and is a former sport science coordinator for UK Disability Athletics. Jones has coedited two books and has authored or coauthored over 110 peer-reviewed journal articles and 12 book chapters, covering change-of-direction biomechanics, assessment and development of change-of-direction speed, and strength diagnostics.

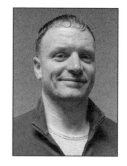

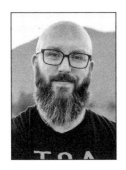

Robert C. Linkul, MS, CSCS,*D, NSCA-CPT,*D, FNSCA, is the owner of TOA (TrainingTheOlderAdult.com), a personal training studio and online continued education provider for fitness professionals in Shingle Springs, California. Linkul is an internationally known continuing education provider for fitness professionals, with his area of expertise being in resistance training strategies for the older adult with physical limitations. Linkul's master's degree is in personal training. He is the 2012 winner of NSCA's Personal Trainer of the Year Award winner, is a 2017 NSCA fellowship inductee, and was selected for the 2021 NSCA board of directors.

Rhodri S. Lloyd, PhD, CSCS,*D, FNSCA, is a professor of pediatric strength and conditioning and the head of the Centre for Applied Sport Science & Medicine at Cardiff Metropolitan University. His research focuses on the influence of growth and maturation on athletic development and injury risk reduction in youth populations. He has published more than 170 peer-reviewed manuscripts, 35 book chapters, and three textbooks on the topics of pediatric strength and conditioning and long-term athletic development. He has been recognized nationally and internationally for his contributions to the field, and in 2021 was made a fellow of the NSCA.

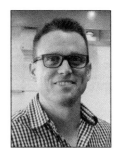

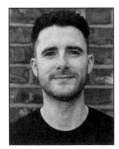

John J. McMahon, PhD, CSCS,*D, is the director of research and education at Hawkin Dynamics. He is also an honorary associate professor of sport and exercise biomechanics at the University of Salford, where he previously worked for 10 years as a researcher and educator. McMahon has coauthored more than 90 journal articles, 17 book chapters, and two books. He has spoken at multiple international conferences, spanning the fields of strength and conditioning, sport biomechanics, and sport science. In 2023, he was named Educator of the Year by the NSCA. McMahon is also a member of NSCA's Foundation Grant Committee.

Gavin C. Pratt, MExSc, is currently the director of strength and conditioning at the UFC Performance Institute. He has been a strength and conditioning coach for over 25 years. Previously, he worked in China with the UFC Academy program and with Shanghai Research in Sports Science across a six-year span; he was the performance manager for Exos, managing a team of coaches and physiotherapists to help drive the Shanghai team to their most successful Chinese National Games in decades. He served as the head of strength and conditioning for numerous Olympic-based sports, including boxing, handball, swimming, and fencing.

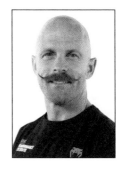

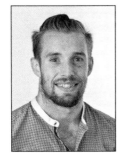

Nicholas Ripley, PhD, CSCS,*D, RSCC, is a lecturer of sport science and strength and conditioning at the University of Salford. He has extensive applied experience across a range of sports, working with numerous professional teams, semiprofessional teams, and individuals. Ripley is holds the Certified Strength and Conditioning Coach with Distinction (CSCS,*D) and Registered Strength and Conditioning Coach (RSCC) credentials from the NSCA. Ripley is also a member of the executive council of the NSCA Lacrosse Special Interest Group. Nicholas is current combat sport athlete, competing in grappling-based sports, and has represented Great Britain.

Josh L. Secomb, PhD, CPSS, is a lecturer in strength and conditioning at the University of Newcastle and is the strength and conditioning coach for Ice Hockey Australia. His research focuses on evaluating and enhancing the physical capacities that underpin technical skill execution and athlete availability in sport. He has over 10 years of experience as a strength and conditioning coach and sport scientist, working across a variety of professional and Olympic team and individual sports, as well with tactical athletes and adolescents. His overarching goal is to elevate practitioner knowledge in order to facilitate evidence-informed decision-making regarding athlete preparation.

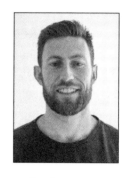

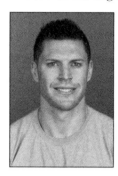

Bobby Smith, MS, CSCS,*D, RSCC*D, is the owner and cofounder of Reach Your Potential Training (RYPT), a sport performance company based out of Tinton Falls, New Jersey. Since opening its doors 12 years ago, RYPT has had over 6,000 registrations and has developed three educational products. Smith has traveled around the country presenting and teaching coaches the RYPT system. Prior to starting RYPT, Smith was a two-sport athlete at Monmouth University, earning All-Conference honors as a running back and Division I All-American honors in the javelin. Smith continued competing after college and won the 2008 Olympic trials in the javelin.

Douglas M. Tvrdy, DPT, OCS, CSCS, is a physical therapist at Madonna ProActive in Lincoln, Nebraska, where he works with orthopedic and sports medicine patients and operates RunWell, a running mechanics and training program. He has held the Certified Strength and Conditioning Specialist (CSCS) credential for 20 years, and he has been certified as an orthopedic specialist in physical therapy for over 15 years. He has published peer-reviewed articles in the *Journal of Strength and Conditioning Research* and *NSCA Coach*, and he serves as an expert reviewer for *Sports Health* and *Physiotherapy Research International*. He was named an NAIA National Scholar-Athlete in football for Hastings College.

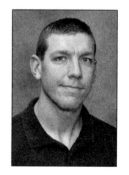

Contributors to the Previous Edition

Jeffrey M. McBride, PhD, CSCS

Mike R. McGuigan, PhD

Sophia Nimphius, PhD, CSCS

Jeremy M. Sheppard, PhD, CSCS, RSCC*E

Adam Storey, PhD

N. Travis Triplett, PhD, CSCS,*D, FNSCA

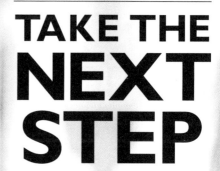
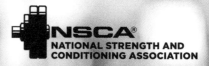
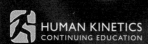